MEDICAL
INTELLIGENCE
UNIT

TRAUMA 2000

STRATEGIES FOR THE NEW MILLENIUM

Edited by:

Richard L. Gamelli, M.D.
and
David J. Dries, M.D.

Loyola University Medical Center
Chicago, Illinois

R.G. LANDES COMPANY
AUSTIN

R.G. LANDES COMPANY
Austin / Georgetown

TRAUMA 2000
Strategies for the Millenium

Submitted: April 1992
Published: July 1992

Production Manager: Terry Nelson
Copy Editor: Constance Kerkaporta

Please address all inquiries to the Publisher:
R.G. Landes Company
909 South Pine Street
Georgetown, TX 78626
or
P.O. Box 4858
Austin, TX 78765
Phone: 512 863 7762
FAX: 512 863 0081

ISBN 1-879702-13-4

FOREWORD

"We've Come a Long Way Baby" was the title of John Davis' presidential address to the American Association for the Surgery of Trauma. It seems appropriate that one of John's proteges (R.G.) has coauthored a monograph on the cutting edge developments in the care of the injured.

Forty years ago, most of the scientific activity in trauma care was limited to retrospective reviews of various clinical problems. While the problems of shock, fluid and electrolyte balance and metabolic response were the interests of some of the greatest surgical scientists in the world, their application to injury focused primarily upon the effects of surgery and anesthesia, the more controlled insult of an elective operation. There was little or no interest in accident scene care, transport vehicles, injury scores or a systems approach to patient problems. Similarly, newer methods of monitoring cardiopulmonary function, cell biology, and nutritional manipulation were in their infancy or as yet unknown.

If trauma was the neglected disease of modern society it was also the (forgotten) step child of Academic Medicine. Distinguished surgeons regularly viewed the injured patient as an unwelcome intrusion upon their other clinical or educational responsibilities. It is not surprising that basic scientists found little support for their interest in the pathophysiology of injury and repair. The public and their elected representatives in government were far more concerned with supporting research into the leading "killers" such as heart disease, cancer, and stroke. They tended to consider accidents as inevitable and issues of survival or disability largely predetermined by the injury itself rather than where or by whom care was given.

Several wars and the efforts of many have combined to change this picture. While much more needs to be done, it is apparent that most citizens now realize that accidents are preventable and that proper treatment makes a difference. An increasing number of medical school surgical departments, hospitals and practitioners realize that injury prevention and treatment are an important part of our educational and health care systems. At the same time researchers are applying a myriad of scientific developments to the known and the unknown of injury.

This monograph by Dries and Gamelli represents the current state of developments in many of these areas. The authors have been selected for their acknowledged role in many of these developments or their application of them to various clinical problems. It offers both a chance to "catch up" for those understandably overwhelmed by the explosion of knowledge in injury-related research, but also points the way to areas of need and directions in which needs may be met. In reviewing the progress that has been achieved in a relatively short time, one feels that the best is yet to come.

Robert J. Freeark, MD
Professor and Chairman
Department of Surgery
Loyola University Medical Center

CONTENTS

1. Trauma Care Systems 1
   Thomas J. Esposito

2. The Future of Trauma Scoring 15
   Howard R. Champion

3. Resuscitation Solutions 20
   Gail T. Tominaga, Kenneth Waxman

4. Myocardial Depression 30
   William R. Law

5. The Pathophysiology and Treatment of the
   Acute Respiratory Distress Syndrome 36
   Richard P. Richardson, William G. Cioffi

6. Inhalation Injury: Pathophysiology and Treatment 44
   Ronald H. Miles, David J. Dries, Richard L. Gamelli

7. The Immune Consequences of Trauma: An Overview 64
   David J. Dries

8. Effects of Trauma on T- and B-Cell Function 74
   Edward Abraham

9. Cytokines and Posttraumatic Sepsis 81
   James P. Filkins

10. Neutrophil Function in the Imflammatory Diseases
    of Trauma and Burn Injury 85
    Joseph S. Solomkin, Robert C. Bass

11. Immune Modulation 91
    David L. Dunn

12. Biological Response Modification: An Emerging
    Therapy in Critical Illness 101
    Timothy G. Buchman

13. Nutritional Support of the Injured Patient 106
    Robert C. Morris

14. Bacterial Translocation and Gut Barrier Failure 112
    Mark R. Mainous, Edwin A. Deitch

15. Sepsis and Glucose Transporters 121
    Cecilia A. Hofmann

16. Acute Phase Proteins 127
    Michael E. Gottschalk

17. Intracellular Calcium Regulation: Derangements
    During Septic Injury 131
    Mohammed M. Sayeed

18. Wound Healing 139
    Richard L. Gamelli

19. Immune Control of Wound Healing 146
    Mark C .Regan, Adrian Barbul

20. Growth Factors in Wound Healing 151
    Thomas A. Mustoe

21. The Current Status of Skin Substitutes 156
    John C. Fitzpatrick, William G. Cioffi

22. Treatment of Endotoxic Shock in the Young Trauma Victim:
    Immunotherapy and Prophylaxis 162
    Masakatsu Goto, Toyokazu Yoshioka, W. Patrick Zeller

23. Hemostasis in the Trauma Patient 167
    *Jeanine M. Walenga, Areta Kowal-Vern,
    Jawed Fareed, Richard L. Gamelli*

24. Hematopoietic Response 179
    Thomas P. Paxton, Richard L. Gamelli

25. Issues in Geriatric Trauma 191
    David J. Dries, Richard L. Gamelli

CONTRIBUTORS

Edward Abraham, M.D.
UCLA School of Medicine
10833 Le Conte Ave.
Los Angeles, CA 90024
Chapter 8

Adrian Barbul, M.D.
Sinai Hospital of Baltimore
2401 W. Belvedere Ave.
Baltimore, MD 21215
Chapter 19

Robert C. Bass, M.D.
Univ. of Cincinnati
231 Bethesda Ave.
Cincinnati, OH 45267
Chapter 10

Timothy G. Buchman, M.D.
Johns Hopkins Univ.
600 N. Wolfe St./Halsted
612
Baltimore, MD 21205
Chapter 12

Howard R. Champion, M.D.
Washington Hospital
    Center
Washington, DC 20010
Chapter 2

William G. Cioffi, M.D.
Surgical Research Institute
Ft. Sam Houston
San Antonio, TX 78234
Chapter 5, 21

Edwin A. Deitch, M.D.
LSU Medical Center
Shreveport, LA 71130
Chapter 14

David J. Dries, M.D.
Loyola Univ. Medical Center
2160 S. First Ave.
Maywood, IL 60153
Chapters 6, 7

David L. Dunn, M.D.
Univ. of Minnesota
Minneapolis, MN 55455
Chapter 11

Thomas J. Esposito, M.D.
Loyola Univ. Medical Center
2160 S. First Ave.
Maywood, IL, 60153
Chapter 1

Jaweed Fareed, M.D.
Loyola Univ. Medical Center
2160 S. First Ave.
Maywood, IL 60153
Chapter 23

James P. Filkins, M.D.
Loyola Univ. Medical Center
2160 S. First Ave.
Maywood, IL 60153
Chapter 9

John C. Fitzpatrick, M.D.
Surgical Research Institute
Ft. Sam Houston
San Antonio, TX 78234
Chapter 21

Robert J. Freeark, M.D.
Loyola Univ. Medical Center
2160 S. First Ave.
Maywood, IL 60153
Foreword

Richard L. Gamelli, M.D.
Loyola Univ. Medical Center
2160 S. First Ave.
Maywood, IL 60153
Chapters 6, 18, 23, 24, 25

Masakatsu Goto, M.D.
Loyola Univ. Medical Center
2160 S. First Ave.
Maywood, IL 60153
Chapter 22

Michael E. Gottschalk, M.D.
Loyola Univ. Medical Center
2160 S. First Ave.
Maywood, IL 60153
Chapter 16

Cecilia A. Hoffman, Ph.D.
Hines VA Hospital
Hines, IL 60141
Chapter 15

Areta Kowal-Vern, M.D.
Loyola Univ. Medical Center
2160 S. First Ave.
Maywood, IL 60153
Chapter 23

William R. Law, Ph.D.
University of Ill. at Chicago
840 Wood St.
Chicago, IL 60612
Chapter 4

Mark R. Mainous, M.D.
LSU Medical Center
Shreveport, LA 71130
Chapter 14

Ronald H. Miles, M.D.
Loyola Univ. Medical Center
2160 S. First Ave.
Maywood, IL 60153
Chapter 6

Robert C. Morris, M.D.
Loyola Univ. Medical Center
2160 S. First Ave.
Maywood, IL 60153
Chapter 13

Thomas A. Mustoe, M.D.
Northwestern Univ.
    Medical School
707 N. Fairbanks Ct.
Chicago IL 60611
Chapter 20

Mark C. Regan, M.D.
Sinai Hospital of Baltimore
2401 W. Belvedere Ave.
Baltimore, MD 21215
Chapter 19

Richard P. Richardson, M.D.
Surgical Research Institute
Ft. Sam Houston
San Antonio, TX 78234
Chapter 5

Mohammed M. Sayeed, Ph.D.
Loyola Univ. Medical Center
2160 S. First Ave.
Maywood, IL 60153
Chapter 17

Joseph S. Solomkin, M.D.
Univ. of Cincinnati
231 Bethesda Ave.
Cincinnati, OH 45267
Chapter 10

Gail T. Tominaga, M.D.
Univ. of Calif.-Irvine
    Medical Center
101 City Drive South
Orange, CA 92668
Chapter 3

Jeanine M. Walenga, Ph.D.
Loyola Univ. Medical Center
2160 S. First Ave.
Maywood, IL 60153
Chapter 23

Kenneth Waxman, M.D.
Univ. of Calif-Irvine
    Medical Center
101 City Drive South
Orange, CA 92668
Chapter 3

Toyokazu Yoshioka, M.D.
Loyola Univ. Medical Center
2160 S. First Ave.
Maywood, IL 60153
Chapter 22

W. Patrick Zeller, M.D.
Loyola Univ. Medical Center
2160 S. First Ave.
Maywood, IL 60153
Chapter 22

CHAPTER 1

TRAUMA CARE SYSTEMS

Thomas J. Esposito

INTRODUCTION

Injury is responsible for the death over 150,000 U.S. citizens annually and disables over 400,000.[1] A number of studies have shown that up to 35% of these deaths can be considered preventable when the severity of injury, appropriateness and timeliness of care is analyzed.[2] This alarming rate of preventable death has been shown to be greatly reduced with the institution of trauma care systems.[3] While similar studies do not currently exist for preventable disability, it can safely be assumed that the rate of preventability and impact of trauma care systems is similar.

A trauma system deals with a continuum of care from prevention of injury and acute care of injury that does occur, to rehabilitation and return to society. Without a system, the level and quality of care rendered may vary on a regional basis or even on a daily or hourly basis within the same region. A system attempts to minimize these variations by setting and maintaining standards of trauma care and coordinating its consistent delivery. The goals and objectives of a trauma care system are to decrease the incidence of trauma, assure optimal and equitable care for all trauma victims, prevent unnecessary death and disability from trauma, contain cost and assure quality of trauma care throughout the system. A trauma system comprises both patient care and societal components. The patient care components include access, prehospital care, hospital care and rehabilitation. The societal components include prevention, education, research, economics and quality.[4]

In order to provide an effective system of trauma care, a state or region must have a fully functional EMS system. Enabling legislation should exist for the development of the trauma system component of the EMS system. Legislation should also exist empowering a lead agency with the authority to administrate the trauma system, set system standards and monitor and maintain adherence to those standards. Responsibilities of this trauma system lead agency include establishing, coordinating and evaluating the following: criteria for prehospital triage; standards for prehospital care (including training and certification of personnel and equipment); guidelines for and integration of transportation and communication; minimum standards for trauma care facilities; a process for accreditation, evaluation and censure of these facilities; and interfacility transfer protocols. Finally, the lead agency must be responsible for determining the adequacy and quality of care. In order to do this, it must coordinate centralized collection and analysis of data related to system operation, patient care and outcome. The lead agency is also responsible for tracking system costs and reporting system results to the public and private sector.

In a 1988 study by West et al,[5] only two states, Maryland and Virginia, were considered to have all essential components of a regional trauma system in place on a statewide basis. Pennsylvania now is also considered to meet these criteria. Eighteen states and the District of Columbia either have incomplete statewide coverage or lack essential components. Twenty-nine states have yet initiated a process of trauma center identification at the time of this study. The National Highway Traffic Safety Administration (NHTSA) has instituted a Technical Assistance Program by which a state is evaluated against a set of ten standards of EMS excellence. The findings from this program reveal there are no fully functional trauma systems in any of the 29 states (including Maryland and Pennsylvania) that have been evaluated to date.[6] Despite minor discrepancies between standards used by the West study and NHTSA, it is unfortunate, but safe to say there are no statewide trauma systems in America today which meet all standards. There is sufficient evidence to show that fragmented components of trauma systems are operating in isolation.

Trauma care and trauma care systems encompass controversial medical, emotional and political issues that often divide the various factions involved with the increasingly broad field of health care delivery. Dealing with variations in geography, population density, demographics, local and regional resources, personnel and politics while balancing cost effectiveness, equity and quality of care presents complex problems. However, if this major public health threat is to be overcome, these issues must be addressed and resolved.

PATIENT CARE COMPONENTS

ACCESS

The concept of trauma system access is commonly considered to involve communication technology such as the establishment of a universal 911 emergency services telephone number. Other interventions include placement of roadside emergency call boxes and in some areas, such as Australia, equipping transportation and agricultural vehicles with emergency beacons which automatically alert EMS personnel in the event of a crash. This has received particular attention in the development of rural trauma systems. The death rate from injury in rural settings is considerably higher than in urban areas. The factors of population density, climate and topography contribute to late discovery and complicate access to the system, potentially contributing to this increased death rate. The concept of restricted access, however, must be considered in a broader sense than just technological communication devices if the problem is to be addressed properly and ultimately resolved.

A trauma system requires many interdependent components to be functional and effective. The major component of any system is a sufficient pool of personnel who are committed to and educated in the care of the injured patient. The most abundant resource in this regard is the public. They must be educated through public service announcements and educational programs in how and when to access the system. The Seattle experience with bystander CPR training has successfully impacted survival in out of hospital cardiac arrest.[7] This experience should be extended to the problem of injury with consideration of training the public in first responder techniques of airway management, hemorrhage control and patient immobilization. Such a program is currently being developed and tested by NHTSA. This may have particular benefits in rural systems where EMS response times are often lengthy.

Failure to establish and maintain effective trauma systems and trauma centers obviously restricts access to care for trauma patients. This problem has primarily been associated with economic and reimbursement factors.[8] However the next leading cause identified in several studies[9,10] is lack of physician participation and support. This is especially true at nonteaching suburban facilities which provide most trauma care, and rely more heavily on "on call" physicians. There appears to be great reluctance on the part of institutions as well as health care providers to care for trauma patients.[9,11,12] This reduces the supply of appropriate trauma care resources and restricts access. If the problems of system failure and access are to be adequately addressed, the etiology of this reluctance to treat these patients must be identified and strategies to eliminate it formulated. This may involve attitudinal assessment among institutional and individual trauma care providers and further dissemination of factual information which would dispel any myths responsible for this reluctance.

PREHOSPITAL CARE

TRANSPORTATION

The concept of the "golden hour" characterizes the time frame in which definitive care should be provided to the major trauma victim in an effort to prevent unwarranted morbidity and mortality.[13] Taking into account the realities of geography and demographics, this "hour" is not always practical or possible. Many systems outline acceptable limits of response time for the delivery of care to the trauma patient. In urban areas this may range from 5-8 minutes; in suburban areas, from 10-15 minutes; in rural areas 45 minutes; and in wilderness areas, approximately 1-1/2 hours. Regions of EMS and initial acute care facility responsibility must be delineated in a way which provides the victim with optimal access to timely care.

Organized transportation of the injured from the field to the hospital can be traced to the time of Napoleon. War has continued to spur refinements in this aspect of injury care which have been employed in the civilian sector. The most notable of these is aeromedical transport. This is commonly associated with the helicopter, although fixed wing aircraft and aquatic vessels also have a place in the transport arena.

The concept of helicopter transport has to some degree come to be synonymous with, and even thought to define, a trauma system. This is far from accurate. The optimal means of patient transportation is dictated by clinical condition, distance to definitive care, accessibility of incident scene and weather conditions. In most settings, particularly urban, ground transportation by appropriately equipped ambulances usually affords the most efficient means of transport. In more remote areas and in some congested

urban and suburban areas, aeromedical transport is appropriate and often necessary. Options include dispatch of a helicopter to the scene; rendezvous with ground providers at a field site distant from the scene of incident; stabilization at an initial facility with interfacility transfer by air. Helicopters are employed in most instances of aeromedical transport but for distances greater than 150 miles, fixed wing aircraft are more practical. Guidelines for aeromedical transport must be established in each system based on variation in personnel, facilities, climate and topography. The number and distribution of ground ambulances, EMS personnel with various levels of training, acute care facilities and helicopters should be a function of system design and configured to minimize response and transport times.

There has been a rapid increase in the presence of helicopters in EMS systems. Many are hospital based, others are operated by municipal agencies or private companies. Many, unfortunately, are used as marketing tools with little regard for actual need, coordination of dispatch, integration of function with other aeromedical and ground services or patient care standards. A trauma system lead agency should serve to avoid such situations. The lead agency provides oversight and direction preventing inappropriate use of resources and political issues from compromising patient care and system function.

PERSONNEL

There are a number of arrangements by which prehospital care is provided ranging from volunteer to private and municipal agency coverage. The personnel employed by these agencies vary widely in their degree of training. These levels of training may range from first responder status to Emergency Medical Technician (EMT) and EMT-paramedic. These are nationally recognized classifications with national standards. Many systems recognize nonstandardized classifications which are intermediate. Levels of training relate to field interventions which are capable of being performed by the individual provider. However, actual performance of these interventions varies widely among systems and often depends on local policy rather than standard training level classification of providers. A number of systems require minimum levels of additional trauma training for prehospital providers. An example is completion of the Prehospital Trauma Life Support (PHTLS) or Basic Trauma Life Support (BTLS) courses.

Adequate patient volume to maintain skills, prehospital provider "burn out" and "rust out," demanding and costly requirements for continuing education and recertification are issues which trauma systems must deal with. This is of particular concern among rural and volunteer providers. These factors can negatively affect the pool of prehospital providers and system access.

TRIAGE

The term triage is derived from the French *word* trier, meaning to sort or cull out. The concept, applied to trauma systems, attempts to assure that the right patient arrives at the right type of facility in the right amount of time. Identification of major trauma victims who will require specialized and intensive trauma care based on their presentation at the incident scene is crucial. The goal of triage criteria is to allocate resources appropriately and save lives. Application of these triage criteria attempts to minimize the rates of overtriage and undertriage.

Overtriage directs minimally injured patients to specialized facilities identified to treat the most serious cases and thereby inappropriately taxes their resources. Conversely, undertriage directs patients who may in fact be in need of sophisticated trauma care to hospitals which are not optimally capable of doing so. This heightens the potential for preventable death and disability.

A certain degree of patient misclassification producing overtriage and undertriage is expected in any system. Overtriage is somewhat more desirable from a patient survival standpoint. This is only true to the point where it does not overburden the resources of the system. High overtriage rates impact quality of patient care and the ability to deliver appropriate care to those who are most in need of it.

The accurate identification of high risk major trauma victims at the scene is difficult. No tool has been developed that can accurately and consistently identify these patients. Adverse field

conditions, limited resources and the need to make rapid assessments compound the problem. A number of scoring systems and criteria for trauma facility triage have been recommended to assist prehospital providers in the task of field triage. The Revised Trauma Score (RTS) is based purely on physiologic criteria.[14] The system advocated by the Committee on Trauma of the American College of Surgeons assesses not only physiologic response but injury anatomy, injury mechanism and comorbid factors.[4] These are the most widely used triage tools in U.S. trauma systems. The objectivity, validity and reliability of such tools is currently under debate. The selection of optimal triage criteria for a particular system is dependent upon prehospital provider training, medical control and the rates of over and under triage which are considered acceptable for that system.

MEDICAL CONTROL

An integral facet of any trauma system is physician involvement in establishing, directing and monitoring emergency medical care. This is more commonly known as medical control. There is wide regional variability in the policies, procedures and authority of medical control of EMS systems. Three phases of medical control have been proposed.[15] These are: prospective, immediate and retrospective. The prospective phase consists of developing treatment protocols and policies, training and certificating prehospital providers, establishing communication, transfer and transport networks, as well as delineating guidelines for recording and collecting data. The immediate or "on line" phase encompasses supervision of EMS units through monitoring communications or direct communication with field providers. The retrospective phase of medical control consists of reviewing field run sheets and emergency department care. This attempts to identify errors in individual care or inadequacies in system policies. Medical control is commonly administered by an emergency physician or trauma surgeon. Policies and procedures should be uniform within regions and in congruence with system standards.

Regardless of prehospital system design and operation, minimum standards must be set taking into account the current distribution and training of prehospital providers as well as proximity to trauma facilities, availability of medical control and air transport. The system should be flexible enough to allow and encourage variation above the minimum standards. However the goal of any system should be the elimination of such variation and continuous upgrading of the minimum standards to the highest level which is realistically achievable.

HOSPITAL CARE

Formal identification of facilities with the commitment and capability to provide optimal acute and rehabilitative trauma care is essential in any true trauma system. Currently, many systems can be classified as "exclusive." This type of system recognizes a limited number of hospitals as being "trauma centers." Optimally, these centers are distributed regionally such that volume and resources are conducive to delivery of specialized and consistent quality care associated with improved outcomes. These types of systems involve rapid transport and bypass of hospitals which are not identified as trauma centers, despite the fact they may be closer to the scene of the injury. This type of system is espoused by many urban practitioners of trauma medicine. The "exclusive" system may be well suited to populated areas with an abundance of health care facilities. However, even in these settings, it has met with problems associated with politics, prestige and finances.

Even when it works well, an exclusive system is not always possible or feasible in rural and remote settings. Hence, for a number of reasons there has been a shift in emphasis to the concept of an "inclusive" system. This recognizes the capabilities of all health care facilities to treat trauma patients according to standards which take into account facility resources and commitment. A role for every provider is defined.

Inclusion rather than exclusion of these facilities allays some of the concerns brought about by exclusion. More importantly however, it provides education of providers in acute management and early transfer; establishes lines of communication, transfer protocols and policies between facilities offering different levels of care;

and should establish reasonable standards of care for all facilities based on role and capability. All facilities are then expected to maintain these standards which are monitored and evaluated. Inclusion in the system may also afford the opportunity to obtain funding for basic resources.

In many ways, this may be more effective than bypass policies in impacting patient outcome. However, it is the system which by setting standards, monitoring adherence to them and implementing appropriate changes based on findings of that monitoring program that affects outcome, not so much whether the system itself is inclusive or exclusive in nature.

Criteria for hospital resources required for consideration as a trauma center have been developed by a number of organizations. The American College of Surgeons Committee on Trauma guidelines[4] are the most widely used. Under this system, hospitals are classified level I, II or III. Level I and II hospitals possess the greatest degree of resources and the highest ability and commitment to provide optimal care to the most severely injured. Level I centers additionally have a major commitment to education and research. Level III centers possess fewer resources but provide maximum quality care commensurate with these resources. Again, standardized transfer agreements and protocols to level I or II institutions from level III institutions are fundamental to optimal care.

In establishing guidelines for the qualifications of a health care facility to be considered as a recognized trauma care provider, many systems must adjust such generic requirements to meet a particular system's unique qualities. Several systems, including Oregon's, have developed criteria for a level IV hospital that provides resuscitation and stabilization of the severely injured prior to transfer to a higher level hospital. The state of Washington has gone one step further in creating standards for a category of level V facilities which do not necessarily need to be hospitals. These may be small clinics or free standing Emergency Centers. The level IV and V concept are at this point still experimental and no data is available to assess their efficacy.

Several systems have recognized the entity of pediatric trauma centers, burn centers and other specialty centers such as eye trauma and reimplantation centers. These centers have different criteria and requirements for development, implementation and evaluation, that address trauma care unique to those specialized patient populations and injuries.

Recognition of trauma care facilities currently revolves around three accepted concepts. These are: categorization, verification or designation. Self proclamation of trauma center status does occur; however in a true system such practices cannot exist. The lead agency of the system must officially be responsible for the process of recognition. Categorization is the least restrictive form of recognition and does not provide a mechanism for ensuring initial or continuing commitment standards; it merely categorizes a facility's resources and capabilities. Verification evaluates resources and capabilities as well as affirms that these are used appropriately for trauma patients. Verification, however, again does not assure standards will be consistently met. Designation limits the number of facilities recognized, and requires application, evaluation and approval. Designation involves a contractual agreement between the facility and the lead agency to maintain system standards. Many systems will use verification by independent site reviewers as the basis for subsequent designation.

Verification independent of lead agency recognition of that verification, should be essentially meaningless in a true and optimally functioning system. Each recognition scheme has particular advantages and disadvantages for any given system. Although associated with much resistance by health care institutions and providers in many systems, designation is generally regarded to be the most effective and best method of ensuring adherence to standards and provision of quality trauma care.

Rehabilitation has uniformly not been an integrated component of trauma care even in the most sophisticated of systems. It is estimated that only one in ten severely injured Americans has access to a rehabilitation service after initial treatment.[1] Currently no system has a formal process of rehabilitation service identification. Standards for trauma rehabilitation or triage and transfer protocols from acute care to rehabilitation services are also not found in any current trauma systems. The state of Washing-

ton is the first system to plan on doing so; however, this has not been implemented.

In the proposed Washington system, standards for rehabilitation facilities and services as well as triage guidelines to them have been set. Adult and pediatric services are designated from level I to level III. As part of designation, these facilities will be required to collect and submit patient data to the state. This data from the rehabilitation phase will be linked with acute care and prehospital data to provide the potential for meaningful longitudinal and functional outcome analysis and system evaluation. If successful, this will be a landmark accomplishment which will advance our knowledge of injury control and trauma system operations.

The concept of interfacility transfer to a higher level of care is well defined and established in most true systems. The concept of "down triage" or "back transfer" from facilities providing a higher level of care to those providing a lesser intensity of care is not. This may be appropriate to patient and system needs at any point in the patient's clinical course. There are advantages as well as disadvantages to such a strategy. This would serve to continually allocate resources appropriately. Level I trauma center beds would not be occupied by a preponderance of patients who, after initial evaluation and treatment, can be adequately cared for at a level III or IV type facility. This may have some negative continuity of care and financial implications. Such policies, though, might foster a sense of cooperation between facilities and physicians. They may lessen the fear of losing patients and prestige which concerns some community physicians and hospitals. These concerns sometimes impede transfers to trauma centers; lessening them would facilitate care at appropriate facilities. "Back transfer" may also offer positive psychosocial affects on patients and families who are separated. Before such policies and protocols are implemented, studies must be done to assess their cost effectiveness and impact on outcome, as well as on the appropriate timing of such transfers.

Quality Assurance/Improvement

A system of trauma care assures that quality care is consistently delivered. This is accomplished by monitoring system function and patient outcomes. Specific problems are identified and targeted for improvement. The system, as it matures, should strive to continually improve the overall quality of care. This requires a process of evaluation involving all participants and components.

A trauma system should be able to demonstrate the impact made on the patients it serves. System managers must be able to evaluate resource utilization, operational policies, procedures and protocols. An effective system evaluates itself against preestablished standards and objectives so that improvements in service can occur. Nationally accepted norms for major trauma patient outcome do exist[16] and many systems use these as a basis for patient outcome analysis. Each system must, again, set criteria for what constitutes quality care and acceptable outcome. It must also determine the cost benefit ratio of achieving that level of quality. The issues of patient and provider confidentiality, as well as protection from liability and inappropriate litigation related to this process, must be addressed. The limits of confidentiality must be clearly defined, preferentially in statute, if QA/QI efforts are to be effective.

DATA COLLECTION AND MANAGEMENT

Data collection and management is the foundation upon which any successful trauma care system is built. Data may come from a variety of sources. These include: law enforcement records, crash reports, death certificates, EMS records, hospital and rehabilitation charts and even insurance records. Many individual hospitals as well as some states have merged various aspects of this data into what is commonly known as a trauma registry. These registries incorporate varying degrees of information from the aforementioned sources pertaining to trauma patients. However, they generally focus on information from hospital and limited prehospital sources. The concept of a trauma registry, if it is to be effective on a systemwide basis, must be broadened in scope to that of an information system.

Trauma information systems provide the capability for total evaluation of trauma care systems through linkage of multiple databases.

This includes injury control and epidemiology, patient care, quality assurance, resource utilization and cost. They also serve to support and evaluate medical research and education. Trauma information systems, however, cannot be all things to all people. A primary mission of the information system must therefore be decided upon by a lead agency. Once this mission is set forth, the key questions which must be answered to accomplish the mission must be ascertained. With key questions having been elucidated, the data necessary to provide those answers can be identified. This is the most rational and effective way to design such an information system.[17] A focus on one area, such as patient care and quality assurance, does not necessarily preclude the ability to ascertain information in other areas such as epidemiology and prevention. There must however be a focus which dictates the major thrust of data collection.

System registries and hospital registries often have a different focus. As a result these two types of registries will collect different data on different types of providers and patients. If a system wide information bank is to be successful, it must have a clear purpose yet be flexible enough to integrate particular needs of all participants. The data set decided upon must not be so large as to be burdensome to those who are responsible for collecting, submitting and analyzing it. Only that data which is necessary to answer key questions should be collected. The data set can always be modified and expanded as system needs change. An overwhelming data set will ultimately affect the accuracy and completeness of data collection and predispose the information system to failure.

Inclusion criteria (case selection criteria) which identify patients to be included for analysis must be defined. These criteria are set in accordance with the purpose of the information system. For example, an injury information system might include cases of drowning and poisoning; a trauma information system would only include patients sustaining trauma. A major trauma information system might include a limited set of trauma patients and implicit in such an information system is the definition of major trauma. An EMS information system would seek information on all patients serviced by EMS providers in addition to the injured. This decision involves difficult distinctions, yet it is imperative that they be made. Preferably this is done by the lead agency in consultation with users and contributors to the information system who are participants in the trauma system.

In its purest form, an information system must collect data on those patients meeting inclusion criteria even if they do not come under the care of a system provider. This is the only way to obtain accurate information on overtriage and undertriage as well as compare the effectiveness of system versus nonsystem care. A final element in maintaining a useful and successful centrally administered trauma system information data base is to acknowledge and encourage local data contributors. This involves designing a system which is flexible enough to allow collection of data which may be pertinent locally but not at the central level. It also behooves the central repository to facilitate submission of data in formats which will not require great expenditure of resources and finances for collection and submission. Many systems rely on the hospital based trauma registry at a local, regional or statewide level. Data sets can and should differ between hospitals, regions and states. However, inclusion criteria and definitions, such as those for urban and rural locations, and complications, such as renal failure and pneumonia, often differ as well. This can make comparison of data between these different registries difficult and inaccurate. Currently the American College of Surgeons (ACS) is formulating minimum and optimum data sets in conjunction with the Joint Commission for Accreditation of Health Care Organizations (JCAHO) and the Centers for Disease Control (CDC). While neither the CDC or the ACS data set is ideal, it is hoped that a consensus on the information to be obtained will serve as a template upon which a national registry is built. Individual hospitals and local, regional and state systems can add to this standard template as they require for their individual needs and interests.

A number of commercial registry software packages are available from various vendors. Care should be taken in purchasing any commercial software or in designing "home-grown" registries. Registry managers must take into account the data elements which may be required to be submitted to a national repository. Also of note

is that the JCAHO is currently beta site testing approximately 12 quality indicators of trauma care. These indicators will require all hospitals treating trauma patients to show at the time of their JCAHO review that these indicators of quality care are continually monitored and met. This will require that all hospital trauma registries capture the data elements necessary to evaluate these indicators. In addition to collecting the appropriate data which is required nationally, it must be collected in a format which will allow uncomplicated export to a central repository. These are important considerations when purchasing or custom designing trauma registry software.

The data collection process must be validated through its own quality assurance/improvement program. This involves tracking the accuracy and completeness of data. Data elements which are persistently missing must be evaluated and the etiology of their absence sought. Often these data elements are too specific and may need to be considered for elimination from the data set. If deemed to be absolutely essential, strategies to improve collection and education of data contributors as to the importance of these data are necessary.

Few if any trauma system registries incorporate long-term data from the rehabilitation phase of trauma care. Many rehabilitation facilities do collect data on patients, but this has not routinely been integrated with data from the prehospital and acute care hospital phases. The most commonly used rehabilitation data set is the Uniform National Data Set for Medical Rehabilitation (UDS).[18] While somewhat extensive, a subset of pertinent data from the UDS should be identified and incorporated into trauma system registries.

The amount and nature of financial data to be collected from all phases of care should be decided upon in each system. This allows estimation of system operation costs, unreimbursed care, costs of certain interventions and specific injuries. Analysis of these data can be used to set health care policy, cost/charge structures and long-term strategic plans.

Integration and analysis of these data should be the goal of future trauma system data collection and management efforts. Only when outcomes are evaluated through a systems approach, considering all phases of care and finance, can one expect to accurately identify the causes of trauma, evaluate the impact of the system on outcome and address the associated mortality and morbidity of injury effectively.

SOCIETAL COMPONENTS

Societal components of a trauma system include public information, education and prevention. Additional components include research, economics and legislation.

Public awareness and education regarding the magnitude of injury, its preventability and the EMS and trauma systems is essential in a trauma system. This aspect is often neglected. Public information and education efforts must serve to enhance the public's role in the system, its ability to access the system and the prevention of injuries. In many areas, trauma care providers from various phases of care act as a clearing house for information on trauma system access. They may also present injury prevention programs. This ultimately leads to better utilization of trauma system resources and improved patient outcome.

Prevention may be the single most important societal component and therefore trauma systems must develop prevention strategies which will bring about effective control of injury. Providers system wide must work with business organizations, lay groups and the public at large to enact these strategies. Information gleaned from system wide trauma registry data is extremely useful for targeting the appropriate geographic areas for specific injury prevention strategies. While trauma prevention may be the most difficult goal to achieve in a trauma system, it may prove to be the most cost effective intervention.

Prevention strategy can take the form of primary, secondary and tertiary interventions. Primary strategies attempt to prevent the event itself from occurring, i.e., lobbying for gun control laws. Secondary prevention strategies seek to lessen the severity of injuries which do occur, e.g., promoting seatbelt and bicycle helmet use or sponsoring car seat loaner programs. Finally tertiary prevention strategies seek to minimize the consequences of injuries which have been incurred (promoting prompt EMS, trauma center and rehabilitative care). Strategies can take an active or passive form. Active strategies require cooperation and participation of the individual in order to be protected, e.g., participation in MADD, SADD seminars. Passive strategies are automatic and require no participation or any special response from the individual, such as automatic license revocation for drunk driving. Passive strategies tend to be more effective although program evaluation in the area of prevention is rare due to complexities of research design and lack of outcome and followup data.

There are many groups within communities which sponsor prevention programs aimed at various injuries. Many of these programs sponsored by these various groups and organizations represent duplicative efforts and redundant expenditure of resources. Perhaps the greatest role of a trauma system in the future will be to identify, coordinate and integrate these programs. This will promote a focused and cost-effective method of injury prevention.

In addition to public education, trauma systems must strive to educate trauma care professionals. This educational initiative must encompass magnitude and preventability issues with the medical community as well as patient care. Many health care professionals do not believe a problem exists in their locale.

The personnel who provide trauma care within a system are often the most abundant resource for that system. This is particularly true in rural areas. At least one study of rural trauma care concludes that the single most important improvement in patient care would arise from increased educational efforts aimed at small town trauma care providers.[19] Innovative strategies for provider education employed by some systems have included concept of mobile training units, video interactive programs and subsidies to underwrite Advanced Trauma Life Support (ATLS) course expenses or locum tenens coverage for physicians taking the course. Evaluation of trauma registry data should yield valuable information as to the focus for—and areas most in need of—such educational programs. The effectiveness of both conventional and experimental educational tools can also be evaluated with the aid of registry data.

RESEARCH

Despite the magnitude of injury as a public health problem in America today, injury related research is allotted only 2% of the national health care research budget.[1] Only recently has the Centers for Disease Control (CDC) developed a division of Injury Control. This division has sponsored a National Injury Control Conference. The major purpose of this conference, and the activities at the CDC preceding it, was to set a national agenda for injury control in the 1990s. The position paper from this conference on trauma care systems has identified several areas of research to be emphasized.[20] These include the study and evaluation of cost effective measures for trauma care systems, comprehensive evaluation of reimbursement issues and identification and evaluation of methods to provide optimal trauma care in rural settings. Also mentioned are the identification and study of urban trauma care problems and the study of ethical moral and legal dilemmas facing trauma care. These include removal of artificial life sustaining technology, organ donation and procurement and defining and dealing with "lethal injury".

System Funding

Trauma systems are expensive to develop and maintain. The costs associated with hospital readiness and system monitoring can be quite burdensome to states and regions that are facing financial constraints. Some states, in order to encourage system development and ensure system viability, have included language in statutes to partially or fully offset costs associated with trauma system development, implementation and operation.

A number of different funding methods have been tried including surcharges on vehicle registration, drivers license application or renewal. Surcharges on the 911 universal telephone access number or additional surcharges on moving violations have also been implemented in some areas. "Sin" taxes on alcohol and firearms have also been proposed. Each of these mechanisms places the cost of providing trauma care on those who use the system most.

Given dwindling reimbursement from third party payers or governmental agencies, a stable mechanism to ensure system funding is essential. While the funding mechanisms in many regions or states may be similar, the distribution of funds varies significantly. It is imperative that these funds be dedicated to the trauma system. Trauma systems supported through the general funds of a state or county are subject to significant reductions in funding level at the whim of legislators or as a result of budget crises. States with examples of funding legislation related to trauma systems can be found in Florida, California, Washington, Pennsylvania and Texas.[21]

Legislation

Both national and state legislation dealing with trauma systems is increasing with the realization of need and effectiveness of these systems in controlling injury. The Trauma Care Systems Planning and Development Act (PL 101-590) was approved by Congress and signed into law by the President in November 1991. This marks a significant advance in the recognition of injury control as a national priority. Under the provisions of the new law, states will be awarded grants to be used in developing, implementing and monitoring state wide trauma systems. Portions of these grants may be used to offset uncompensated trauma care. The law also establishes an advisory committee to assist the Secretary of Health and Human Services in assessing the nation's trauma care needs and developing a model national trauma system plan. In addition, there is provision for a national emergency medical system and trauma care clearing house to assimilate and disseminate information on trauma care as well as supply technical assistance to those states requesting it. Finally, the law establishes funding for research and programs that seek to improve rural emergency medical services. While the bill was originally budgeted at $60 million it has only been funded for $5 million. Even this small amount represents a commitment to systematize and improve trauma care nationally.

As a result of national initiatives, many states are now looking to establish trauma systems and to develop trauma legislation. The importance of comprehensive trauma legislation in system planning and implementation cannot be understated. The National Highway Traffic Safety Administration (NHTSA) has conducted a study of trauma system legislation.[21] In that review, 34 states were noted to have existing legislation and one with legislation pending. There are varying degrees of specificity to each of the state's legislation. Of those reviewed, the most comprehensive and complete statutes are found in California, Washington, Illinois, Texas and Florida.

Several elements have been identified as key in designing successful model trauma legislation. Those elements include the need to designate a lead governmental agency; to integrate the trauma system within an already functioning EMS system; to plan for the orderly movement of trauma patients to trauma facilities; to standardize care within the system both in the prehospital and in the hospital setting; to collect data and evaluate system performance measured against preestablished standards and patient outcome; to provide a form for quality assurance and quality improvement such that the information is protected within the system; and finally to allow the system to grow by securing a steady source of funding necessary for system development and system maintenance. In order to take into consideration the needs of different communities, statutes should be broad in scope covering the essentials mentioned above. This allows for the more detailed system refinements to be developed in the regulatory rather than the statutory process.

TRAUMA SYSTEM DEVELOPMENT

Developing and establishing a trauma system is a major challenge to any state or community. The process is a lengthy one fraught with many challenges.[22] It often requires redistribution of patients as well as medical and economic resources. It also requires public and legislative support and public education. Steps involved in the process include a needs assessment phase, identification and empowerment of a lead agency, development of standards which would include triage criteria and a process for trauma care facility recognition. An implementation phase then follows during which the standards and

facilities become operational under the direction of the lead agency. The evaluation phase completes the process through the assessment of standards, ongoing needs and quality assurance/improvement efforts.

The needs assessment phase is essential for winning public and professional support for a trauma system. It is also helpful in identifying the current state of trauma care, setting standards and identifying phases of care and geographic locations which may need special attention. Historically, needs assessment has focused around using various methods to estimate preventable deaths. Autopsy studies as well as studies looking at all available clinical records have been reported.[2] The latter approach yields information on the timing and adequacy of prehospital and hospital care. The combination of clinical review and autopsy studies produce the greatest amount of useful information. Autopsy rates for trauma related deaths vary greatly between and within states. The quality of examination is also quite variable. Both these factors make such autopsy studies difficult to accomplish in most states. The state of Washington has taken a unique and much broader approach to needs assessment which truly attempts to evaluate trauma care as a continuum.[23]

Once the need for a trauma system has been established a second priority is to delegate legal authority for the development and operation of such a system. This step requires legislation that empowers such an agency as the authoritative body. This agency may be public or private. Of the 21 states with active trauma programs 15 delegate authority for program administration and development to the state emergency medical services office. The state of Pennsylvania delegates that authority to a private trauma systems foundation. The lead agency is charged with developing criteria for the trauma system, identifying and recognizing the appropriate facilities to care for these patients, establishing a trauma registry and establishing quality assurance/improvement programs. It is imperative that this agency have legislative authority thus avoiding legal repercussions. Exemplary trauma system legislation which includes identifying a role and responsibility for a lead agency is felt to exist in the states of Washington, Texas, Virginia, Pennsylvania, Florida and California.[21]

During the implementation phase, the lead agency must set and institute standards and establish the process for trauma care provider recognition. The recognition process and system standards should be applied to prehospital and rehabilitation providers as well as to cute care facilities. Centralized data collection and analysis also begins during this phase. At this point decisions must be made as to the inclusive or exclusive character of the system being developed. Decisions on standards, the recognition of providers and data collection must be made in consultation with representatives of provider agencies and interested parties from all phases of trauma care. In order to foster committed participation in the system, providers must feel they have adequate input into the development process. These decisions must also be made with consideration of the current state and variation of trauma care resources and practices. Standards which are set at a level which cannot be realistically achieved initially, as well as failure to build a constituency, will risk system failure at the outset.

The final and perhaps most important step in establishing a trauma system is the evaluation and modification phase. This is driven by quality assurance and improvement activities based on data collection and analysis. A trauma information system (registry) is essential to document the epidemiology and demographic characteristics of injury in a given community, region or state; to aid ongoing need and resource assessment; and to support quality improvement activities. This completes the loop by identifying new problems to be assessed and by developing strategies to address those problems which are then implemented and again evaluated. A trauma system must be a dynamic entity that responds to the needs of the community it serves, both provider and consumer. This process requires continual assessment of the various components within the trauma system.

The EMS Division of the National Highway Traffic Safety Administration sponsors two programs which aid in the development of new trauma systems and the assessment of existing systems and regional trauma care resources. The Technical Assistance Program permits states to utilize highway safety funds to support the technical evaluation of existing and proposed Emergency Medical Services programs and assists with the development of integrated EMS programs that include comprehensive systems of trauma care. The assessment team is composed of individuals who have demonstrated expertise in EMS development and implementation. The team evaluates each state on ten standard components. In addition to assessing the effectiveness of each component individually, significant consideration is given to the interrelationship of the components producing a comprehensive and integrated system of emergency and trauma care. The team then compares the status of EMS in the state to NHTSA standards and makes recommendation on how the state might achieve those optimal standards.

A second program sponsored by NHTSA is the Development of Trauma Systems (DOTS) seminar program. This seminar is aimed at individuals who might play key leadership roles in trauma system development and operation. The eight hour seminar provides the participant with the conceptual framework around which a trauma system can be developed. Issues pertinent to planning and implementation, operation and evaluation of regional trauma systems are discussed.

Finally the American College of Surgeons sponsors a site evaluation and verification program. This program is offered to hospitals who wish to have their trauma care capability verified by an independent organization. While this program is quite helpful, verification by the ACS does not constitute designation as a trauma center. Only a lead agency with legislative empowerment can designate a facility. A number of state and regional trauma systems do use a ACS verification as a basis for system designation.

TRAUMA SYSTEM FAILURE AND BARRIERS TO DEVELOPMENT

Although no existing trauma systems meet all criteria necessary to be considered truly comprehensive and fully functional, many do approach these optimal standards. A number of these existing systems are, however, failing. Many more potential systems are being stifled by barriers to development. As previously discussed, the reasons for this are commonly attributed to finances and lack of provider reimbursement. While problems with reimbursement cannot be denied, other factors related to tradition, politics, government, society and medicine contribute as well. These are perhaps more difficult to identify and solve. The financial as well as these other factors need further examination. Solutions to problems in systems that are operating must be found. Potential problems and barriers must be identified and addressed in the planning phase of new systems.

Regionalization and concentration of trauma care at specialized facilities increases resource utilization and unreimbursed charges at these facilities. The concepts of back triage and inclusive systems may aid in lessening this burden and foster shared responsibility. Estimation of trauma care costs and reimbursement before system implementation and provider recognition will allow system planners and facility administrators to know at the outset what participation as a trauma care provider will mean financially. This will also allow estimation of funding levels for the system that will be necessary. This may prevent a high provider dropout rate once the system is operational.

Lack of physician commitment has been shown to be a prevalent factor in trauma center closure. Nearly 40% of surgeons prefer not to care for trauma patients.[11] However some perceptions associated with this reluctance, such as increased medicolegal risk, are not substantiated. There is a great need for dissemination of accurate data to allay this concern. Other concerns such as negative impact on private practice and increased time commitment must be further investigated if physician commitment is to be improved.

Lack of evaluation and meaningful analysis of central trauma registry data has also contributed to dysfunctional trauma systems. This problem often stems from lack of registry purpose and data collection only for the sake of data collection. A more serious problem revolves around failure of the system data repository to report useful information back to contributors. This gives little incentive for them to submit accurate data and no opportunity to realize the importance of collection efforts and to put data to use. Options allowing collection of additional data which is locally pertinent by individual

providers and the local analysis of this data is key to system success.

Finally, failure of the lead agency to be empowered or to use that empowerment effectively has also caused many systems to falter. Seeking the advice and participation of a broad based constituency of trauma care providers can often help identify and deal with allies and opponents. This is best accomplished through an advisory panel composed of representatives of various trauma care provider and consumer groups. For example if a state hospital association is not consulted prior to formulating a plan for trauma care facility recognition, then the plan can obviously be expected to be met with resistance. If a trauma registry is designed without the input of prehospital providers and emergency department staff then data collection is fraught with problems. Only when all participants understand and feel part of system development and operation can it be successful.

In summary a trauma system organizes and integrates trauma care resources within a geographic area. The system maintains and continually evaluates standards of care throughout all phases—prevention through rehabilitation. Successful operation of a trauma system involves the complex intermingling of multiple societal and patient care components as well as personalities and politics. Many of the problems associated with failure to develop and maintain functional trauma systems are predictable and surmountable. Institution of systematized care has been shown to decrease preventable death from trauma. It is crucial that trauma systems continue to be developed, maintained and refined if the associated mortality and morbidity of injury is to be effectively controlled.

REFERENCES

1. National Academy of Science: Injury in America, A Continuing Health Problem. Washington: National Academy Press, 1985.
2. Cales RH, Trunkey DD. Preventable trauma deaths: A review of trauma care systems development. JAMA 1985; 254:1059-1063.
3. Shackford SR, Hollingsworth-Fridlund P, Cooper GF et al. The effect of regionalization upon the quality of trauma care as assessed by concurrent audit before and after institution of a trauma system: A preliminary report. J Trauma 1986; 26:812-820.
4. Committee on trauma. Resources for optimal care of

the injured patient. American College of Surgeons, Chicago 1990.

5. West JG, Williams MJ, Trunkey DD et al. Trauma systems current status future challenges. JAMA 1988; 259:3597-3600.

6. National Highway Traffic Safety Administration. Technical assistance program statewide EMS assessments: A compilation of findings. Washington, DC 1991.

7. Thompson RG, Hallstrom AP, Cobb LA. Bystander initiated cardiopulmonary resuscitation in the management of ventricular fibrillation. Ann Int Med 1979; 90:737-740.

8. Champion HR, Mabee MS. An American crisis in trauma care reimbursement. Washington, DC 1990.

9. Trauma care: Lifesaving system threatened by unreimbursed costs and other factors. U.S. General Accounting Office, Washington, DC 1991.

10. Dailey JT, Teter H, Soderstrom CA, Provenzano G. Trauma center closures: A national assessment. J Trauma 1991; 31:1026.

11. Esposito TJ, Maier RV, Rivara FP et al. Why surgeons prefer not to care for trauma patients. Arch Surg 1991: 126:292-297.

12. Richardson DJ, Miller FB. Will future surgeons be interested in trauma care: Results of a resident survey. J Trauma 1991: 31:1037.

13. Cowley RA. The resuscitation and stabilization of major multiple trauma patients in a trauma center environment. Clin Med 1976; 83:14.

14. Champion HR, Sacco WJ, Copes WS. A revision of the trauma score. J Trauma 1989; 29:623-629.

15. McSwain N. Medical control—what is it? J Am Coll Emerg Phys 1978; 7:114.

16. Champion HR, Copes WS, Sacco WJ et al. The major trauma outcome study: Establishing national norms for trauma care. J Trauma 1990: 30:1356-1365.

17. Cales RH, Kearns ST. Concepts. In: Johnston JB, ed. Trauma Registers. Trauma Quarterly 1989; (5): 1-8.

18. Hamilton BB, Granger CV, Sherwin FS et al. A uniform national data system for medical rehabilitation. In: Fuher MJ, ed. Rehabilitation Outcomes: Analysis and Measurement. Baltimore: PH Brookes Publishing Co, 1987.

19. Krob MJ, Cram AE, Vargish T et al. Rural trauma care: A study of trauma care in a rural emergency medical services region. Ann Emerg Med 1984; 13:891-895.

20. Executive Summaries: Third Injury Control Conference. Position paper on trauma care systems. J Trauma 1992; 32: 127-129.

21. Cooper GF. Comprehensive trauma system legislation: An overview. US Dept Transp NHTSA, Washington DC, 1991.

22. Esposito TJ, Lazear SE, Maier RV. Trauma care systems development: Evolution and current trends. In: Maull KI, ed. Advances in Trauma and Critical Care, 1991: 115-131.

23. Esposito TJ, Nania J, Maier RV. State trauma system evaluation: A unique and comprehensive approach. Ann Emerg Med 1992; 21:351-357.

CHAPTER 2

THE FUTURE OF TRAUMA SCORING

Howard R. Champion

Injury severity scoring mechanisms are as essential for trauma as are grading or staging for any other disease. Many physiologic and anatomic trauma scores are in use today. While there is much debate about their relative merits, these scores have the potential to greatly impact future resource allocation and reimbursement determinations and quality of care assessment methodologies.

PHYSIOLOGIC INDICES: USE IN TRIAGE

The severity of a patient's injury, reflected in vital signs (blood pressure and respiratory rate) and level of consciousness, and extent and type of injury are factors in determining the optimum treatment and transport strategy to be used. Physiologic scores with these elements, e.g., the Glasgow Coma Scale (GCS) and the Revised Trauma Score (RTS), have been widely used in trauma triage for many years and have proven valuable in facilitating accurate patient assessment (on-scene and en route to definitive care) by nonphysician emergency personnel.

ANATOMIC INDICES: USE IN COMPARATIVE STUDIES

Anatomic indices, which require complete and accurate diagnoses, have limited use for field triage because a complete diagnosis is generally unavailable until definitive diagnosis or autopsy. The value of anatomic scores is that they permit evaluation and classification of the damage associated with the injury, activities that are crucial in trauma system evaluation and outcome assessment. To varying degrees anatomic scoring systems, e.g., the Abbreviated Injury Scale (AIS), Injury Severity Score (ISS) and Anatomic Profile (AP) are predictive of patient outcome, which makes them essential elements in the combination indices discussed below.

COMBINATION INDICES: USE IN OUTCOME EVALUATION

Although both physiologic and anatomic scores are continually being re-evaluated and improved, it is combination indices that hold the most promise in characterizing injury severity because they are more predictive of patient outcome. Combination indices allow injury severity to be quantified for epidemiologic studies, comparisons among patient cohorts and quality assurance. For effective scientific study of trauma and unfortunately because such scales are beginning to be used in defining reimbursement and in extramural quality of care assessments, these indices must be made to perform to the best of their ability.

CURRENT DEMANDS OF TRAUMA SCORING

Ideally, injuries are grouped and classified to provide a method of grading injury severity that controls for case mix differences among various patient populations with disparate combinations of injuries (enabling epidemiologic comparison as well as comparison of patient outcome over time and changes in patient care), to permit quality assurance review relative to patient outcome and process of care, and to provide a method for imposing financial accountability for treatment and for estimating the costs of various injuries and combinations of injuries. These issues and how they relate to resource allocation and reimbursement are discussed below.

RESOURCE ALLOCATION

Trauma scoring could become a major determinant in resource allocation. As the costs of medical care continues to rise, variations in practice patterns and outcomes have sparked increasingly fierce competition among healthcare providers and public demand for more efficient, effective healthcare services. Current economic trends have resulted in the emergence of quality assurance as a pivotal force for cost containment, with important legal ramifications. For example, some malpractice insurance carriers require that their clients provide quality assurance documentation and correct identified practice deficiencies, often with the result of increased malpractice premiums. In this context, trauma severity scores facilitate standardization of patient data in order to impose accountability for treatment and to estimate the costs of various (including multiple) injuries and combinations of injuries of varying severity.

IMPROVEMENTS IN OUTCOME-ORIENTED RESEARCH

Most contemporary outcome-oriented research has focused exclusively on patient mortality. TRISS, for example, the mainstay of the Major Trauma Outcome Study (MTOS), is a combination index that uses the RTS (physiologic index) and ISS (anatomic component) to characterize injury severity and estimate patient survival probability (Ps). TRISS-generated probabilities of survival are utilized in the preliminary outcome-based evaluation (PRE) to support quality assurance activities. PRE identifies patients with unexpected outcomes—patients with seemingly nonfatal injuries who died (TRISS-estimated Ps > .05)—and those with typically lethal injuries who survived (TRISS-estimated Ps < .05) whose cases may be worthy of quality assurance review.

Limitations of TRISS's anatomic component prompted the development of A Severity Characterization of Trauma (ASCOT), which relies instead on the AP and weights the RTS variables according to etiology of injury. This gives ASCOT greater prognostic power than TRISS with regard to patient mortality, and makes ASCOT likely to become a robust predictor of other important outcomes. For example, AP component D, not used in predictions of survival probability because it is a summary score of relatively minor injuries, may be used in the future in impairment outcome predictions because it includes many injuries that are likely to have long-term effects. Statistically valid impairment and severity outcome predictions in turn have direct implications for resource allocation because they relate to length of hospital and intensive care unit (ICU) stay, and, subsequently, reimbursement.

Incomplete Data

In an ideal situation, a complete description of anatomic injury, obtained from surgery, CT scan or postmortem examination would be available for every trauma patient. Lacking this, only patients with all data required by TRISS or ASCOT have traditionally been included in statistical quality assurance studies. This excluded a large number of patients, at first because few trauma registries had been established and more recently because increased use of paralytic agents and ventilation in prehospital care often makes it impossible to obtain the necessary scores. Two essential elements of quality assurance, used both in TRISS and ASCOT, are the z and W statistics, which are used to compare patient outcomes of a particular institution with an accepted norm. The z statistic compares the actual numbers of survivors in a trauma center with the number expected based on current norms. The W statistic indicates the degree of variance from the expected norm of survivors per 100 patients.

For optimum quality assurance, facilities should include all consecutive patients in their analyses. Exclusion of patients with missing variables introduces a statistically significant bias into the results of these outcome evaluations. For example, patients excluded from analysis due to lack of data have a mortality rate twice that of included patients. The actual degree of bias depends on the extent of injury of excluded patients, i.e., exclusion of any unexpected deaths or survivors can bias z and W to a large degree.

STATISTICAL BOUNDING TO DETERMINE BIAS

To mitigate the bias, whether large or small, bounds for z and W that show the impact of incomplete patient data are currently being developed. Bounding W is simple, but bounding z raises a complex mathematical optimization issue that may be resolved via statistical modeling in computerized trauma registries. Although it is always preferable to have complete patient data, these bounding techniques will prove useful in quantifying the effect of missing data that could have been obtained, but for whatever reason, e.g., patient in extremis or patient transferred from nontrauma center, were not. To account for intubated or therapeutically paralyzed patients whose lack of data is considered unavoidable, new bounding methods are being developed which will contribute to improved reliability of research and quality assurance efforts.

REIMBURSEMENT

Inadequate reimbursement for trauma care has become a threat to the existence of trauma centers and the concept of the regional trauma network. Improvements in outcome and resource use prediction have the potential to lead to more appropriate payment mechanisms for trauma which may help alleviate the current crisis in trauma care reimbursement.

An example of an injury classification scheme used for reimbursement that is particularly ill-suited for trauma is the much-debated Diagnosis Related Group (DRG) concept. Introduced in 1983 by the Health Care Financing Administration in an effort to contain costs, this prospective payment system collapses all of an individual patient's various diagnoses into the single most severe or complex diagnosis and assigns a predetermined average length of stay (LOS) and associated fixed amount for reimbursement. Because DRGs do not take into account the severity of injury and the necessarily higher costs of trauma care, trauma centers and other institutions that accept trauma patients are reimbursed at 0-50% of the actual costs of the services they perform.

Use of DRGs has reduced the ability of trauma centers to withstand the growing economic burden of uncompensated care that has already forced many centers to close. An alternative, Patient Management Categories (PMCs), recently was introduced as a potential substitute for DRGs. Like DRGs, however, PMCs use the International Classification of Diseases (ICD) nomenclature, a poor method of characterizing injury severity. Furthermore, PMCs use LOS and treatment in their characterization, variables that can be affected by so many factors, e.g., inappropriate treatment or changing standards of care, that their relationship to the injury is far from direct. Injury cannot be classified by treatment.

The unique nature of trauma care presents ongoing problems associated with reimbursement in that (1) trauma care differs from nontrauma care even for the same procedures (because of associated injuries and intervening conditions such as hemorrhagic shock); (2) the morbidity that surrounds trauma may be poorly related to the extent of a single injury; and (3) trauma care entails a multidisciplinary effort. Current and proposed codes do not provide an accurate picture of the many services that are required for the trauma patient. An equitable reimbursement policy requires the following: (1) that the codes account for the condition of the patient, including the injuries sustained, the severity of physiological derangement at presentation and the multiplicity and additive effect of the injuries, age, etc.; (2) a fair assignment of relative work values that accounts for all physician work involved in trauma care; and (3) timely payment and encouragement of efficiency and effectiveness of care. A new reimbursement methodology is desperately needed that accomplishes the above, i.e., diagnostically based Trauma Related Groupings that utilize recognized trauma-specific guidelines.

Furthermore, the high cost of trauma care (approximately three times the cost of other types of hospital care) and the burgeoning ranks of the unemployed have created an ever-widening gap known as uncompensated care. Uncompensated care and inadequate reimbursement have created an impossible economic situation that has resulted in the closure of more than 40 trauma centers in the past three years alone.

ICU INDICES

In recent years, significant efforts have been and continue to be made to incorporate severity indices into the ICU, but these indices still fail the needs of both ICU patient and physician, i.e., they provide the least information where it is needed most for outcome prediction.

The Acute Physiology And Chronic Health Evaluation (APACHE) classification system was developed to create a better methodology for measuring case mix among ICU patients and to facilitate research on ICU resource utilization and quality of care. The

most recent version of this system, APACHE III, is better suited than its predecessor for outcome comparison. However, it is still based on a relatively small database and its predictive capabilities for surgical patients has yet to be adequately demonstrated by sophisticated statistical testing.

The future of ICU indices will no doubt depend on innovative use of technology, i.e., manipulation of computer data at the patient's bedside. State-of-the-art ICUs already allow physician access to information on vital organ function via bedside computer. Soon prognoses will be able to be computed based on the patient's primary condition, vital organ indices on a given day and time and any trends regarding the patient's condition over the past three- to five-day period. Appropriate integration of the most current patient information and the slope of change has the potential to significantly raise the predictive capability of ICU indices. The combination of sophisticated mathematical modeling and bedside computer generation of data will, in the mid-to-late 1990s, considerably facilitate the use and value of ICU indices for surgical patients.

TECHNICAL IMPROVEMENTS IN SCORING

While current methods of classifying injury are probably robust enough to be a data substratum for the quality assurance/peer review process, they have proven inadequate to quantify the severely injured, multiple trauma patient for purposes of resource allocation and cost reimbursement. As cost accounting, marginal costs associated with individual patients, and the need for services to cover direct costs become increasingly burdensome to hospital and trauma center administrations, it will become more critical that injury severity classifications correlate with the resources needed for optimum treatment. Caution must be used, however, to avoid the use of these scores to in any way encourage the use of "economic triage." Furthermore, as outcome research shifts from mortality to other outcomes such as impairment and quality of life, the flexibility to move from one scale to another using the same database becomes important.

While the perfect characterization of injury severity may never be found, it is reasonable to expect trauma scores to be improved to their maximum potential, e.g., mitigating the bias created by missing data by determining bounds for z and W, and to be used appropriately (unlike DRGs). Failing this, trauma research and the regional trauma network concept face an increasingly uncertain future.

SELECTED READING

1. MacKenzie EJ. Injury severity scales: Overview and directions for future research. Am J Emerg Med 1984; 2:537.

2. Champion HR, Sacco WJ, Hannan DS et al. Assessment of injury severity: The Triage Index. Crit Care Med 1980; 8:201.

3. Champion HR, Sacco WJ, Carnazzo AJ et al. The Trauma Score. Crit Care Med 1981; 9:672.

4. Champion HR, Sacco WJ. The Trauma Score as applied to penetrating injury. Ann Emerg Med 1984; 13:6.

5. Champion HR, Sacco WJ, Hunt TK. Trauma severity scoring to predict mortality. World J Surg 1983; 7:4.

6. Morris JA, Auerbach PS, Marshall GA, et al. The Trauma Score as a triage tool in the prehospital setting. JAMA 1986; 256:1319.

7. Baker SP, O'Neill B, Haddon W Jr et al. The Injury Severity Score: A method for describing patients with multiple injuries and evaluating emergency care. J Trauma 1974; 14:187.

8. Copes WS, Champion HR, Sacco WJ et al. The Injury Severity Score revisited. J Trauma 1988; 28:69.

9. Champion HR, Sacco WJ, Lepper RL et al. An anatomic index of injury severity. J Trauma 1980; 20:197.

10. Knaus WA, Draper EA, Wagner DP et al. APACHE II: A severity of disease classification system. Crit Care Med 1985; 13:818.

11. Champion HR, Sacco WJ. Trauma severity scales. St. Louis: Mosby Year Book Inc., 1986.

12. Hamilton BB, Granger CV, Sherwin FS et al. A uniform national data system for medical rehabilitation. In: Fuhrer MJ, Baltimore: Paul H. Brookes, 1987.

13. Shackford SR, Hollingsworth-Fridlund P, McArdle M et al. Assuring quality in a trauma system—the medical audit committee: composition, cost, and results. J Trauma 1987; 27:866.

14. Champion HR, Copes WS, Sacco WJ et al. A new characterization of injury severity. J Trauma 1990: 30:539.

15. Champion HR, Copes WS, Sacco WJ et al. The Major Trauma Outcome Study: Establishing national norms for trauma care. J Trauma 1990: 30:1356.

16. Champion HR, Mabee MS. An American crisis in trauma care reimbursement. Emerg Care Q 1990; 6:65.

17. Civetta JM. Evaluation of APACHE II for cost containment and quality assurance. Ann Surg 1990; 212:266.

18. Karmy-Jones R, Copes WS, Champion HR et al. Results of a multiinstitutional outcome assessment: Results of a structured peer review of TRISS-designated unexpected outcomes. J Trauma 1992: 32:196.

CHAPTER 3

RESUSCITATION SOLUTIONS

Gail T. Tominaga

Kenneth Waxman

INTRODUCTION

Intravenous fluid therapy has been the mainstay of prehospital and emergency center management of postinjury shock for the last half of this century. The majority of acutely ill or injured patients require volume replacement as part of their resuscitation. These include patients suffering from hemorrhage, trauma and acute abdominal events. Aggressive fluid resuscitation is generally the initial therapy for these fluid deficits.

There are many indicators of adequate fluid resuscitation. However, clinical signs such as heart rate, blood pressure and urinary output are not very reliable. Shock can be defined as a state in which tissue oxygenation is inadequate to meet metabolic demands. The major goal of resuscitation of seriously ill and injured patients is to provide sufficient oxygen to meet their metabolic requirements. Multiple factors following shock states alter oxygen transport at the tissue level so that increased oxygen delivery is necessary to meet these increased metabolic demands. The ideal end point of fluid resuscitation should be optimization of oxygen delivery and oxygen consumption.

Various resuscitative fluids are currently available and can be classified as crystalloid solutions, colloid solutions or blood substitutes. Colloids can be natural such as albumin or synthetic such as hetastarch and dextran. Because of the limited availability of blood and blood products as well as concerns over infectious and immunologic risks, there has been increasing interest placed on blood substitutes, such as perfluorochemicals and stroma free hemoglobin. This chapter will review the various resuscitation solutions currently available for clinical use and oxygen-carrying solutions under investigation. Finally the future of resuscitation solutions will be discussed.

CRYSTALLOIDS

A crystalloid is any solution of crystalline solids dissolved in water. Dextrose solutions essentially provide free water because dextrose is metabolized rapidly. Hence, dextrose solutions are ineffective plasma expanders.

Saline solutions are distributed into the extracellular space which represents about 33% of total body water. Once equilibrium of the intravascular and extravascular spaces occurs, approximately 25% of normal saline infused remains in the vascular space. In addition, the use of normal saline may result in hypernatremia and hyperchloremic acidosis. For this reason, Ringer's lactate solution is often preferred when massive crystalloid infusions are administered since it has a slightly lower sodium content and contains sodium lactate which is metabolized to bicarbonate. In general, crystalloids are used to expand the volume of the entire extracellular fluid space, including the interstitial space and the plasma volume. Half normal saline solutions may be indicated in dehydration with hypernatremia, but are less effective plasma expanders.

HYPERTONIC SALINE

Recently there has been increased interest in hypertonic saline treatment of hemorrhagic shock. In the military setting with the need to limit volume, weight and amount of supplies, logic encourages development of a smaller volume but equally effective solution for fluid resuscitation. Hypertonic saline can increase plasma and interstitial volume by recruiting intracellular water. However, this effect is transient and correlates with the equilibration of sodium in the extravascular compartment. The beneficial hemodynamic effects of hypertonic saline are increased systemic blood pressure, increased cardiac output, improved oxygen transport and increased mesenteric and coronary blood flow. In addition, hemodynamic response to hypertonic saline may be augmented by a vagal pulmonary reflex that leads to selective musculocutaneous vasoconstriction resulting in shunting of blood to vital organs.[1] This reflex is thought to be dependent on the presence of high concentration of sodium ions in the interstitium. Hypertonic saline has also been reported to increase myocardial contractility and cause precapillary dilation.

Several studies have reported that hypertonic saline resuscitation compared favorably to lactated Ringer's injection and normal saline resuscitation when hemodynamic parameters were measured. However, Krausz et al demonstrated that the infusion of hypertonic saline within 15 minutes of hemorrhagic shock resulted in increased bleeding, hypotension and early death in an uncontrolled hemorrhagic shock model in animals.[2] Many questions remain with respect to use of hypertonic solutions. Furthermore, comparative human studies demonstrating survival benefit with hypertonic saline have not yet been reported.

Clinical studies have used a maximum volume of 250 ml and a maximum concentration of 7.5% NaCl solutions. Theoretically, larger volumes of this concentration can cause hypernatremia and hyperosmolarity. In addition, fluid shifts from the intracellular to the intravascular compartments can lead to intracellular dehydration. This may have a deleterious effect upon organ function such as brain function after traumatic or ischemic cerebral insult. However, this effect may also be of benefit after head injury as hypertonic saline has been demonstrated in animal models to reduce intracranial pressure.

COLLOIDS

Colloids refer to suspensions of particles with molecular weights larger than those of crystalloids. Colloids maintain plasma volume because particles in the colloid solution are large enough to resist movement through the normal capillary membrane into the interstitial space. Natural colloids include 5% and 25% albumin solutions. The 5% solution remains largely within the vascular space when the capillary membrane is intact so that it represents a natural plasma expander. The hyperoncotic 25% solution effectively pulls fluid from the interstitial space so that it may be preferred in edematous patients. Synthetic colloids include hetastarches and dextran solutions which will be described in more detail later.

HYPERTONIC SALINE WITH DEXTRAN

Posthemorrhage hemodynamic improvement after a bolus of hypertonic saline with no added colloid is short lived. A more sustained effect has been shown with a solution of 7.5% NaCl in 6% dextran-70. A U.S. multicentered trial demonstrated that the infusion of 250 ml of 7.5% NaCl in 6% dextran is to be as effective as standard resuscitation solutions in the prehospital management of traumatic hypotension.[3] This solution was found to have minimal adverse effects. However, no significant improvement in overall survival was shown. Vassar et al demonstrated the requirement of smaller volumes of hypertonic saline/dextran-70 compared to lactated Ringer's solution for prehospital resuscitation. In addition, there was a trend for improved survival in head-injured patients and possible benefits in penetrating trauma patients.[4] Hypertonic saline/dextran has also been studied in burn patients and found to be only transiently effective in treating burn shock.[5]

Dextran

Dextrans are polysaccharides produced by the conversion of sucrose into long glucose polymers by the bacterial enzyme dextransucrase. Clinically used dextrans are produced by the bacterium *Leuconostoc mesenteroides*. The molecules produced by the bacteria are very large, with molecular weights of several million daltons. For intravenous infusion, partial acid hydrolysis produces dextran fractions within specific weight ranges. Two dextran solutions are most widely used, a 6% solution with an average molecular weight of 70,000 (dextran-70) and a 10% solution with an average molecular weight of 40,000 (dextran-40 or low molecular weight dextran). The dextrans can be efficiently produced in large quantities and stored for many years at room temperature either in powdered form or in solution.[6]

Dextran is mainly secreted unchanged in the urine. The rate of renal excretion depends on the molecular size with smaller dextran molecules being excreted rapidly and larger molecules excreted very slowly. Dextran molecules not excreted in the urine slowly diffuse into the interstitium where uptake into the reticuloendothelial cells and slow metabolism

to carbon dioxide occur.[7] Reticuloendothelial cell dysfunction as a result of this uptake has been postulated, but the clinical implication of this remains unproven.

The plasma half-life of dextran solutions depends on their molecular size. Dextran-40 is excreted more rapidly than dextran-70, but dextran-40 solutions have a higher oncotic effect per gram infused and, thus produce a more pronounced plasma volume expansion.

In addition to plasma volume expansion, dextran solutions have antithrombotic effects. This is probably mediated by inhibition of platelet and leukocyte aggregation as well as augmentation of blood flow in the microcirculation. Since a major pathophysiologic deficit following shock is decreased microcirculatory blood flow, the administration of dextrans to patients in shock may offer therapeutic advantage. This effect may be mediated by two mechanisms: (1) the viscosity of blood is decreased by hemodilution; (2) low molecular weight dextran specifically inhibits erythrocyte and platelet aggregation within the capillaries and, thus, may reverse or prevent intravascular sludging.

Anaphylactic reactions to dextran occur in 0.03%-0.07% of patients[8] and may be severe or even fatal. These reactions usually occur during infusion of the first 100 ml. Close monitoring during the initiation of dextran infusion is suggested.

Dextran affects normal coagulation in a dose related fashion. Low doses of dextran (less than 1.5 grams per kg body weight) are not associated with clinical bleeding, but platelet adhesiveness and plasma levels of clotting factors are decreased. Larger doses of dextran have been associated with significant bleeding complications. Such consideration limits its use in perioperative or bleeding patients to 1,000 to 1,500 ml in 24 hours. Precipitation of acute renal failure has been associated with significant bleeding complications although this is controversial. Renal failure following dextran use is usually reported when renal perfusion is reduced or when preexisting renal damage is present. Hence, it is not recommended in patients with renal insufficiency.

Another potential problem reported with

dextran infusion is subsequent difficulty in blood crossmatching. This effect may be due to the adherence of the dextrans to antigens on the red cell membrane. This problem can be avoided by obtaining a blood specimen for crossmatching prior to infusion.

Dextrans are effective plasma expanders with efficacy equal or superior to albumin. A number of studies have shown this plasma volume expansion with subsequent hemodynamic improvement.

Low molecular weight dextran has also been used effectively as a plasma substitute for priming in extracorporeal circulation. Dextrans have also been studied and used as possible effective modalities in treating patients with myocardial ischemia, cerebral ischemia, peripheral vascular disease and in maintaining vascular graft potency.

HYDROXYETHYL STARCH

Starch is the energy storage polysaccharide of plants and is analogous functionally and structurally to glycogen, the energy storage polysaccharide molecule of animals. Starch is composed of two types of glucose polymers: amylose, a linear molecule, and amylopectin, a highly branched molecule that structurally resembles glycogen. Amylopectin is well tolerated when infused intravascularly into animals but is rapidly hydrolyzed enzymatically, with a half-life of only 20 minutes. Modification of the starch molecule by hydroxyethylation, creating hydroxyethyl starch (HES), has made it less susceptible to amylase hydrolysis and hence more stable within the plasma6[5]

There are several types of HES solutions, characterized by their average molecular weight and degree of substitution. The first developed solution, hetastarch, has a large mean molecular weight (69,000; range 10,000 to 100,000) with a wide range. This has implications when considering elimination of HES from the vascular space. Smaller molecules are excreted unchanged into the urine whereas larger molecules slowly diffuse into the interstitium where slow enzymatic degradation occurs. In normal subjects, HES is almost completely cleared from the plasma

within two days (half-life is 17 hours), yet only about 50% of the HES is eliminated from the body. The remaining HES is eliminated very slowly and much of the initial dose persists for weeks after infusion in the reticuloendothelial cells.

Pentastarch is a less highly hydroxylated HES with a lower mean molecular weight than hetastarch. As a result it is more rapidly eliminated from the tissues after infusion. Theoretically there is less risk of reticuloendothelial impairment with pentastarch.

HES appears to be extremely well tolerated with relatively infrequent and mild side effects. Allergic reactions to HES are uncommon; unlike dextran, HES is not antigenic. In one large series, the incidence of allergic reactions to HES was 0.085% (in 16,405 infusions) compared with 0.011% (in 60,048 infusions) for albumin infusion.[8] There were no fatal anaphylactic reactions to HES reported in this study.

The only clinically important adverse effect of HES infusion appears to be some impairment of coagulation which seems to be dose related. Low doses have no effect on coagulation, whereas moderate doses (20 ml per kg) may transiently decrease platelet counts, decrease fibrinogen levels, prolong prothrombin time and partial thromboplastin time. Platelet function, including adhesiveness, remains intact.[9] Although these effects may be measured, there is no evidence of clinical bleeding problems with HES infusions of as much as 20 ml per kg. There have been no controlled human studies of larger infusions with HES, but studies of animals have shown increased incisional bleeding, increased intraoperative blood loss and spontaneous serosal bleeding when very large doses of HES are infused.[10]

A problem of unclear significance with HES infusion is an occasional elevation of the serum amylase level. It is unclear if this hyperamylasemia is the result of subclinical pancreatitis, if HES acts as a physiologic stimulant to pancreatic amylase secretion or if it results in amylase aggregation.[11] It is known that amylase-starch complexes form and can increase serum amylase to more than twice the normal values over a period of several days. Unlike dextrans, HES does not interfere with blood crossmatching, and there is no apparent adverse effect on renal function.

HES has been well studied for its efficacy as a plasma volume expander. HES (60% solution in saline) increases plasma volume from 71% to 230% of the volume infused.[9] The colloid osmotic pressure is increased significantly following HES infusion, which explains the ability of HES to expand the plasma volume by more than the infused volume. The colloid osmotic pressure remains elevated two to five days following HES infusion, corresponding to the plasma half-life of HES.

In comparative studies of fluid therapy, infusing 6% HES solutions has increased central venous pressure, pulmonary capillary wedge pressure, cardiac output and ventricular stroke work, with efficacy equivalent to that of 5% albumin infusion. There have been no reported bleeding problems in these studies including perioperative patients. HES has also been successfully used as a priming solution for cardiopulmonary bypass.

HES has similarities and differences compared to dextran. Both dextran and HES effectively raise colloid osmotic pressure and plasma volume, though the plasma volume increase may be greater and somewhat more sustained following infusion of higher molecular weight dextrans. Dextrans are more useful agents in decreasing blood viscosity and increasing microcirculatory blood flow and thus have advantage as antithrombotic agents and as therapy for microcirculatory flow disturbances. HES, on the other hand, appears to be associated with fewer adverse effects, including a lower incidence of anaphylaxis, fewer bleeding problems and no adverse renal effects.

CRYSTALLOID VERSUS COLLOID

Crystalloid solutions have been shown to be effective but relatively inefficient plasma volume expanders. They are inefficient because once infused intravascularly they distribute over the entire extracellular fluid space of which only a relatively small portion is the plasma volume. Large volumes of crystalloid fluids need to be infused to result in effective plasma volume expansion which can lead to generalized edema. Many studies have indicated that about three times more fluid is required for resuscitation when crystalloid rather than colloid solutions are administered. Colloid fluids contain larger molecules that diffuse relatively slowly across the semipermeable capillary membranes. Hence, colloids are primarily distributed in the intravascular space. However, the main disadvantage of colloid use remains their cost. Current 1992 cost to our hospital is $42.00 for 500 ml 5% albumisol, $21.00 for 50 ml 25% albumisol, $37.50 for 500 ml hetastarch, $12.79 for 500 ml dextran-40, $20.32 for 100 ml dextran-70. In comparison, crystalloid costs are much less at $0.65 for 1 liter normal saline and $0.80 for 1 liter lactated Ringers.

PERFLUOROCHEMICAL EMULSIONS

Fluoridation of hydrocarbons generates a biologically inert liquid with high oxygen solubility. This differs from hemoglobin in that hemoglobin combines with oxygen whereas oxygen is dissolved in perfluorochemical (PFC) emulsions. Oxygen is thereby supplied to tissues via simple diffusion after delivery by perfluorochemical emulsions. Its potential use as a blood substitute has been delayed because it requires suspension in an emulsion suitable for intravascular infusion.

In 1965 Clark et al[12] demonstrated that a mouse could survive when completely submerged in a PFC liquid equilibrated with oxygen at 1 atmosphere. In 1967, Sloviter and Kaminoto[13] made a PFC emulsion with albumin and found that isolated, perfused brain preparations could be maintained with this emulsion as well as with blood. In1968, Geyer et al[14] performed the first successful total exchange transfusions with rats using a PFC emulsion made from perfluorotributylamine (FC47). There were, however, significant problems with these early emulsions, including prolonged tissue retention times (half life 895 days) and pulmonary and hepatic toxicity.

During the 1970s, an improved emulsion, "Fluosol-DA 20%" (Fluosol),[15] was developed. This emulsion is 20% PFC by weight and contains 7 parts perfluorodecalin for short tissue dwell time and 3 parts perfluorotripropylamine for improved emulsion stability. Poloxamer 188 (Pluronic F-68) and egg yolk phospholipid are added as emulsifying agents, and hydroxyethyl starch is added to increase oncotic pressure. Fluosol must be stored frozen and infused within 24 hours of thawing.

Perfluorochemical emulsions are eliminated unchanged through the airways. The particle size of Fluosol-DA emulsion has a mean diameter of 0.1 microns. This small size allows elimination through the alveolar membrane. There is also some uptake of PFC emulsions by the reticuloendothelial cells. The half-life of Fluosol is dose dependent. At a dose of 10 ml per kg, the circulatory half-life is approximately 8 hours; at a dose of 20 ml per kg, the plasma half-life is about 17 hours. Trace amounts of Fluosol are present in the liver and spleen for up to 80 days posttreatment. Accumulation of perfluorocarbons occurs upon repeated administration. Therefore, administration more than once every six months is not recommended.

Because the oxygen dissolved in PFC emulsions is not bound as it is to hemoglobin, the amount of oxygen transported depends on the partial pressure of oxygen in the arterial blood (PaO_2) Although PFCs have about 20 times the solubility for oxygen as plasma, significant volumes of oxygen are still only dissolved at high PaO_2 values. Thus the clinical use of PFC emulsions requires good pulmonary function and high inspired oxygen concentrations. An advantage of this relatively low "affinity" of PFC for oxygen is that nearly all oxygen dissolved in PFC at arterial oxygen tensions will be released to peripheral tissues at tissue oxygen tensions.

PFC emulsions improve peripheral blood flow by plasma volume expansion and possibly by improved microcirculatory flow. The small PFC emulsion particles (1/70th the size of erythrocytes) may flow through constricted areas of the microcirculation not accessible to erythrocytes. This may improve peripheral tissue oxygenation both by delivering oxygen dissolved in the PFC and by increasing plasma flow and delivery of the oxygen dissolved in plasma.

Fluosol was given to normal volunteers and tested in clinical trials in Japan in 1978.[16] It was first used in the United States in 1979, and limited trials have been performed, largely in anemic and bleeding patients who refused blood on religious grounds. Mitsuno and co-workers[17] reported that Fluosol infusion did result in significant plasma volume expansion. Tremper and Waxman et al[18,19] reported a small series of anemic patients who had some improvement in oxygen delivery and oxygen consumption following Fluosol administration.

A number of adverse effects have been possibly related to administering PFC emulsion. These include transient leukopenia, elevated liver function tests, increased pulmonary arterial pressures, transient hypotension and pulmonary failure. It appears likely that an emulsifying agent in Fluosol, poloxamer 188, may be responsible for some of these adverse effects via activation of the complement system.[20]

The clinical usefulness of currently available PFC emulsion as a blood substitute has not been well established. A number of limitations of these solutions appear to be problematic. First, the volumes of PFC emulsion that have been infused have been limited, and with these volumes only a relatively small amount of oxygen can be dissolved. Therefore its oxygen-transporting capability is limited. Second, the plasma half-life is relatively short. The stability of the current emulsion limits the shelf-life, even when stored frozen. Third, in order to dissolve significant volumes of oxygen in Fluosol, very high PaO_2 tensions must be achieved and adequate pulmonary function and high inspired oxygen concentrations are necessary. Finally, a number of possible adverse effects following Fluosol administration have been reported. Most of these limitations may be improved upon when a better, biologically inert surfactant becomes available.

There are potential therapeutic uses for PFC emulsions other than as blood substitutes. The most promising of these is in the use as coronary artery angioplasty perfusate. Anderson et al demonstrated significantly prolonged time to onset of angina, duration of chest pain and subjective evaluation of chest pain when Fluosol was infused through the central lumen of the angioplasty catheter in 29 patients with single vessel disease and good cardiac function.[21] Cowley et al evaluated the use of Fluosol in 38 high risk cardiac patients (defined as those with unstable angina, history of recent myocardial infarction, severe left ventricular dysfunction, multivessel disease or high risk lesions). Cardiac output declined less in Fluosol treated patients as compared to controls. No adverse side effects attributable to Fluosol were noted.[22] Hence, intracoronary perfusion of Fluosol during angioplasty may ameliorate or prevent procedural ischemia in high-risk cardiac patients.

Other possible uses of perfluorochemicals include radiation therapy enhancers, drug delivery solvents, radiologic contrast medium and for the acute treatment of myocardial or cerebral ischemia.

A second generation perflurooctylbromide emulsion is under development as are other perfluorohydrocarbon emulsions. Potential exists for these improved solutions to be very effective resuscitation fluids.

Stroma-Free Hemoblobin

Hemoglobin solutions offer several potential advantages as resuscitative fluids. These include oxygen carrying capacity at normal oxygen tensions, no blood typing, low viscosity, oncotic activity and no antigenicity. The two major drawbacks of hemoglobin solutions are the short plasma half-life and the high oxygen affinity (low P50 value) of the purified hemoglobin.

The initial problems with hemoglobin solutions was renal toxicity. This has now been shown to be primarily due to erythrocytic stromal components of the hemoglobin preparation, not the hemoglobin itself. In addition, stroma of red cell membranes has been shown to initiate blood coagulation and the complement systems. This has led to the development of stroma-free hemoglobin solutions, which are highly purified hemoglo-

bin solutions, with erythrocytic membrane fragments removed.[5]

The preparation of hemoglobin solutions generally consists of hemolysis of washed, outdated human red blood cells (RBC), purification by crystallization and washing and reconstitution for storage in solution or in dry form. While these preparations are relatively stable, there is gradual breakdown to methemoglobin when they are stored at room temperature. Shelf life is greatly prolonged if stroma-free hemoglobin is stored frozen. Newer concepts include the use of nonhuman hemoglobin, i.e., bovine,[23] or the preparation of pure human hemoglobin using recombinant technology.[24]

A major problem with the stroma-free hemoglobin preparations is increased affinity for oxygen compared with that of erythrocytes. The oxygen half-saturation (P50) of stroma-free hemoglobin solutions varies from 12 to 16 torr compared with 26 to 27 torr for fresh blood. This increased oxygen affinity, depicted by the left shifted oxygen dissociation curve, is due to the loss of tetrameric hemoglobin, lack of 2,3-diphosphoglycerate (2,3-DPG), and a higher pH compared with the intracellular erythrocyte pH. This increased affinity for oxygen by stroma-free hemoglobin solutions could lead to inadequate release of oxygen in the tissues, despite adequate circulating volumes of oxygen. By reacting hemoglobin with pyridoxal 5' phosphate the P50 has been demonstrated to increase to 23 to 26 torr. In addition, hemoglobin has been encapsulated with 2,3-DPG in liposomes, simulating erythrocytes. The liposome encapsulated hemoglobin (LEH) have a normal hemoglobin dissociation curve.[25]

Another problem with stroma-free hemoglobin solutions is their relatively rapid clearance from the vascular space due to uptake by the reticuloendothelial system and renal excretion. In experimental studies, stroma-free hemoglobin solutions have a plasma half-life of two to four hours. Furthermore, the rapid loss of hemoglobin has been associated with a significant osmotic diuresis which can result in intravascular volume depletion. To counter these effects, hemoglobin has been complexed to form larger molecular weight species. A disadvantage of these techniques is that they tend to further lower the P50. By modifying hemoglobin with 3,5 dibromosalicyl-bis-fumarate to form a beta-beta cross linked structure complexed with pyridoxal 5' phosphate and polymerized, the P50 is increased. This molecule has a P50 of 32 torr and a prolonged intravascular half life. In addition, the liposome encapsulated hemoglobin solutions (LEH) with coats of lecithin and cholesterol have been reported to increase intravascular half-life to 16 to 24 hours. The inclusion of carbohydrate components such as gangliosides into the liposomal bilayer results in increased circulation times. As a result, these ganglioside-containing liposomes may exhibit a reduced impact on the reticuloendothelial system.

The LEH solutions have been shown to increase plasma half-life and can carry oxygen sufficient to sustain life, but safety has not yet been proven. The development of a commercial blood substitute will only be possible after the safety, efficacy and toxicity issues have been thoroughly studied. However, hemoglobin solutions continue to have great potential for further development.

FUTURE

It is exciting to speculate about the future of fluid resuscitation. One possibility is the use of altered colloid solutions. Hetastarches can be further modified to attain prolonged intravascular retention. By varying molecular weights and degree of hydroxyethylation, very specific starches can be produced. In addition, hypertonic saline solutions mixed with colloid solutions may prove beneficial. Studies are currently in progress using 6% saline in dextran-70. Whitley et al[26] has recently demonstrated the need for smaller amounts of fluid when resuscitation was performed with hypertonic saline combined with 10% pentastarch. These combination solutions appear to prolong the effect of hypertonic saline.

A second possibility is in the development of oxygen carrying fluids. Work on perfluorochemicals and stroma-free hemoglo-

bin solutions is ongoing. These solutions may prove extremely beneficial as immediately available blood substitutes which do not require blood typing and eliminate the risk of disease transmission.

A third possible route of development is the addition of pharmaceutically acting agents to existing resuscitative fluids. Damage sustained to tissues following trauma and hemorrhagic shock may in part be due to reperfusion injury. There is rapidly growing evidence indicating that oxidants play a major role in producing microvascular and parenchymal damage associated with reperfusion of ischemic tissues. Pretreatment with antioxidant enzymes or oxygen metabolite scavengers have been shown to be protective in animal studies. The possible addition of these enzyme/scavengers, i.e., superoxide dismutase, catalase, deferoxamine, xanthine oxidase inhibitors, allopurinol, to resuscitation fluids may decrease the tissue insult sustained during reperfusion after hemorrhagic shock. Rhee et al has demonstrated an improvement in survival after hemorrhagic shock with the addition of superoxide dismutase to the resuscitation fluid in an animal model.[27]

Pentoxifylline, a methylxanthine, used to improve microcirculatory flow in peripheral vascular disease has also been shown to be an antagonist of tumor necrosis factor. Coccia et al has demonstrated improvement in survival after hemorrhagic shock with the addition of pentoxifylline to resuscitation fluid in an animal model.[28] This drug may prove beneficial in resuscitation of hemorrhagic shock. However, the intravenous form is not yet available in the United States.

ATP-MgCl has been shown to produce a number of beneficial effects following organ ischemia and simple hemorrhagic shock in animal models.[29] Further studies with ATP-MgCl may be warranted, although a hypotensive effect of ATP-MgCl infusion makes this difficult. Similarly calcium channel blockers are of potential benefit as they may protect cells from injury, but they too may cause hypotension early after injury.[30]

In addition, many inflammatory mediators have been found to have an important role in the microvascular injury found after trauma and tissue ischemia. These include tumor necrosis factor, interleukin-1 (IL-1), interleukin-2 (IL-2), interleukin-6 (IL-6) and platelet activating factor (PAF). TNF, IL-1, and IL-6 have been reported to be important mediators of inflammatory responses in trauma. The depression of IL-2 synthesis has been demonstrated to represent a major dysfunction within the cascade of immunologic defects induced by mechanical and thermal trauma.[31] The partial restoration of IL-2 synthesis by indomethacin suggests that blockade of the cyclooxygenase pathway as an immunomodulating therapy may reverse some of the immunologic abnormalities in multiple trauma patients. A complex interaction between PAF and cytokines occurs in traumatic states, the exact mechanism of which is unclear, leading to the acute phase reaction and circulatory collapse. PAF antagonists are potentially useful in treating shock because of their ability to inhibit deleterious PAF/cytokine autogenerated feedback processes. Many antibodies, inhibitors, and enhancers of these inflammatory mediators are under investigation, some of which may prove useful as agents to add to resuscitative fluids.

Finally, the concept of aggressive fluid resuscitation in trauma prior to definitive treatment has been recently questioned. As early as 1918, Cannon et al[32] proposed that bleeding was related to blood pressure and full fluid resuscitation to a normal blood pressure may cause more bleeding in the presence of surgical bleeding. Mattox has performed a preliminary randomized trial in penetrating trauma patients comparing no prehospital fluid administration to prehospital fluid resuscitation.[33] The study demonstrated an increase in survival in those patients receiving no prehospital fluid resuscitation. Although this study demonstrated a benefit without prehospital fluid resuscitation, larger studies need to be performed. It is important to note that the study population was restricted to penetrating trauma and transport times were short. There may be deleterious results if this is applied to patients with long transport times or to the blunt trauma patient. The patient sustaining blunt trauma, in general, has more global tissue injury. With inadequate fluid resuscitation, the patient may become acidotic, initiating the catecholamine response as well as inflammatory responses. This may cause additional harm to the traumatized patient. However, the restriction of prehospital fluids may prove beneficial in the penetrating trauma patient with short transport times.

Thus, not only the nature of fluid resuscitation but its indications and volume need further investigation. The result of working towards answers to these questions will be better resuscitation fluids leading to improved survival from shock and trauma.

References

1. Rocha-e-Silva M, Negraes GA, Soares AM et al. Hypertonic resuscitation from severe hemorrhagic shock: Patterns of regional blood flow. Circ Shock 1986; 19:165-175
2. Krausz MM, Landau EH, KIin B, Gross D. Hypertonic saline treatment of uncontrolled hemorrhagic shock at different periods from bleeding. Arch Surg 1992; 127:93-96.
3. Mattox KL, Maningas PA, Moore EE et al. Prehospital hypertonic saline/dextran infusion for posttraumatic hypotension. Ann Surg 1991; 213(5):482- 491.
4. Vassar MJ, Perry CA, Gannaway WL, Holcroft JW. 7.5% sodium chloride/dextran for resuscitation of trauma patients undergoing helicopter transport. Arch Surg 1991; 126:1065-1072.
5. Onarheim H, Missavage AE, Kramer GC, Gunther RA. Effectiveness of hypertonic saline-dextran 70 for initial fluid resuscitation of major burns. J Trauma 1990; 30(5):597-603.
6. Waxman K, Tremper KK, Mason GR. Blood and plasma substitutes—plasma expansion and oxygen transport properties. West J Med 1985; 143:202-206.
7. Atik M. The uses of dextran in surgery: A current evaluation. Surgery 1969; 65:548-562.
8. Ring J, Messmer K. The incidence and severity of anaphylactoid reactions to colloid volume substitutes. Lancet 1977; 1:466-469.
9 Korttila K, Grohn P, Gordon A et al Effects of hydroxyethyl starch and dextran on plasma volume and blood hemostasis and coagulation. J Clin Pharmacol 1984; 24: 273.
10. Karlson KE, Grohn P, Gordon et al. Increased blood loss associated with administration of certain plasma expanders. Surgery 1967; 62:670-678.
11. Kohler H, Kirch W, Horstmann HJ. Formation of high molecular aggregates between serum amylase and colloidal plasma substitutes. Anaesthesist 1977; 26:623-627.

12. Clark LC, Gollan F. Survival of mammals breathing organic liqueds equilibrated with oxygen at atmospheric pressure. Science 1966; 152:1755.

13. Sloviter HA, Kaminoto T. Erythrocyte substitute for perfusion of brain. Nature 1967; 216:458.

14. Geyer RP, Monroe RG, Taylor K. Survival of rats totally perfused with a fluorocarbon-detergent preparation. In: Norman JC, ed. Organ Perfusion and Preservation. New York: Appleton-Century-Crofts, 1965:85.

15. Yokoyama K, Yamanouchi K, Watanabe M et al. Preparation of perfluorodecalin emulsion: An approach to the red cell substitute. Fed Proc 1975; 34:1478.

16. Ohyanagi H, Toshima K, Sekita M et al. Clinical studies of perfluorochemical whole blood substitutes: Safety of Fluosol-DA (20%) in normal human volunteers. Clin Ther 1979; 2:306-312.

17. Mitsuno T, Ohyanagi H, Naito R. Clinical studies of a perfluochemical whole blood substitute (Fluosol-DA)—summary of 186 cases. Ann Surg 1982; 195:60-69.

18. Tremper KK, Friedman AE, Levine EM et al. The preoperative treatment of severely anemic patients with a perfluorochemical ozygen-transport fluid, Fluosol-DA. N Engl J Med 1982; 307:277-283.

19. Waxman K, Tremper KK, Cullen PF et al. Perfluorocarbon infusion in bleeding patients refusing blood transfusions. Arch Surg 1984; 119:721724.

20. Vercellotti GM, Hammerschmidt DE, Craddock PR et al. Activation of plasma complement by perfluorocarbon artificial blood: Probable mechanism of adverse pulmonary reactions in treated patients and rationale for corticosteroids prophylaxis. Blood 1982; 59:1299-1304.

21. Anderson HV, Leimgruber PP, Roubin GS et al. Distal coronary artery perfusion during percutaneous transluminal coronary angioplasty. Am Heart J 1985; 110:720-726.

22. Cowley MJ, Snow FR, Disciascio G et al. Perflourochemical perfusion during coronary angioplasty in unstable and high-risk patients. Circulation 1990; 81:(suppl VI)27-34.

23. Lee R, Atsumi N, Jacobs EE et al. Ultrapure, stroma-free, polymerized bovine hemoglobin solution: Evaluation of renal toxicity. J Surg Res 1989; 27:407-411.

24. Hoffman SJ, Looker DL, Roehrich JM, Cozart PE et al. Expression of fully functional tetrameric human hemoglobin in Escherichia coli. Proc Nat Acad Sci USA 1990; 87(21):8521-8525.

25. Rabinovici R, Rudolph AS, Ligler FS et al. Liposome-encapsulated hemoglobin: An oxygen-carrying fluid. Circ Shock 1990; 32:1-17.

26. Whitley JM, Prough DS, Brockschmidt JK et al. Cerebral hemodynamic effects of fluid resuscitation in the presence of an experimental intracranial mass. Surgery 1991; 110(3):514-522.

27. Rhee P, Waxman K, Clark L, Tominaga G, Soliman MH. Superoxide dismutase polyethylene glycol improves survival in hemorrhagic shock. Am Surg 1991; 57(12):747-750.

28. Coccia MT, Waxman K, Soliman H et al. Pentoxifylline improves survival following hemorrhagic shock. Crit Care Med 1989; 17(1):36-38.

29. Chaudry IH, Sayeed MM, Baue ARP. Effect of adenosisne triphosphate-magnesium chloride administration in shock. Surgery 1974; 75:220-227.

30. Horton JW. Calcium-channel blockade in canine hemorrhagic shock. Am J Physiol 1989; 267(5):R1012-1019.

31. Faist E, Mewes A, Baker CC et al. Prostaglandin E_2 (PGE_2) dependent suppression of interleukin 2 (IL-2) production in patients with major trauma. J Trauma 1987; 28(8):837-848.

32. Cannon WB, Fraser H, Cowell EM. Preventive treatment of wound shock. JAMA 1918; 70(9)618-621.

33. Martin RR, Bickell W, Mattox KL et al. Prospective evaluation of preoperative volume resuscitation in hypotensive patients with penetrating truncal injuries—preliminary report. J Trauma 1991; 31:1033.

CHAPTER 4

MYOCARDIAL DEPRESSION

William R. Law

In the efforts to achieve cardiovascular stability in trauma victims, myocardial depression remains a deadly obstacle. Why has the search for the cause (and resolution) of myocardial depression eluded us? Perhaps because we are looking for a singular, primarily effector where there are actually many that lead to the outcome of what is loosely referred to as myocardial depression. This is compounded by the problem that there is no consensus with regard to definition.

To some purists myocardial depression requires demonstration that the intrinsic contractile capability of the heart, that is, inotropic status independent of humoral and neural support or inhibition, is impaired. This is difficult to demonstrate in a clinical setting, and neglects broader definitions that include relevant conditions of myocardial impairment that are just as problematic. In many patients myocardial depression simply means that cardiac output is below expected values for a given preload. Administration of fluids to such patients may raise pulmonary arterial wedge pressure (PAWP), but have little impact on cardiac output. It is also expected that a normally responsive patient will demonstrate an increase in cardiac output after administration of a positive inotropic agent, such as dobutamine or dopamine, yet patients exhibiting myocardial depression often respond poorly or not at all to inotropic agents. Manifestation of any of these factors, intrinsic inotropic defect, adrenergic unresponsiveness or reduced output at a given preload, individually or collectively, may classify a patient as exhibiting myocardial depression. Each deserves discussion.

Cardiac Chamber Dynamics

In the patient that has received adequate quantities of crystalloid and/or colloid fluids, myocardial depression may be suggested when pulmonary arterial wedge pressures become elevated with little or no concomitant increase in cardiac output. In cases of blood loss the rationale for administration of fluids, either crystalloid or colloid, is clear—restore circulating volume. But circulatory shock may present in septic or burn patients wherein no immediate blood loss is apparent. Although there is some loss of vascular volume through extravasation, losses of peripheral vascular reactivity and myocardial depression alone can be responsible for the circulatory shock seen in these patients. Advances in monitoring cardiac chamber dynamics under these conditions have permitted acknowledgement of the various conditions that can lead to this presentation. It is expected that increasing left heart filling pressure will lead to increased cardiac output in a normally responding heart, in accordance with Starling's Law of the heart. If this does not occur, one might suspect a defect in cardiac contractile capability. This may be so, but other possibilities must be considered.

The common use of pulmonary arterial wedge pressure as an index of left heart filling pressure, and thus, preload, presumes two things that may not hold true in trauma or burn victims. First, it is expected that changes in left heart filling pressure appropriately reflect changes in preload, or end-diastolic volume. This is so only as long as compliance ($\Delta V/\Delta P$) of the ventricle remains the same. However, compliance may decrease, and left heart filling pressures would climb rapidly with small changes in end-diastolic volume. In such a case a relaxation, rather than contractile, defect is indicated. If compliance increases, large increases in end-diastolic volume can occur with relatively small changes in left heart filling pressures so that monitoring filling pressures alone can be deceiving. This can be observed in fluid resuscitated endotoxemia models.

Intravenous administration of endotoxin has been used extensively as a model of hypodynamic sepsis and is characterized by hypotension, reduced cardiac output and maintained or elevated systemic vascular resistance.[2] The hyperdynamic profile can be observed after intravenous endotoxin administration if accompanied by fluid administration.[1,18] Abel and Beck[1] demonstrated that when cardiac output was maintained at a constant, pre-endotoxin level with additional volume administration, dogs that received intravenous *E. coli* endotoxin demonstrated reduced systemic vascular resistance, rather than the elevated resistance commonly observed during endotoxin shock.[2] Teule et al[18] found that 90 minutes after intravenous endotoxin administration dogs demonstrated characteristic hypodynamic profiles. After this 90 minute period fluids were given, resulting in a hyperdynamic state with some restoration of arterial blood pressure, elevation of cardiac output and depression of systemic vascular resistance. This is similar to the responses reported in other models of sepsis by Show and Wolfe[16] and Natanson et al.[10,11]

Figure 1 illustrates left ventricular car-

diac loops from a normal dog. The X-axis is LV diameter (obtained with sonomicrometry), and the Y-axis is time-matched LV pressure. Movement in time is counterclockwise. Mean left atrial blood pressures (LAP) were measured directly (catheter in the left atrium) before (Panel A) and after fluid administration (Panel B). Saline infusion (to LAP = 7.2 mmHg) resulted in small changes in both end-diastolic and end-systolic diameter values. The amount of fluid required to obtain this LAP was 500 ml. Mean arterial pressure was unaltered and cardiac output moderately elevated (1.8 to 2.1 L/min) with only a small decrease in systemic vascular resistance (70.6 to 60.4 mmHg/L/min). The cardiac pressure-diameter loop presented in Figure 2, Panel A was obtained in a dog before it was given a slow infusion of *E. coli* endotoxin (1 mg/kg over 1 hour). Left atrial pressure (LAP) was 6.6 mmHg. At the end of the endotoxin infusion (Panel B) the depression in developed LV pressure and the reduced chamber size are evident. The decrease in end-diastolic diameter indicates a reduction in preload at this time as does the reduced LAP (3.3 mmHg).

Similar findings during hypotensive endotoxin shock have been reported by our laboratory[6,7] and others.[18] At 90 minutes postendotoxin, normal saline was infused IV, and loops recorded when LAP reached 5.1 and 6.9 mmHg (Panels C and D, respectively). The volume required to achieve the 6.9 mmHg LAP was 2.5 L, five times that required in the control dog. The primary effects of this fluid infusion was on the end-diastolic diameter which increased dramatically. Systemic vascular resistance, which had fallen slightly (from 64.1 to 53.6 mmHg/L/min) after one hour of endotoxin infusion, fell dramatically during saline infusions (18.7 and 15.6 mmHg/L/min at LAP = 5.1 and 6.9 mmHg, respectively). Despite the rise in left ventricular pressure, mean arterial pressure remained reduced (77 and 71 mmHg at LAP = 5.1 and 6.9 mmHg, respectively). Similar effects have been reported in septic patients by Parker et al,[13] in which the distinction between survivors and nonsurvivors was the increase in compliance in the heart of survivors. Under these circumstances it is easy to see how filling pressures do not appropriately reflect true preload (end-diastolic volume). Experiments like these have helped describe myocardial depression more accurately. When end-diastolic volumes are elevated so easily and left heart pressure development does not follow, little doubt is left that myocardial depression is present.

Another presumption made when using PAWP is that it appropriately reflects left heart filling pressure. Under most circumstances this is true. However, increases in pulmonary interstitial fluid pressure may develop, as in patients demonstrating adult respiratory distress syndrome (ARDS), and

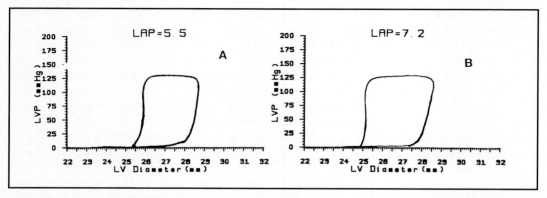

Fig. 1. Cardiac pressure-diameter loops from a control dog before (Panel A) and after left atrial pressure (LAP) was raised with fluid administration. Movement in time is counterclockwise. Left atrial pressures are indicated.

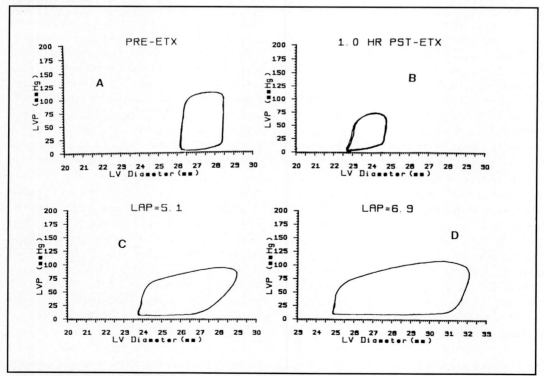

Fig. 2. Cardiac pressure-diameter loops from a dog that received endotoxin. Data in panel A were obtained prior to 1 mg/kg E.coli endotoxin infusion. After infusion of endotoxin over one-hour data in panel B were obtained. Panels C and D were obtained after left atrial pressure (LAP) was raised with fluid administration. Movement in time is counterclockwise. Left atrial pressures are indicated.

may render PAWP inaccurate because the pulmonary vasculature exhibits Starling resistor phenomena. Increases in interstitial pressure can cause partial or complete occlusion of outflow tracts, especially in the circuit involved in the "wedge" and thus interfere with the accurate measurement of left atrial filling pressure with this method. Administration of fluids may even appear to be increasing PAWP without adequately reflecting left heart filling pressure because fluid movement out of the vascular compartment and into the interstitium can be accelerated by the leaky capillary phenomenon commonly seen in these patients. This can exacerbate increases in interstitial pressure and further belie the meaning of the PAWP obtained. Under these circumstances true preload may not be adequately increased by fluid administration so a conclusion of myocardial depression could be premature.

It is becoming clear that judging adequacy of resuscitative efforts with fluids by monitoring blood pressures or cardiac output alone or in combination can be very misleading in patients wherein myocardial depression may or may not be involved. More direct measures of ventricular dynamics are now available to help elucidate the underlying problem when cardiac output is low despite normal to high PAWP. The technology to monitor ventricular volume or dimension is available but has not been used extensively for this particular problem. Ultra-fast (CINE) CT images are being examined as a non-invasive means of determining ventricular diameter, cardiac output and myocardial perfusion.[21,22] Radionuclide gated blood pool scanning combined with standard thermodilution cardiac output measurements have been useful in demonstrating decreases in LV ejection and increased LV end-diastolic volume in septic patients.[13] While these techniques are useful, they may be unfeasible at sites that do not possess the necessary equipment or may be inadequate under circum-

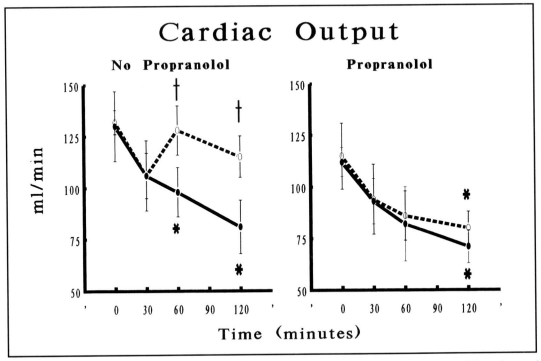

Fig. 3. Cardiac output (ml/min) in rats that received endotoxin with saline treatment (solid circles and lines) or naloxone treatment (open circles, broken lines; 4 mg/kg + 2 mg/kg*hr). The left side shows results in rats that did not receive propranolol, the right side, rats that received propranolol (1 mg/kg+1 mg/kg/hr). Values are means ±SEM. *Significant difference from within group baseline (t=0); p≤0.05 t. Significant difference between naloxone treated and untreated group at corresponding time; p≤0.05.

stances where on-line measurement of chamber dynamics is more desirable. Although a more invasive technique, the recently developed volume conductance catheter[5] can update measurement of left ventricular volume quickly enough to obtain on-line determinations of left ventricular volume, and it is far less costly than an ultra-fast CT scanner. As these methods become better characterized, they have the potential to significantly enhance diagnostic capability.

Adrenergic Unresponsiveness

Administration of positive inotropic agents such as dobutamine or dopamine generally follows if the response to fluids is unsatisfactory. The goal is to improve cardiac function by stimulation of cardiac beta-adrenergic receptors without causing undo alpha-adrenergic vasoconstriction in peripheral tissues. However, diminished adrenergic responsiveness is another factor that can be present when myocardial depression is manifested.[3]

The reduction in adrenergic responsiveness has been thoroughly investigated in animal models of sepsis and septic shock[15,17] and many causal factors have been identified. Of those that have been described, an inhibitory interaction discovered between opioid receptors and adrenergic receptors may permit reversal of the phenomenon. Originally, naloxone, an opioid receptor antagonist, was thought to hold great possibilities for the treatment of septic shock. However, clinical trials of naloxone used alone were unimpressive, but at the time, little was known about the physiological mechanisms of action in shock for this drug. New evidence suggests that naloxone can reverse the loss of cardiac and vascular responses to adrenergic activity during septic shock. Changes in cardiac output during septic shock in rats are presented in Figure 3. Propranolol was administered to one group of animals (right panel) to determine the influence of endogenous beta-adrenergic support to cardiac output in this experiment. The left panel are data from animals that did not receive propranolol (adrenergically intact). Naloxone-treated animals are designated by the open circles and hatched lines in both groups. Cardiac output fell to

comparable levels in all animals that did not receive naloxone, but in the adrenergically intact group naloxone treatment attenuated this effect. However, under beta-blockade with propranolol, the protective effects of naloxone on cardiac output were not seen. Thus it appears that opioid receptor blockade interacts with and enhances the effects of beta-adrenergic actions, and that without an intact adrenergic receptor system opioid receptor blockade is ineffective. It can also be seen from this figure that the heart demonstrated some unresponsiveness to beta-adrenergic stimuli. Plasma catecholamines are elevated during endotoxin shock. Expecting that they would confer some cardiac support, one would expect that beta-blockade with propranolol would cause an even greater fall in cardiac output during endotoxin shock. Yet, no difference in cardiac output depression was observed between the rats that received propranolol and those that did not, suggesting that the circulating catecholamines were having no effect, even without beta-blockade. Naloxone, in addition to requiring an intact beta-adrenergic system, also can be said to reverse this adrenergic unresponsiveness in the heart.

There is some clinical data that corroborates this phenomenon. In patients that were not responding to either fluids or dopamine Swinburn et al[3] found that naloxone administration improved cardiac output and blood pressure. This suggested that patients that were unresponsive to inotropic intervention became responsive after naloxone administration. The potential for such targeted use of opioid receptor blockade has led efforts to reevaluate the use of opioid receptor blockade when myocardial depression is accompanied by diminished adrenergic responsiveness.

Determining the Cause

Identifying the cause of myocardial depression has been difficult. Lefer[8] suggested a circulating myocardial depressant factor (MDF) based on experiments wherein sera from animals in shock (hemmorhagic, splanchnic occlusion and endotoxin shock) was shown to depress contractile function when placed in media surrounding isolated cat papillary muscles. Attempts to characterize this MDF were relatively unsuccessful, and for a time interest waned. The concept was recently rekindled when Reilly et al[14] reported that sera from septic patients caused in vitro depression of spontaneously beating rat myocardial cells when the sera was added to the medium. Using this in vitro assay they found that the rat myocardia cell depression correlated well with in vivo depression of ejection fraction in the source patients.

The identity of the causative factor, or substance, is still unknown, and it may well be found that any one of a number of substances released during shock may effect such myocardial depression. Endotoxin, a component of the cell wall of gram negative bacteria, was once thought to be common pathway factor leading to myocardial depression, but it now appears that it is just one of several substances that lead to the release of other, secondary mediators. Prime candidates that are now being examined include tumor necrosis factor (TNF) and interleukins 1, 2 and 6.[9,19,20]

Antibodies to endotoxin have been shown to afford some degree of protection[23] but must be given early to avoid generation of significant quantities of the secondary mediators. Where that cannot be accomplished, advances in the development of antibodies to TNF or the interleukins may make these available for wide spread use,[4,12] but much more work must be done to demonstrate efficiency and safety of such therapy.

References

1. Abel FL, Beck RR. Canine peripheral vascular response to endotoxin shock at a constant cardiac output. Circ Shock 1988; 25:267-274.
2. Altura BM, Lefer AM, Schumer W. Handbook of Shock and Trauma, New York: Raven Press, 1983.
3. Hackshaw KV, Parker GA, Roberts JW. Naloxone in septic shock. Crit Care Med 1990; 18:47-51.
4. Hinshaw LB, Tekamp-Olson P, Chang AC et al. Survival of primates in LD100 septic shock following therapy with antibody to tumor necrosis factor (TNFα). Circ Shock 1990; 30:279-292.
5. Kass DA, Yamazaki T, Burkhoff D et al. Determination of left ventricular end-systolic pressure-volume relationships by the conductance (volume) catheter technique. Circ 1986; 73:586-595.
6. Law WR, McLane MP, Raymond RM. Effect of insulin on myocardial contractility during canine endotoxin shock. Card Res 1988; 22:777-785.
7. Law WR, McLane MP, Raymond RM. Insulin and

8. Lefer AM. Role of a myocardial depressant factor in the pathogenesis of circulatory shock. Fed Proc 1970; 29:1836.
9. Natanson C, Danner RL, Elin RJ et al. Role of endotoxemia in cardiovascular dysfunction and mortality. J Clin Invest 1989; 83:243-251.
10. Natanson C, Danner RL, Fink MP et al. Cardiovascular performance with E coli challenges in a sanine model of human sepsis. Am J Physiol 1988; 254:H558-H569.
11. Natanson C, Fink MP, Ballantyne HK et al. Gram-negative bacteremia produces both severe systolic and diastolic dysfuntion in a canine model that simulates human septic shock. J Clin Invest 1986; 78:259-270.
12. Ohlsson K, Bjork P, Bergenfeldt M et al. Interleukin-1 receptor antagonist reduces mortality from endotoxin shock. Nature 1990; 348:550-552.
13. Parker MM, Shelhamer JH, Bacharach SL et al. Profound but reversible myocardial depression in patients with septic shock. Ann Int Med 1984; 100:483-490.
14. Reilly JM, Cunnion RE, Burch-Whitman C et al. A circulating myocardial depressant substance is associated with cardiac dysfunction and peripheral hypoperfusion (lactic acidemia) in patients with septic shock. Chest 1989; 95:1072-1080.
15. Romano FD, Jones SB. Beta-adrenergic stimulation of myocardial cyclic AMP in endotoxic rats. Circ Shock 1985; 17:243-252.
16. Shaw JHF, Wolfe RR. A conscious septic dog model with hemodynamic and metabolic responses similar to responses of humans. Surg 1984; 95:553-561.
17. Smith LW, Winbery SL, Barker LA, McDonough KH. Cardiac function and chronotropic sensitivity to ß-adrenergic stimulation in sepsis. Am J Physiol 1986; 251:H405-H412.
18. Teule GJJ, Den Hollander W, Bronsveld W et al. Effect of volume loading and dopamine on hemodynamics and red-cell redistribution in canine endotoxin shock. Circ Shock 1983; 10:41-50.
19. Urbaschek R, Urbaschek B. Tumor necrosis factor and interleukin 1 as mediators of endotoxin-induced beneficial effects. Rev Infect Dis 1987; 9:S607-S615.
20. Waage A, Brandtzaeg P, Halstensen A et al. The complex pattern of cytokines in serum from patients with meningococcal septic shock. J Exp Med 1989; 169:333-338.
21. Wolfkiel CJ, Ferguson JL, Chomka EV et al. Determination of cardiac output by ultrafast computed tomography. Am J Physiol Imag 1986; 1:117-123.
22. Wolfkeil CJ, Ferguson JL, Chomka EV et al. Measurement of myocardial blood flow by ultrafast computed tomography. Circ 1987; 76:1262-1273.
23. Zeigler EJ, Fisher CJ, Sprung CL et al. Treatment of gram-negative bacteremia and septic shock with HA-1A human monoclonal antibody against endotoxin. N Engl J Med 1991; 324:429-436.

beta-adrenergic effects during acute endotoxin shock: myocardial interactions in vivo. Cardiovasc Res 1990; 24:72-80.

CHAPTER 5

THE PATHOPHYSIOLOGY AND TREATMENT OF THE ACUTE RESPIRATORY DISTRESS SYNDROME

Richard P. Richardson
William G. Cioffi

INTRODUCTION

Acute respiratory distress syndrome (ARDS), which results from a diverse set of etiologies culminating in pulmonary damage, produces a characteristic progressively severe form of respiratory failure. ARDS can be caused by direct damage to the lungs, e.g., smoke inhalation, trauma or pneumonia, or by blood-borne mediator(s) arising from an area of inflammation remote from the lungs. Whatever the insult, the ARDS clinical presentation of hypoxemia and decreased pulmonary compliance is a common occurrence in the surgical intensive care unit. A 7% incidence and 41% mortality in critically ill or traumatized patients emphasizes the importance of ARDS as well as the need for further research.

This chapter will provide an overview of ARDS covering briefly its pathophysiology and putative mediators. The focus, however, will be on treatment, both conventional and experimental, that is being used and developed for ARDS.

PATHOPHYSIOLOGY

The hallmark of ARDS is a change in alveolar capillary permeability. All pulmonary insults, either directly or via mediators, alter the integrity of alveolar capillary membranes resulting in the accumulation of interstitial and alveolar fluid as well as increased lymph flow. The extravasated fluid diminishes pulmonary compliance, alveolar volume and oxygen diffusion from alveolus to capillary. Clinically, this is manifested by dyspnea, tachypnea, hypoxemia and an increasing shunt fraction which almost invariably necessitates mechanical ventilation. The decreasing pulmonary compliance commonly associated with an increasing shunt fraction often necessitates higher ventilating pressures, increased FiO_2 and greater minute ventilation which may exaggerate the histopathologic changes of ARDS and even induce such changes de novo. The alveolar and interstitial exudates predispose to bronchopneumonia which further damages pulmonary architecture. If ARDS is prolonged and severe, the inflammatory process may cause permanent damage as a consequence of pulmonary fibrosis.

Damage of the alveolar capillary can occur with a number of disease processes. Smoke inhalation, which presents a myriad of toxic compounds to the lungs, typifies direct damage to the alveolar capillary membrane. In most cases, however, the damage appears to be the result of a cascade of biochemical reactions stemming from a traumatic or inflammatory event remote from the lungs.

A potential mediator of ARDS in many instances is the lipopolysaccharide (LPS) component of the outer membrane of gram-negative bacteria which is presumed to initiate a constellation of biochemical responses.The gross disruption of natural physical barriers by trauma and subsequent iatrogenic instrumentation provides an obvious avenue for the systemic introduction of bacterial lipopolysaccharide. LPS may not necessarily originate from an exogenous source but in fact may possibly emanate from the host's own bacterial flora. This subtle mode of lipopolysaccharide exposure, termed bacterial translocation, involves the transepithelial migration of bacteria from the gut to regional lymphatic tissue and then possibly the portal circulation and reticuloendothelial system of the liver and spleen. In a variety of animal models, a number of conditions are associated with translocation including trauma, hemorrhagic shock, bowel bacterial overgrowth, immunodeficiency syndromes and loss of epithelial integrity secondary to inflammatory bowel disease, radiation, physical trauma or total parenteral nutrition. However, the clinical relevance of these observations has yet to be proven.

Lipopolysaccharide administration to human volunteers results in early plasma elevations of interleukin-1 and tumor necrosis factor (TNF) as well as a marked granulocytopenia. The granulocytopenia subsequently shifts to a profound granulocytosis which correlates temporally with a rise in plasma cortisol. Endothelium exposed to LPS expresses increased numbers of neutrophil adherence receptors which when combined with LPS-induced granulocytosis results in large numbers of neutrophils marginating in the pulmonary vasculature. Complement activation secondary to insults such as trauma, sepsis or inflammation also enhances lung injury by promoting neutrophil aggregation, activation and adherence to endothelium. The C_{5a} product of the activated complement cascade appears to induce neutrophil aggregation and adherence although its action alone is probably not sufficient to produce ARDS.

Neutrophils, when activated, can damage pulmonary capillaries by elaborating enzymes such as elastase, collagenase, lysozymes and cathepsins. Such enzymes are capable of altering the basement membrane to increase permeability. In addition to directly damaging alveolar capillaries, neutrophil enzymes can induce release of a wide range of other mediators such a histamine that increase capillary permeability. Another possible mode by which the neutrophil promotes ARDS is by the generation of toxic oxygen radicals such as superoxides. These compounds can directly damage lung capillary endothelium as well as the pulmonary interstitium. Activated neutrophils that have marginated in the pulmonary vessels can damage the alveolar-capillary interface by local release of superoxides. Systemic production of superoxides is usually due to reperfusion of tissue that has, during a period of ischemia, increased xanthine oxidase activity which then liberates excessive amounts of toxic oxygen radicals. The superoxides can also indirectly damage lung capillaries by inhibiting antiproteases thereby making the capillaries more susceptible to proteolytic degradation.

The cyclooxygenase and lipooxygenase pathways of arachidonic acid metabolism have been implicated in the genesis of ARDS. Thromboxane A_2 and PGF_2-alpha are products of the cyclooxygenase pathway and potent vasoconstrictors. Such vasoconstrictor activity may account for the microvascular thrombosis and pulmonary hypertension of ARDS. Vasoconstrictors of the lypooxygenase pathway are also produced and include leukotrienes C_4, D_4 and E_4. Leukotriene B_4 promotes endothelial adherence of neutrophils and increases capillary permeability as well as superoxide production.

Platelet activating factor (PAF) has also been studied as a mediator of ARDS. It is a phospholipid metabolite that amplifies the cyclooxygenase and lipooxygenase pathways, promotes platelet and neutrophil aggregation and enhances superoxide generation. In addition, it increases systemic and pulmonary vasoactivity as well as permeability.

The peptide mediators elaborated by monocytes and macrophages are termed monokines and include interleukin-1 (IL-1) and tumor necrosis factor (TNF). Both of these monokines are endogenous pyrogens and play a possible role in ARDS initiation by their varied effects. TNF stimulates neutrophil degranulation and endothelial adherence, increases prostaglandin production and enhances procoagulant activity. IL-1 has similar effects on prostaglandin synthesis and procoagulant activity. Both monokines are induced by endotoxin and each can enhance monocyte-macrophage release of other inflammatory mediators such as interleukin-6 as well as the potent neutrophil chemoattractant interleukin-8.

TREATMENT

The therapeutic options for ARDS can be conveniently grouped into two categories. The first includes all efforts to limit or eradicate the source of alveolar capillary damage while the second class of therapy provides cardiopulmonary support as the lungs heal. There are conventional and experimental modes of both forms of therapy.

The incidence, severity and duration of ARDS can be minimized by prompt, physiologically-based management of traumatized and/or critically ill patients. Prevention of shock, debridement of nonviable tissue, rapid stabilization of fractures, elimination of sources of sepsis, drainage of abscesses and appropriate antibiotic therapy are mainstays of critical care and can prevent or stem the alveolar capillary damage that occurs with ARDS.

Novel efforts to overcome factors responsible for ARDS have included attempts to block or suppress the possible biochemical mediators. Monoclonal antibodies to the inflammatory cytokines have been effective in various animal models of infection and sepsis. Studies of monoclonal antibodies to LPS have been interpreted as effecting improved survival in a subset of patients with septic shock and gram-negative bacteremia but no overall

benefit was evident. The activation of the complement system, as discussed previously, has been implicated as a possible initiator of ARDS. Experimentally, the severity of lung injury can be diminished following burns or trauma by prior depletion of complement. The clinical use of steroids to block activation of the complement cascade, however, has been disappointing. Platelet and white blood cell aggregation, which is accentuated in ARDS, can be inhibited by pentoxifylline in vitro, but no clinical trials have yet employed this compound.

Similarly in experimental studies, depletion of neutrophils before a traumatic insult attenuates the extent of pulmonary damage. The injurious oxygen radicals generated by neutrophils have been the focus of studies examining antioxidants and xanthine oxidase inhibitors. In addition, the monoclonal antibody 60.3, which is directed to the leukocyte adherence glycoprotein CD 18, has been used in attempts to block the adherence of neutrophils to endothelium. Experimental studies have shown promising results for these compounds but currently there is no supporting clinical evidence.

Products of the cyclooxygenase and lipooxygenase pathways are also potential mediators of ARDS. Although some experimental evidence suggests that cyclooxygenase pathway inhibition with the nonsteroidal antiinflammatory agent ibuprofen does block thromboxane A_2 formation, such action has not been translated into clinical utility. Likewise, inhibitors of the lipooxygenase pathway as well as leukotriene receptor antagonists have shown promise experimentally but clinical data are lacking. Prostaglandin E_1 (PGE_1) has been administered to ARDS patients because of its potent vasodilatory actions. PGE_1 reduces both pulmonary and systemic vascular resistance while augmenting cardiac output but also increases the pulmonary shunt of ARDS and has no effect on survival. As noted above, antibodies and antagonists to PAF and the monokines IL-1 and TNF have shown effectiveness in laboratory studies but clinical corroboration of those effects is lacking.

The administration of multiple agents to effect ARDS mediator blockade has shown promise in a porcine model of sepsis-induced

ARDS. A combination of cyclooxygenase, histamine and serotonin inhibitors (ibuprofen, cimetidine, diphenhydramine, ketanserin, and methylprednisolone) has been shown to significantly diminish pulmonary capillary permeability while abrogating hypoxemia and cardiovascular deterioration. Similar results have been obtained with the combination of ibuprofen, cimetidine and diphenhydramine. Thus, in contrast to single agent therapy, the use of a polypharmacy of mediator inhibitors may ultimately provide an effective ARDS treatment regimen.

Understanding the pathophysiology of ARDS is critical for the implementation of therapy best able to compensate for the inherent gas exchange abnormalities. As discussed previously, alteration of alveolar capillary integrity and permeability allow alveolar and interstitial fluid accumulation. Hypoxemia from pulmonary shunting and diminished lung compliance result, usually necessitating mechanical ventilation.

The hyperdynamic cardiac status that accompanies ARDS can often be attributed to the underlying insult such as trauma, infection, inflammation or septic shock. However, ARDS itself can invoke a hyperdynamic response. The significant shunt of ARDS provides a reduced area of functional alveolar-capillary interface. Increased pulmonary blood flow to nonshunted lung compensates totally or partially for the shunt and therefore, a higher cardiac output must be maintained in ARDS to insure an appropriate level of effective pulmonary blood flow.

Cardiac output is dependent upon preload, myocardial contractility, and afterload. Critically ill or traumatized patients are often hypovolemic which is associated with a reduced ventricular end-diastolic volume. Such a reduction in preload will, if myocardial contractility and afterload are fixed, cause a fall in cardiac output. Adequate intravascular volume is required for treatment of ARDS and if uncertainty arises concerning an individual's volume status, a pulmonary artery catheter must be placed to permit measurement of cardiac output and pulmonary vascular pressures.

A reduction of myocardial contractility is common in shock and septic states. Lipopo-

lysaccharide (LPS), acid-base disturbances, coronary atherosclerosis and intrinsic myocardial disease can contribute to diminished myocardial contractility. Biventricular failure often accompanies ARDS, in part, because of the increased pulmonary vasoconstriction and resistance. Inotropic agents that are not vasoconstrictive or have some pulmonary vasodilatory effect are useful in this setting. However, vasodilation of the pulmonary vascular tree may only accomplish greater perfusion of nonventilated regions and increase the shunt. Thus inotropic agents with vasodilatory capacity must be used judiciously by balancing increased cardiac output with increased shunt.

The third determinant of cardiac output is afterload. Vasoconstriction compromises cardiac output which in turn reduces effective pulmonary flow. Determination of both pulmonary and systemic vascular resistances is possible with pulmonary artery catheterization, and such measurements allow optimization of afterload by vasodilator therapy as necessary.

The use of a pulmonary artery catheter in patients with ARDS also enables one to measure vascular filling pressures and cardiac output and to calculate both pulmonary and systemic vascular resistance. The catheter also provides a means of obtaining mixed venous blood samples for determining mixed venous oxygen saturation and calculation of oxygen consumption. Finally, the implementation of mechanical ventilation imposes its own respiratory and hemodynamic consequences. This impact of mechanical ventilation can be assessed by pulmonary artery catheterization which permits careful adjustment of ventilator settings to optimize cardiopulmonary function.

Providing an adequate hemoglobin concentration is another important aspect of ARDS therapy as is the recognition and treatment of alkalosis which shifts the oxygen-hemoglobin dissociation curve to the left thereby impeding oxygen dissociation in the nutrient vessels to tissue. Since hemoglobin concentration is the crucial determinant of the oxygen content of blood and the shunt of ARDS reduces effective pulmonary blood flow, provision of an adequate hemoglobin concentration enhances oxygen delivery in a compromised cardiopulmonary system. The risk of transfusion-related hepatitis and HIV infection, however, has prompted study of blood substitutes such as fluorocarbons and stroma-free hemoglobin. Fluorocarbons are inert chemicals that have a high solubility for respiratory gases. Studies of fluorocarbons as blood substitutes have shown that they are immiscible with blood and therefore must be prepared as an emulsion to prevent embolization. Such emulsions must be stored frozen and require patients to inspire high oxygen concentrations to ensure adequate oxygen delivery to the periphery. The intravascular half-life is short ranging from 7.5 to 22 hours depending on the volume administered and fluorocarbons are taken up by and persist in the reticulo-endothelial system (RES). The long-term toxicity of these compounds is unknown. Further investigations are needed to clarify the clinical utility of fluorocarbons. Stroma-free hemoglobin has also been studied as a blood substitute but problems with its use have included its transient intravascular existence, impairment of the reticuloendothelial system, difficulty in sterilization, vasoconstrictor activity, nephrotoxicity, neurotoxicity (retinal axonal degeneration and impaired maze performance in rats) and excessively high oxygen affinity. However, newer methods of preparation including ultrafiltration and polymerization have been reported to eliminate many of these adverse effects. A recent clinical trial of stroma-free hemoglobin in children showed no complications associated with its administration.

Mechanical ventilation is the mainstay of supportive care in ARDS as the lungs recover. The goal of such therapy is to reduce the ventilation-perfusion mismatch of ARDS which is usually accomplished by increasing airway pressure. The accumulation of interstitial and alveolar fluid diminishes pulmonary compliance necessitating an increased airway pressure to deliver a fixed ventilatory volume. Associated with the use of elevated airway pressures is a greater risk of barotrauma and resultant pneumothorax, especially as pressures increase above 40 cm H_2O. In addition, positive pressure ventilation has been associated with pulmonary parenchymal dam-

age at relatively low peak airway pressures. In baby pigs, peak airway pressures of 40 cm H_2O alone induced changes similar to ARDS consisting of interstitial congestion and thickening, interstitial lymphocyte infiltration, hyaline membrane formation, alveolar hemorrhage, alveolar neutrophil infiltration, emphysematous change and organized alveolar exudates. Higher airway pressures can cause hemodynamic compromise not only as the result of tension pneumothorax but by impairment of right heart filling secondary to the transmission of the increased intrathoracic pressure.

The application of positive end-expiratory pressure (PEEP) is a common means of increasing mean airway pressure and functional residual capacity (FRC) to ensure adequate oxygenation. PEEP is defined as maintenance of above-atmospheric pressure at the end of expiration. The beneficial effects of PEEP include redistribution of fluid from alveolus to interstitium and recruitment of respiratory bronchioles and alveoli previously closed secondary to ARDS damage and loss of surfactant. The resultant increase in FRC provides increased alveolar surface area at end-expiration for gas exchange with increased oxygenation of blood. The significant hemodynamic consequences of PEEP, which include diminished cardiac output due to reduced cardiac inflow volume (preload), necessitate measurement of all relevant cardiopulmonary parameters (blood oxygen saturation, cardiac output, etc.) on a scheduled basis and after each change in PEEP level. In addition routine plotting of pressure-volume curves assists in the determination of optimal PEEP settings.

Conventional modes of mechanical ventilation utilize time-controlled, volume-controlled and pressure-controlled ventilators. Time-controlled ventilators terminate respiration after a preset time interval while volume-controlled ventilators cease inspiration after delivery of a predetermined volume. Inspiration is stopped with pressure-controlled ventilators when a preset airway (or ventilator conduit) pressure is reached. PEEP can be used with all three types of mechanical ventilation. In addition, assist-control, intermittent mandatory ventilation (IMV) or synchronized intermittent mandatory ventilation (SIMV) can be applied. The assist-control mode allows the patient to initiate a machine-generated breath by an attempted inspiration that produces a pressure that is negative in relation to baseline or end-expiratory pressure. A backup rate can be imposed in the event the number of attempted inspirations would not provide adequate ventilation. IMV allows spontaneous breathing without ventilator assistance but delivers machine breaths at a set regular rate. The SIMV mode is similar to the assist-control mode except that it allows the patient to breath spontaneously between machine-delivered breaths. Again, if the patient fails to initiate an adequate number of breaths, a backup rate is imposed.

Newer methods of mechanical ventilation are being developed in response to the limitations of conventional mechanical ventilation. Inverse ratio pressure-controlled ventilation (IRV) is one experimental mode being studied. Conventional modes of mechanical ventilation use inspiratory/expiratory (I:E) ratios comprised of a short inspiratory period and a long expiratory period. IRV I:E ratios can range from 1:1 to 4:1 significantly prolonging inspiratory time and decreasing expiratory time. Improvement in blood oxygenation is often seen with implementation of IRV which has been attributed to better recruitment of alveoli and enhanced gas diffusion. IRV is associated with higher PEEP and intrathoracic pressures than ventilation techniques employing conventional I:E ratios. These adverse effects of IRV can significantly impair venous return, reduce cardiac output and result in serious hemodynamic consequences.

Asymmetric lung disease can often be treated more effectively by simultaneous independent lung ventilation (SILV). This method employs the use of a double-lumen endotracheal tube and two ventilators which provide independent flow to each lung. SILV is potentially useful in asymmetric ARDS, lobar pneumonia, unilateral lung contusions, persistent unilateral atelectasis and bronchial stump leaks. The use of independent lung ventilation allows tailoring of PEEP, tidal volumes, ventilatory pressures, inspiratory and expiratory times and ventilatory modes to each lung as related to its distinct pathology. Pressure volume curves are generated for each lung and after each ventilator change, arterial and mixed venous blood gases and cardiac output should be determined. The disadvantage of the technique is the small diameter of each of the lumina of the double-lumen endotracheal tube which raises airway resistance and impedes clearance of secretions.

Conventional mechanical ventilators typically provide a tidal volume larger than the dead space to ensure adequate gas exchange. Several novel techniques have been developed that effect gas exchange using small tidal volumes and high ventilatory frequencies. The methods have been termed high frequency ventilation (HFV) and have the theoretic advantage of providing adequate gas exchange with lower peak airway pressures. HFV modes include those that apply the ventilatory pressure changes to the chest wall or pleural surface directly or those that generate the pressure changes at the airway opening. The difficulty in the former technique has been the application of the ventilator to the body wall or pleural surface. Thus, the most common mode used today generates the pressure changes at the airway opening.

The four types of HFV that are applied to the airway opening are high frequency positive pressure ventilation (HFPPV), high frequency jet ventilation (HFJV), high frequency oscillation (HFO) and combined high frequency ventilation (CHFV). HFPPV utilizes compressed gas for inspiration and then allows passive exhalation at a frequency of 60-120 breath/min, tidal volumes of 3-5 ml/kg and I:E ratios of less than 0.3. Exhalation is also passive in HFJV which delivers 100-600 breaths/min at high pressure via a small bore cannula. The tidal volume delivered is usually 3-4.5 ml/kg but is difficult to measure because it includes gas entrained from the surrounding airway. HFO uses both active inspiration and active exhalation to deliver tidal volumes of 1-3 ml/kg at 1-20 Hz. Finally, CHFV superimposes an HFV rate on conventional volume-controlled or pressure-controlled ventilatory volumes and rates. CHFV also includes modes where HFV is periodically interrupted to allow return of airway pressures to baseline levels.

HFV has been used with success as salvage therapy in patients with ARDS refractory to conventional mechanical ventilation (CMV). In one prospective clinical trial, 35 refractory patients treated with CHFV were compared with a similar group of 88 subjects that received CMV alone. A 23% survival was observed in CHFV patients who were clinically and physiologically similar to ARDS nonsurvivors treated only with CMV. CHFV was associated with lower peak airway pressures and a higher oxygen delivery/consumption ratio.

Despite its efficacy as salvage therapy, the use of HFV prophylactically in patients at risk for ARDS has been disappointing. At present there are no clinical trials that show a benefit of prophylactic HFV over conventional mechanical ventilation when mortality, airway pressures, incidence of barotrauma or number of days in the intensive care unit are examined. In addition, the level of hemodynamic compromise with HFV is similar to that observed with conventional mechanical ventilation although synchronizing HFV with ventricular systole has shown some promise in preventing depression of cardiac output. Results with HFV have been far more encouraging when it has been used prophylactically in burn patients with inhalation injury. In such patients, HFV was associated with a significantly lower incidence of both pneumonia and mortality as compared to recent historic controls. Currently, HFO can only be applied to neonates because of technological limitations associated with the oscillating diaphragm at higher tidal volumes. Development of an adult HFO utilizing an alternating electromagnetic field to oscillate the diaphragm is in progress and may provide additional benefits to ARDS patients. HFV has been shown to reduce chest infections and hospital stay while improving postoperative arterial oxygenation following thoracic procedures when compared to conventional ventilation using a double-lumen endotracheal tube and unilateral lung collapse. Finally,

HFV has been used with some success as salvage therapy in cancer patients with tracheal or bronchial disruption where conventional means of ventilation were inadequate for support.

Many nonconventional means of oxygenation and CO_2 removal in patients with severe ARDS are currently being studied. Extracorporeal membrane oxygenation (ECMO) utilizes a closed extracorporeal circuit of blood in contact with a thin membrane that allows blood oxygenation and CO_2 removal. In most instances, conventional mechanical ventilation (CMV) is continued with airway pressures less than 40 cm H_2O and FiO_2 less than 0.5. Although a large prospective randomized trial of ECMO plus CMV versus CMV alone in adult patients demonstrated no difference in survival rates, more recent studies from several centers have shown encouraging results with ECMO in adults. Results have been promising in neonates with lung immaturity where a significant increase in survival time has been documented with use of ECMO, although mortality was unaffected. The limitations of ECMO may be due to the extent of pulmonary and other associated organ failure that may not be reversible.

The technique of extracorporeal CO_2 removal ($ECCO_2R$) also utilizes an extracorporeal blood circuit and membrane but lung motion is minimized in an attempt to limit further pulmonary damage. Tracheal insufflation of 100% oxygen with low frequency (3-5 breaths/min) positive pressure ventilation can provide adequate gas exchange. Several preliminary reports have claimed promising results with this technique but its effectiveness remains unconfirmed.

The extracorporeal circuits of ECMO and $ECCO_2R$ require systemic anticoagulation to prevent thrombotic complications, but hemorrhagic complications can ensue. The application of a heparin coating to the extra-corporeal circuit appears to prevent thrombotic complications while maintaining normal coagulation profiles. Such an advance in ECMO and $ECCO_2R$ should increase the safety of the procedures when they are used in clinical trials.

An intravenous oxygen/carbon dioxide

exchange device (IVOX) has been developed which is inserted into the inferior vena cava through a jugular or femoral venotomy. The device consists of multiple fibers which provide a surface area of approximately 2,000-6,000 cm^2 for gas exchange. Preliminary animal studies have shown an oxygen and carbon dioxide exchange rate of approximately 100 ml/min without hemodynamic impairment or hematologic complications. Clinical trials are planned for subjects with severe pulmonary failure.

Damage and loss of surfactant in patients with ARDS has prompted study of replacement therapy with synthetic surfactant. Administration of synthetic surfactant to premature infants with respiratory distress syndrome has been shown to improve respiratory mechanics, diminish ventilatory support and reduce mortality. In animal models and a few studies of patients with ARDS where damage to the pulmonary architecture is usually more severe, improvement in respiratory mechanics has been attributed to administration of synthetic surfactant. Clinical trials are now needed to assess the potential benefits of surfactant replacement therapy in ARDS.

Finally, liquid ventilation is a novel technique in which fluorocarbons are instilled into the respiratory tree to provide a fluorocarbon-blood interface for gas exchange. A preliminary report in infants with severe respiratory distress showed improvement in oxygenation and lung distensibility although all of the infants ultimately died. Apparently the fluorocarbons are readily removed from the lungs when the therapy is terminated. Further studies are needed to refine methodology, clarify indications for use and document beneficial effects.

Summary

ARDS is a severe and often lethal form of respiratory failure resulting from an insult to the alveoloar-capillary interface. Accumulation of alveolar and interstitial fluid results in hypoxemia and diminished pulmonary compliance. Approaches to treatment include limitation or eradication of the pulmonary insult as well as support of the cardiopulmonary

system as the lungs heal. Treatment is focused on limiting damage and arresting disease progression by prevention of shock, excision of necrotic tissue, early skeletal fracture immobilization, abscess drainage and appropriate antibiotic therapy. Novel approaches have attempted to abrogate the specific effects of postulated mediators although no specific pharmacotherpay exists for ARDS. It is likely that any successful therapy attempting blockade of putative mediators will entail a cocktail of several compounds since no single agent has been shown to be clinically effective. Cardiopulmonary support at present consists of conventional mechanical ventilation (CMV) with careful monitoring of hemodynamic parameters to guide ventilator adjustments. Newer modes of ventilatory support are being developed although none at present have been documented to be superior to CMV except in smoke inhalation injury where prophylactic use of HFV has reduced pneumonia and mortality rates. Continued research on the pathophysiology of ARDS will aid in the development of effective treatment strategies for this deadly syndrome.

Selected Reading

1. Cioffi WG Jr, Rue LW III, Graves TA et al. Prophylactic use of high-frequency percussive ventilation in patients with inhalation injury. Ann Surg 1991; 213:575-82.
2. Corbet A, Bucciarelli R, Goldman S et al. Decreased mortality rate among small premature infants treated at birth with a single dose of synthetic surfactant: a multicenter controlled trial. American Exosurf Pediatric Study Group 1. J Pediatr 1991; 118:277-284.
3. Gattinoni L, Pesenti A, Mascheroni D et al. Low-frequency positive-pressure ventilation with extracorporeal CO_2 removal in severe acute respiratory failure. JAMA 1986; 256:881-886.
4. Greenspan JS, Wolfson MR, Rubenstein SD, Shaffer TH. Liquid ventilation of human preterm neonates. J Pediatr 1990; 117:106-111.
5. Mortenson JD, Berry G. Conceptual and design features of a practical, clinically effective intravenous mechanical blood oxygen/carbon dioxide exchange device (ICOX). International J Artif Org 1989; 12:384-389.
6. Tsuno K, Miura K, Takeya M et al. Histopathologic pulmonary changes from mechanical ventilation at high peak airway pressures. Amer Rev Resp Dis 1991; 143:1115-1120.

CHAPTER 6

INHALATION INJURY: PATHOPHYSIOLOGY AND TREATMENT

Ronald H. Miles
David J. Dries
Richard L. Gamelli

Inhalation injury has been referred to as smoke inhalation injury, smoke poisoning, carbon monoxide poisoning and pulmonary burn. In actuality, an inhalation injury can involve aspects of all of these. A comprehensive definition would include exposure to heat, particulate matter or gases, resulting in asphyxia or clinically evident damage to the tracheobronchial tree.[1] In the setting of a burn, an inhalation injury has a greater effect on mortality than either the age of the patient or the total body surface area of the burn.[2,3] In patients sustaining cutaneous burns and an inhalation injury, mortality has been shown to be 20% to 40% greater than in patients with a similar cutaneous burn but without an inhalation injury. [3,4]

The severity of an inhalation injury is determined by the type and concentration of gases or particulates inhaled, the duration of exposure to the noxious environment and the concomitant presence of other injuries.[5,6] Although an inhalation injury can occur as an isolated event, it much more commonly occurs in association with cutaneous thermal injury. It becomes difficult to differentiate the effects of these two injuries as the cutaneous burn may contribute significantly in its own right to the developing pulmonary pathology.

CLASSIFICATION OF INJURY

Three schemes are most often discussed in the classification of an inhalation injury. These have been based on clinical presentation and symptoms, the anatomic location of the injury or the agents responsible for the injury.

Aub et al[7] in evaluating patients in the Cocoanut Grove fire of 1942 identified four groups of patients based an their clinical response to the initial inhalation insult. Those patients presenting with hypoxia and immediate evidence of respiratory tract injury subsequently died. A second group developed cyanosis, dyspnea and restlessness attributed to the onset of pulmonary edema that developed within hours of exposure. At 24 to 48 hours a group of patients emerged with worsening dyspnea. All were noted to have massive upper airway edema that often required intubation or urgent tracheostomy. The final group of patients developed segmental atelectasis or pneumonia, usually after the second day.

Stone's classification system also is derived from the clinical course often observed after inhalation injury. Three stages were described with progression from respiratory insufficiency to pulmonary edema to bronchopneumonia. Pneumonia, the final stage, developed in all patients who survived longer than 72 hours.[8]

An alternative classification, based on the anatomic location of injury, has been described by Moylan.[9] He described three levels of injury: upper airway, major airway and parenchymal. The upper airway encompasses the nasopharynx and oropharynx to the level of the true vocal cords. Injuries to this region manifest as edema of the larynx within 24 hours. Major airway injuries involve the trachea and large bronchi producing mucosal damage and epithelial desquamation. The most extensive injuries involve damage of the entire respiratory tract including the pulmonary alveoli.

A classification system based on the mechanism of injury has also been proposed.[10] Thermal injury may be due to either dry heat or steam. Hypoxia is secondary to both oxygen consumption by the fire and the generation of carbon monoxide. Chemical irritation may result from the introduction of any number of toxins within the fire environment.

THE INITIAL INHALATION INSULT

From a clinical standpoint it is possible to look at smoke as having essentially four components with pathophysiologic implications. The first of these is simply heat. Although the respiratory system is very efficient at cooling heated air, in a superheated environment it is possible to sustain burns to the upper airway. Secondly, the particulate matter in smoke can cause injury in several ways. Particulates may act either as direct irritants, or if small enough ($<1\mu$), these superheated particles may cause thermal damage in the distal airways.[11] These particles may also transport toxins to the lower airways and alveoli. These toxins may then produce direct damage or become absorbed and subsequently disrupt cellular events. These toxins are likely responsible for many of the early deaths after an inhalation injury.

ENVIRONMENTAL VARIABLES THAT DETERMINE SEVERITY

The most important determinants of an inhalation injury are the type and concentration of the inhaled substances—a direct reflection of the smoke composition, which can be extremely variable. In controlled studies, smoke obtained from burning pine wood yielded 250 toxic byproducts, and over 75 different products of combustion have been identified from polyvinyl chloride.[12-14] The composition of the smoke present in any particular fire thus becomes a function of the fuel being burned (Table 1), the temperature generated and the amount of oxygen present.[6]

The single factor most responsible for the type and concentration of toxic products generated from a given fuel source is the temperature of the burning environment and the rate at which this temperature is reached. As a general rule, when the temperature increases in a fire from 220° C to 1000° C, complex molecules convert to progressively simpler molecules.[15] Hydrocarbons produce carbon monoxide (CO) and carbon dioxide (CO_2), nitrogen-containing compounds produce hydrogen cyanide (HCN) and chlorine-containing compounds produce hydrochloric acid (HCl).[16]

The final variable in determining the composition of smoke is the amount of oxygen present in the fire environment. Smoke is produced through two separate decomposition processes, combustion or pyrolysis. Combustion occurs in the presence of oxygen and can be defined as the oxidation of a substance accompanied by the production of light and heat. When unlimited oxygen is present, complete combustion generates CO_2 and H_2O. If the oxygen is being consumed by the fire faster than it can be supplied, incomplete combustion takes place producing variable

Substance	Source	Estimated lethal concentration in PPM (10 min exposure)
Carbon monoxide	All organic materials	>4000
Hydrogen cyanide	Polyurethane, wool, silk, paper	>350
Acrolein (aldehydes)	Wood, acrylics, cotton, rubber	30-100
Nitrogen dioxide	Cellulose, wood	>200
Ammonia	Nylon, wood, silk, polyurethane	>1000
Hydrogen chloride	Polyvinyl chloride, upholstery	>500
Other halogen acids		
Hydrogen flouride	Teflon	400
Hydrogen bromide	Fire retardants	500
Sulfur dioxide	Rubber	>500
Isocyanates	Polyurethane	>100
Acrylonitrites	Polyurethane	4 *
Hydrogen sulfide	Wool, silk, rubber	300*
Hydrocarbons		
Benzene	Petroleum plastics	>100*
Styrene	Polystyrene	>100*
Phosgene	Polyvinyl chloride	2 *

PPM: parts per million; * Maximum level allowing escape within 30 minutes.
Adapted from Prien and Traber[11]; Terril et al[16]; Chernock and Meehan[58]; Summer and Haponik.[45]

Table 1. Toxic components of smoke.

amounts of carbon monoxide (CO).[17] Pyrolysis, on the other hand, is the simple decomposition of a substance by heat and occurs if there is no oxygen present.

PATHOPHYSIOLOGY

UPPER AIRWAY INJURY

Inhalation injury to the upper airway, in general, is secondary to direct thermal damage or chemical irritation. Inhalation of heated air greater than 150°C produces instantaneous injury to the mucosa of the oropharynx and larynx resulting in edema, erythema and ulceration.[18] Edema formation is secondary to direct microvascular injury, vasoactive inflammatory mediators and oxygen free radicals. Histamine can induce venular endothelial cells to contract and may initiate edema formation.[6]

Depending on the severity of the injury, edema can occur immediately or may not be clinically evident for up to 24 hours. Mucosa lining the hypopharynx, epiglottis and aryepiglottic folds is loosely attached to the underlying tissues and can undergo impressive swelling with little airway impedence.[19] The glottis, being surrounded by cartilaginous rings, is not nearly as tolerant of edema. Glottic swelling is displaced inward, narrowing the airway. In an adult, narrowing beyond 8 mm provides a significant danger of complete airway obstruction.[20] In most cases, upper airway edema resolves over four to five days.[21]

In addition to the direct thermal injury, toxic products present in smoke also damage the upper airway. Water-soluble toxic compounds such as ammonia, hydrogen chloride and sulfur dioxide adhere to mucous membranes forming corrosive acids and alkalies.[22] The end result is cell death, ulceration and further edema. These irritants can also cause extensive bronchorrhea and bronchospasm.[23]

Lower Airway Injury

Injury to the lower airway is produced not only by thermal and chemical injury but may also be the result of asphyxiation.

Thermal Damage. Lower airway injury due to dry heat occurs in less than 5% of patients hospitalized with burn or inhalation injuries.[24] This is due to the inherently low heat-carrying capacity of dry air, and the fact that the moist upper airways effectively dissipate heat. In one study, 300°C dry air introduced into the larynx was cooled to 50°C by the time it reached the trachea.[25] In addition, the vocal cords close reflexively at approximately 150°C to protect against lower airway injury.[26] There are situations, however, where thermal injury to the lower respiratory tract can occur. Smoke contains a great deal of particulate matter, and superheated particles less than 1 μ can gain access to the alveolus and produce direct thermal injury.[11] Steam inhalation can also produce extensive damage to the lower airways. Steam, having 4000 times the heat-carrying capacity of dry air, contains considerably more heat energy. Inhaled steam can easily exceed oropharyngeal heat dissipation, producing direct thermal injury as far as the distal respiratory bronchioles.[25]

Chemical Damage. Injury to the lower airways produced by the inhalation of the wide variety of chemical irritants found in smoke is the most complex and least well understood form of inhalation injury. While individual toxins may produce unique changes, a generalized response of the lower respiratory tract to acute injury has been fairly well characterized. The resulting injury may be at the level of the tracheobronchial tree or the pulmonary parenchyma (encompassing the alveolar capillary interface).

Tracheobronchial Tree Injury. Patients who undergo bronchoscopic examination immediately following an inhalation injury are noted to have tracheobronchial edema, muco-

sal erythema with areas of sloughing and loss of mucociliary activity.[27] An inflammatory exudate rapidly forms and interstitial edema develops. Analysis of this inflammatory exudate has demonstrated high concentrations of thromboxane A_2 (a potent smooth muscle constrictor) and the proteolytic enzyme ß-glucuronidase.[28] The presence of these mediators implies that initial events stimulate neutrophils and activate the arachadonic acid cascade. The pathologic consequence of these events is progressive airway obstruction.

The early development of interstitial edema is at least partly attributable to pathologic changes in the tracheobronchial tree. The edema formation is often attributed to permeability changes in the pulmonary microvasculature; however, there may also be a significant contribution from the bronchial circulation. Studies have demonstrated a tenfold increase in bronchial blood flow after inhalation injury which could alter hydrostatic forces within these vessels. This hyperemic response is thought to be mediated by histamine.[29]

Pulmonary Parenchymal Injury. The initial insult to the tracheobronchial tree causes bronchoconstriction and airway obstruction resulting in alveolar hypoxia and vasoconstriction. Neutrophils present in the lung at the time of initial injury are trapped as a result of this vasoconstriction.[30] Simultaneously, chemical irritants within smoke stimulate pulmonary macrophages to release chemotactic factors, recruiting additional neutrophils to the lung.[31] The neutrophils sequestered in the pulmonary microvasculature are activated and degranulate releasing proteolytic enzymes and oxygen free radicals. These proteolytic enzymes degrade fibronectin and disrupt the interstitial matrix allowing fluids and protein to pass from the interstitial space.[32] Oxygen free radicals enhance this process by inhibiting the anti-protease system.[33]

As the pulmonary injury progresses, neutrophils accumulate in the pulmonary microvasculature. This is thought to occur via release of a neutrophil chemotactic factor by pulmonary alveolar macrophages and by way of activation of the alternate pathway of the complement system. Present evidence suggests that these sequestered neutrophils are responsible for a significant component of the pulmonary parenchymal injury. Activated neutrophils undergo both a lysosomal degranulation with release of proteolytic enzymes and a respiratory burst that generates oxygen free radicals. The oxygen free radicals generated by neutrophils contribute to pulmonary injury in several ways. The inhibition of the antiprotease system by these substances allows the proteolytic enzymes present to destroy more tissue. Oxygen radicals may also act as chemoattractants, recruiting more neutrophils into the pulmonary microvasculature.[31]

Progressive pulmonary parenchymal damage is associated with the development of extravascular lung water and, in severe cases, pulmonary edema and respiratory failure. In neutrophil-mediated lung injury, the mechanism appears to involve an increase in microvascular permeability as evidenced by the observed increases in lymph-to-plasma protein ratios. The changes in pulmonary permeability are believed to be due to endothelial cell injury. Although actual morphologic evidence of damage to the endothelial cells has not been demonstrated, it has been suggested that elevations in lung angiotensin-converting enzyme (ACE), a product of endothelial cells, is indicative of damage.[34]

Damage from Asphyxiants

Asphyxiation, defined as the lack of oxygen and subsequent increase in carbon dioxide, is a major source of morbidity and mortality in fire victims. Inhalation of carbon monoxide is the most frequent immediate cause of death from fires.[5,35] The hypoxia may be due to the consumption of oxygen by the fire or to the inhalation of systemic toxins, particularly hydrogen cyanide (HCN) and carbon monoxide (CO). Although not directly injurious to the tracheobronchial tree, these toxins are systemically absorbed from the lower respiratory tract.

There are several mechanisms by which inhaled CO may produce hypoxia. These include impaired oxygen transportation by hemoglobin, decreased oxygen delivery to peripheral tissues, inhibition of cellular respiration and cardiovascular dysfunction. When CO is inhaled, it rapidly diffuses across the alveolar capillary membrane to bind hemoglobin, forming carboxyhemoglobin. As CO has an affinity 200 times greater than oxygen for hemoglobin, the O_2-transporting capacity of blood may be reduced 50% by the inhalation of smoke with a concentration of only 0.1% CO.[11]

CO also disrupts cellular respiration by interfering with mitochondrial cytochrome oxidase systems. CO competes with oxygen, binding the iron atoms in the ferrous (Fe^{++}) state on cytochrome A_3 which then blocks oxidative phosphorylation.[36]

CO also competes with oxygen in binding other heme proteins, including myoglobin, peroxidase and catalase.[37] It is hypothesized that binding to myoglobin is particularly deleterious to cardiac muscle. Pathologic changes in the heart reported after inhalation of CO include hemorrhage, muscle cell degeneration, leukocyte infiltration and multifocal myocardial necrosis.[38] Cardiac dysrhythmias may be the ultimate cause of death in many cases.[20]

The other systemic toxin that can produce tissue hypoxia is cyanide (CN). There are multiple sources of CN in the fire environment including rubber, polyurethane, silk and nylon. When inhaled, hydrogen CN (the gaseous form of CN) is rapidly absorbed and inhibits cellular metabolism. CN's specific site of action is also directed at cytochrome A_3, where it irreversibly binds iron in the ferric (Fe^{+++}) state,[36] thus blocking cellular respiration one step below the site of CO inhibition.[39] The central nervous system and the heart appear to be most vulnerable to the hypoxia and subsequent lactic acidosis produced by CN.[40]

Features of Specific Irritants

There are a multitude of toxic compounds that produce various aspects of the pathophysiologic pulmonary response after an inhalation injury; however, little is known about the underlying mechanisms that elicit these responses.

Acrolein. Burning wood produces predominantly CO but also yields large amounts of acrolein. Acrolein is a toxic, highly irritating, three-carbon aldehyde. It is lipid-soluble and can therefore gain access to the lower airways and pulmonary parenchyma via inhaled soot particles. The pathologic consequences of inhaled acrolein include pulmonary edema and disruption of pulmonary antibacterial defenses.[11,14] Studies suggest that the formation of pulmonary edema occurs by macrophage-mediated activation of the arachadonic acid cascade, but the underlying events remain incompletely described. [42]

Hydrogen Chloride. Hydrogen chloride, along with phosgene and chlorine, are several of the more toxic products liberated by polyvinyl chloride. Hydrogen chloride is water-soluble and therefore produces much of its damage by adhering to the moist mucous membranes of the upper airway and then liberating a strong acid.[15] In studies evaluating smoke containing HCl, mucosal degeneration, desquamation and intense inflammation of the proximal airways has been observed [43]

Phosgene. Phosgene is a colorless, lipid-soluble gas found in aniline dyes and plastics (including polyvinyl chloride). When it reacts with water, hydrochloric acid is formed. Clinically it produces pulmonary edema, thought to occur from direct alveolar injury.[44]

Chlorine. Chlorine is an extremely irritating, water-soluble gas that produces severe pharyngeal and laryngeal edema. Exudative inflammatory bronchitis can also develop causing plugging of small bronchi and atelectasis.[45]

Hydrogen Cyanide. HCN is produced mainly from burning polyurethane. Inhalation of fumes liberated from polyurethane may cause irritation and pulmonary edema. Pathologic examination reveals vascular congestion and edema fluid that contains fibrin. Large numbers of macrophages are seen although there are relatively few PMN's present.[46]

Ammonia. Ammonia is also released from the degradation of polyurethane, in addition to being a combustion product of both wool and silk. Like chlorine, it is water-soluble and produces severe upper airway edema and desquamation.[47] The lower airways are not always spared, however, as bronchiolitis and alveolar injury have been described.[48]

Nitrogen Oxide. Nitrogen oxides are capable of causing severe tracheobronchial injury. They are lipid soluble and often reach the distal airways. Nitrogen oxide reacts with water in the lower respiratory tract to form nitric acid. The nitrates and nitrites subsequently formed produce direct tissue destruction.[11] Nitrogen dioxide is a powerful oxident that can cause lipid peroxidation, generating oxygen free radicals. Patients who survive the initial insult often develop recurrent symptoms several weeks later for unknown reasons.[49] Absorbed nitrogen oxides also have systemic consequences. Nitrate ions react with hemoglobin to form methemoglobin, nitrite ions cause smooth muscle relaxation and hypotension and nitric acids contribute to systemic acidosis.[11,45]

Sulfur Dioxide. Sulfur dioxide is an irritating, water-soluble gas that is oxidized to sulfuric acid in the presence of water and can cause severe mucosal injury. Pulmonary edema is also seen after SO_2 inhalation and may be a result of direct damage to the alveolar capillary membranes or increased capillary hydrostatic pressure produced by SO_2-mediated venoconstriction.[50]

THE ROLE OF A CUTANEOUS THERMAL INJURY

The interaction of an inhalation injury and cutaneous burn results in a synergy of deleterious effects. The incidence of respiratory insufficiency in patients sustaining an inhalation injury only is about 12% while it is as high as 62% in patients with an associated cutaneous burn. Likewise, overall mortality is estimated at 7% after an isolated inhalation injury but 20-40% in patients sustaining both an inhalation and concomitant cutaneous burn injuries.[34]

In addition, immune system dysfunction is well recognized after cutaneous thermal injury. Changes in cell-mediated immunity and defects in opsonization are well characterized. Diminished levels of circulating immunoglobulin and alterations in the complement pathways have been identified.[51-53] Various cytokines, prostaglandins and endotoxin have been identified as possible mediators of this posttraumatic or postthermal immunosuppressed state[54] and may also play a role in ongoing pulmonary injury. These complex systemic interactions are poorly understood regarding their role in predisposing this patient population to both infection and multisystem organ failure.

POSTINHALATION PULMONARY COMPLICATIONS

Pulmonary complications are the leading cause of significant morbidity and mortality after burn and inhalation injury. Advances in the care and management of the burn patient suffering an inhalation injury has lead to the observation that pulmonary complications, either in the form of infection or respiratory failure, presently account for 20-84% of all deaths.[29,55] This group of patients is at high risk for the development of pulmonary complications as inhalation injury produces not only a direct tracheobronchial insult but sets in motion a series of systemic events with far-reaching consequences. The combination of injuries within this group of patients produces a unique environment within the respiratory system and sets the stage for increased susceptibility to pulmonary infection and respiratory failure.

INFECTION

Pulmonary infections occur in 15-60% of patients hospitalized with an inhalation injury.[55-57] The incidence of pulmonary infection in patients sustaining an inhalation injury increases with cutaneous burn size. Full thickness burns greater than 5% and partial thickness burns greater than 12% are associated with higher rates of pneumonia in patients with an inhalation injury.[58] The development of pulmonary infection in the setting of an inhalation injury has devastating implications. The mortality rate for a documented pulmonary infection in this group of patients is 50-86%.[2,4,29]

The increased risk of developing a pulmonary infection after an inhalation injury is the result of both the local injury and sys-

temic host alterations. The local insult to the tracheobronchial tree creates an environment that is easily seeded by bacteria. Altered respiratory defenses from the direct inhalation insult and systemic immunosuppression from a cutaneous burn can cripple the host and set the stage for a highly lethal pulmonary infection.

LOCAL FACTORS

Ciliary Dysfunction. An immediate effect of an inhalation injury is disruption of mucociliary function, a key element in the host respiratory defense system.[22] Various inhalants, including aldehydes and acrolein, directly suppress muco-ciliary activity.[59] Ciliary dysfunction leads to impaired clearance of debris, secretions and bacteria, leading to airway obstruction. A culture medium of respiratory secretions, necrotic tissue and inhaled debris creates an environment ripe for bacterial seeding.

The Pulmonary Alveolar Macrophage. An important mediator of the host respiratory defense system is the pulmonary alveolar macrophage (PAM). Normal functions of the PAM include phagocytosis, intracellular destruction of microorganisms, transport of these substances from the respiratory tree and detoxification of inhaled materials. Animal studies have documented significantly impaired PAM chemotaxis and phagocytosis after inhalation injury.[60,61]

Cutaneous thermal injury also alters PAM function. Reduced phagocytosis and chemotaxis have been identified after isolated cutaneous thermal injury.[62] This cell population plays a significant role in the initial response of the pulmonary host defense system to invading microbes, and the enhanced susceptibility to pulmonary infection may be partially explained by these findings.

Surfactant. A hallmark of inhalation injury is surfactant damage. Pulmonary surfactant, synthesized by type II pneumocytes, lines the respiratory tree. Its main functions are to reduce alveolar surface tension and prevent alveolar collapse.[63] Nieman et al documented surfactant damage within seconds after smoke exposure in dogs.[64] The immediate manifestation was atelectasis. Recent work has also demonstrated that surfactant may subserve functions beyond simple mechanical stabilization of alveoli. Surfactant regulates the numbers of PAM within the lung, influences PAM chemotaxis and may play an intimate role in preparing PAM for bacterial phagocytosis.[65] Others have shown that surfactant has bactericidal capabilities.[66] In addition, investigators have demonstrated a possible link between surfactant injury and PAM function. PAM harvested from atelectatic lung segments demonstrated diminished phagocytic activity against *Pseudomonas aeruginosa*. Interestingly, normal PAM phagocytosis was restored within hours of lung reexpansion.[67] These findings suggest that alveolar changes, beyond simple collapse, may predispose the lung to infection.

PATHOGENS

The most common pathogens in pulmonary infection occurring after inhalation injury follow a predictable pattern. The initial organisms to colonize the damaged respiratory tree are most often penicillinase-resistant gram positive cocci *(Staphylococcus sp)*. These organisms are cultured within the first four days after injury. By the seventh day after injury gram negative organisms have colonized the tracheobronchial tree. *Pseudomonas sp* are the most common pathogens at this time, followed closely by the KIebsiella-aerobacter group.[29,68,69] Gram negative enteric bacteria such as *E. coli* and *Enterobacter sp* are also cultured at this time.[69-71] These findings implicate the gastrointestinal tract as a potential source of bacterial seeding, possibly via bacterial translocation.[54] The presence of these less virulent organisms also reflect, at least to some extent, the degree of host immunosuppression occurring in this patient population. The overwhelming majority of pathogens in this population arise from endogenous hospital flora. It is important to have a knowledge of the institutional epidemiology of these pathogens when antibiotic therapy is begun.

THE ADULT RESPIRATORY DISTRESS SYNDROME

The patient suffering both an inhalation injury and cutaneous burn is at high risk to develop respiratory failure and the adult respiratory distress syndrome (ARDS). The initial injury triggers a cascade of events that can directly produce, or perpetuate, the pulmonary injury. The same pathophysiologic processes described in the early stages of an inhalation injury are thought to play a major role in the pathogenesis of ARDS.

The incidence of ARDS, when it occurs after an isolated inhalation event, is unknown. However, there is a clear difference between patients that suffer an isolated inhalation injury and those that have an associated cutaneous thermal burn. Patients hospitalized with isolated inhalation injuries usually encounter few respiratory sequelae, and ventilatory support is seldom required.[72] ARDS is rarely encountered in this group of patients.[73] When ARDS does occur after an isolated inhalation event, it is rapid in onset and belies the underlying severe pulmonary parenchymal injury. This direct insult can lead rapidly to the development of ARDS.

An isolated cutaneous burn can also have a significant impact on the respiratory system. In one epidemiologic study the risk of developing ARDS after an isolated cutaneous burn was found to be 2.3%, but when it developed mortality was 50%.[74] In this study there was no attempt to document the presence of an inhalation injury.

Herndon et al have reported that, in patients that sustained both a cutaneous burn and inhalation injury, 25% developed pulmonary edema. In those patients, the mortality rate was found to be 60%. Clark et al reported that respiratory failure requiring mechanical ventilatory support is four times higher in patients with thermal and inhalation injury when compared with patients who had only an inhalation component.[72]

There are a number of factors, both direct and indirect, that have been shown to be associated with the development ARDS.[74,76]

Direct pulmonary injury	Systemic insult
Aspiration	Sepsis bacteremia
Pneumonia	Cutaneous burn
Inhaled Toxins	Shock
(smoke, phosgenes, nitrogen oxides)	(hypovolemic, cardiogenic)
Oxygen toxicity	Disseminated intravascular coagulation
Near drowning	Multiple blood transfusions
	Drug toxicity
	(ethchlorvynol, heroin, acetylsalicylic acid)
	Pancreatitis
	Fat embolism

Adapted from Stevens and Raffin.[80]

Table 2. Factors associated with the development of ARDS.

(Table 2) Regardless of its etiology, ARDS remains lethal. Since the initial description in 1967 by Ashbaugh and colleagues,[77] the mortality rate has remained essentially unchanged at 50-70%.[78]

ENDOGENOUS MEDIATORS OF LUNG INJURY

The initial inhalation insult activates an array of endogenous mediators that may not only cause but perpetuate the acute lung injury.

The Neutrophil. Neutrophil sequestration in the pulmonary microvasculature is a critical and appropriate host defense response, but likely becomes a key component in perpetuating pulmonary parenchymal destruction. The role of the PMN in generalized tissue injury has been extensively reviewed.[79] The neutrophil has also been the focus of acute lung injury in many animal models. Toxic oxygen metabolites, including superoxide anions, hydrogen peroxide, singlet oxygen species and hydroxyl radicals are produced by the intracellular and membrane-bound enzymes of the neutrophil. These highly reactive molecules can rapidly denature proteins, directly damage tissues and disrupt the balance of the pulmonary protease/antiprotease system.[80] Given our current level of understanding, the neutrophil should be viewed as an effector of injury once a "signaling event" has occurred. Pulmonary sequestration of the

PMN is a notable event here for its rapid occurrence after inhalation injury, and may be one of the primary events leading to respiratory failure and ARDS.

The Endothelial Cell. Elevated levels of angiotensin-converting enzyme (ACE) have been found in peripheral blood immediately following inhalation insult suggesting that some form of pulmonary endothelial injury has occurred.[81] Others have demonstrated histologic damage to the pulmonary endothelium after severe inhalation injury.[82] Endothelial cell injury has also been demonstrated after an isolated cutaneous burn. Till et al have shown increased pulmonary capillary permeability (implicating endothelial cell injury) to occur as early as two hours after thermal skin burn in rats.[83]

Although many investigators have focused on the pulmonary endothelial cell as a target of injury, this population of cells might also potentiate lung injury. Pulmonary endothelial cells account for 50% of the entire endothelial cell population within the human body, and their impact as a mediator in ongoing injury could be substantial.[34] These cells propagate platelet aggregation and adherence by the release of von Willebrand factor. Significant quantities of prostaglandin I_2 (prostacyclin) are released by endothelial cells, as are large amounts of thromboxane A_2. Both compounds have significant vasoactive properties and are strong neutrophil chemoattractants.[84]

Endotoxin. The role of sepsis and infection in precipitating respiratory failure and ARDS is well documented. In two major epidemiologic reviews examining predisposing factors in the development of ARDS, infection or sepsis was identified in 31-38% of patients.[74,76] More recently appreciated is that lung injury can be an early manifestation of a systemic inflammatory process culminating in multiple organ failure (MOF).[85,86]

The endotoxin hypothesis links the events of inflammation and sepsis with ARDS and MOF. Endotoxin has been shown to have the capability in vitro to directly injure cultured pulmonary endothelial cells.[87] The mechanism by which this occurs is unknown, but it is likely that it plays a minor role in pulmonary injury. A more important pathway of endotoxin-mediated pulmonary injury involves the neutrophil. Endotoxin can activate the complement system leading to pulmonary sequestration of neutrophils.[88] It is also capable of, in a complement-independent manner, eliciting neutrophil migration into the pulmonary microvasculature via PAM activation.[89] Endotoxin may also facilitate neutrophil "priming," and enhanced release of toxic metabolites and other inflammatory mediators.[90] Intravenous infusion of endotoxin has produced pulmonary injury in sheep, dogs and rabbits.[88]

It is important to emphasize the fact that patients harbor within their gastrointestinal tract a readily available source of endotoxin. The phenomenon of gut bacterial translocation is well characterized after experimental burn injury.[91] Changes in gastrointestinal structure and local hormonal alterations may facilitate the process of translocation. These underlying derangements have prompted investigators to speculate that the gastrointestinal system could be the reservoir that drives the host septic response and can ultimately produce organ dysfunction, ARDS and multiple organ failure.[92]

Tumor Necrosis Factor. Tumor necrosis factor (TNF), a cytokine released by activated monocytes and macrophages, has been recognized as another mediator of inflammation and tissue injury. Investigators have demonstrated increased pulmonary capillary leak in guinea pigs after intravenous TNF infusion.[93] One potential mechanism of this TNF-mediated response is thought to occur after neutrophil activation. TNF has also been demonstrated to be cytotoxic and could produce increased pulmonary vascular permeability by direct pulmonary endothelial cell injury.[94]

Complement. Complement activation is a frequent occurrence in numerous pathophysiologic events and has been demonstrated in many states associated with pulmonary injury. Bacterial sepsis and multiple trauma,[95] cardiopulmonary bypass[96] and hemodialysis[97] have been demonstrated to produce pulmonary dysfunction via complement activation. The burn patient also has well recognized alterations in the complement system during the immediate postburn period.[53] The impact that these alterations in the host complement pathways might have upon the respiratory system is unknown, but investigators hypothesize that this is one reason that the burn patient is at a greater risk to develop pulmonary dysfunction and respiratory failure.[2] The majority of evidence that links complement activation to acute lung injury involves neutrophil-mediated responses which produce pulmonary endothelial cell injury.[98]

Eicosanoids. Eicosanoids are metabolic products generated via the arachidonic acid cascade and include the prostaglandins, thromboxanes and leukotrienes. These compounds have an enormous spectrum of biologic activity and are generated as a consequence of many inflammatory processes.[99] Thromboxane has been found in high concentrations in lung lymph specimens after lung injury in animal models.[84] This potent vasoconstrictor likely has a great impact upon the pulmonary microvasculature and could account for the impressive shunting of blood flow that occurs after some forms of lung injury. There is little doubt that these substances play a role in lung microvascular injury, however the magnitude of this role is currently debated. Voelkel et al have made the point that identification of eicosanoids in models of lung injury could simply be a marker of cellular membrane damage.[100]

Eicosanoids may, in a more indirect fashion, have a greater influence on lung injury. Leukotriene B_4 is a potent stimulator of neutrophil chemotaxis and induction. This compound is also found in high concentrations within neutrophils and macrophages and could therefore serve as an amplifier of the inflammatory response.[101] Arachidonic acid and the prostaglandins also have significant chemoattractant properties and influence the cell surface properties of the neutrophil that allow it to marginate along endothelial cells.[102]

More important roles in mediating lung injury may yet be defined for these inflammatory compounds. Prostaglandin E_2 has recently been reported to play an important regulatory role in the production of tumor necrosis factor by the macrophage. The level at which this regulatory activity appears to take place involves the events of mRNA transcription.[103] Leukotriene B_4 might play a similar role in the coregulation of TNF production.[90] These findings may ultimately describe a more pivotal role for these compounds in mediating cellular injury and organ dysfunction.

Ongoing Pulmonary Damage after Inhalation Injury

Infection. Infection is the most significant risk factor for progressive lung injury. Sittig et al noted bacteremia to occur in 8.4% of 1008 patients with thermal cutaneous injury. The incidence was higher with larger burns and mortality greater.[104] Significant derangements that occur within the pulmonary defense system after an inhalation injury produce a lung that is less able to protect itself from infection. Management strategies must minimize the risk of infection.

Oxygen Toxicity. The inherent toxicity of oxygen has been appreciated for over 30 years. The toxicity of oxygen is related chiefly to three factors: oxygen concentration, duration of exposure and individual susceptibility.[105] There is substantial evidence to support the hypothesis that free radicals and toxic oxygen metabolites are the central components that produce injury.

The pathophysiologic events that occur after exposure to high concentrations of oxy-

gen have been well characterized. Exposure to 100% oxygen produces significant tracheobronchitis by 12 hours and pulmonary interstitial fluid accumulation by 48 hours.[106] In healthy baboons mechanically ventilated with 100% O_2 for 7 days, gas exchange was significantly impaired by day 5. Forty percent oxygen therapy delivered constantly over a one- to two-week period has been shown to produce injury in mitochondrial systems.[107] Management approaches and ventilator support in patients who suffer an inhalation injury and impaired of gas exchange must facilitate efficient oxygen delivery to minimize further pulmonary injury.

Barotrauma. Some form of barotrauma has been estimated to occur in 8-38% of patients who require mechanical ventilation and is felt to be directly related to peak airway pressure (PAP) and positive end-expiratory pressure (PEEP).[108] The patient with ARDS often requires high ventilatory pressures and PEEP to facilitate adequate oxygenation. Obviously, the risk of barotrauma becomes higher in this patient group.[109]

The ongoing effects of barotrauma subject the injured lung to further parenchymal damage and alveolar disruption and delay the healing process. Ventilator therapy must attempt to minimize this form of insult.

Fluid Management. Patients with both a cutaneous burn and inhalation injury have a significantly greater initial fluid requirement over the first 24 to 48 hours when compared with patients suffering only a cutaneous burn injury.[110] However, the smoke-injured lung is less able to protect itself from fluid accumulation with rapid fluid infusion. This has been attributed to a combination of endothelial and epithelial injury, damage to lymphatics and surfactant inactivation.[111] Excessive administration of fluids can lead to further physiologic derangements and impaired oxygen delivery. Investigators have also demonstrated that fluid restriction (in an attempt to avoid pulmonary edema formation), has produced greater accumulation of extravascular lung water, suggesting that underestimation of fluid requirements may also exacerbate the pulmonary injury.[112]

Long-Term Sequelae

Studies in fire fighters have demonstrated few long-term effects of smoke inhalation; only 13% of this population had any detectable airway abnormality by pulmonary function testing, and none of these patients were symptomatic.[113] Reported airway abnormalities include tracheal stenosis, bronchiectasis, bronchiolitis obliterans and endobronchial polyposis.

Tracheal Stenosis. Tracheal stenosis has been noted in up to 10% of patients suffering an inhalation injury.[114] However, all patients in these reports were intubated or had undergone tracheostomy. The development of this complication was directly correlated to the duration of endotracheal intubation.

Bronchiectasis. Bronchiectasis, or chronic dilatation of the bronchi, has been sporadically reported. Patients characteristically present with dyspnea, hypoxia and hypercapnea thought to be secondary to the effects of chronic proximal airway obstruction.[115]

Bronchiolitis obliterans. A rare but devastating complication is the development of bronchiolitis obliterans. This disorder is characterized by obliterative changes of the small bronchioles with varying degrees of peribronchial fibrosis and cellular infiltration. It has been described after inhalation of nitrogen oxides, hydrogen chloride, sulfur dioxide, ammonia, phosgene and chlorine. The pathophysiologic mechanism appears to be related to persistent obstruction of the small airways by cellular debris or exudate. The changes observed with this process appear to be irreversible.[116]

Endobronchial polyposis. A more benign disorder reported after inhalation injury is the development of endobronchial polyposis. Bronchoscopically, numerous polypoid mucosal lesions throughout the trachea and bronchial tree may be noted. Biopsies of these lesions have shown pyogenic granulomas. The pathophysiology of these lesions probably involves the impaction of inhaled superheated particles on the respiratory mucosa with subsequent overzealous formation of granulation tissue. Followup has demonstrated that these lesions become progressively smaller with time.[117]

Treatment

Medical Management Strategies

Treatment protocols have evolved in an attempt to minimize the direct pulmonary sequelae of an inhalation injury. Antibiotics remain the mainstay of treatment in established pulmonary infection. The use of corticosteroids has yielded some interesting historical observations, but septic complications mitigate against their use in patients with an inhalation injury and a cutaneous burn. The incidence of bronchopneumonia and its inherent mortality remain unchanged in the last two decades.[29,118]

Pulmonary Toilet. The cornerstone in the treatment of inhalation injuries remains aggressive pulmonary toilet and strict adherence to infection prevention strategies that minimize respiratory tree contamination. Bronchorrhea can be profuse and host mechanisms to clear secretions are significantly impaired following an inhalation insult. Chest physiotherapy and postural drainage coupled with frequent tracheal suctioning is required. Humidification of inspired gases is an important adjunct in loosening thick bronchial secretions.[57] Bronchoscopy can aid in the removal of bronchial casts and debris. This procedure should be repeated as necessary, and bronchial brushings sent for culture. Although surveillance sputum cultures can be useful, bronchial brush specimens are more likely to document true pulmonary infection.[119]

Antibiotics. Prophylactic antibiotic therapy has been evaluated in an effort to reduce the high incidence of bronchopneumonia following an inhalation insult. Stone et al administered prophylactic penicillin and gentamicin (alone and in combination) to animals after an experimentally produced inhalation injury. There were no differences in mortality or bacteremic episodes when compared to animals not receiving antibiotics, and prophylactic antibiotics played no role in preventing bacterial pneumonia.[120] In fact, prophylactic antibiotic administration has been implicated in the selection of resistant organisms with a significantly worse pneumonic process. Levine et al prospectively studied systemic as well as aerosolized delivery of prophylactic gentamicin in burn patients who also had an inhalation injury. Mortality was identical in both groups, and bacteremia was documented in 75% of patients receiving antibiotics. In addition, the authors noted that resistant organisms emerged in both the burn wound and oropharyngeal secretions.[71]

Steroids. The rationale behind steroid use has stemmed from the potential of these compounds to confer protection to the alveolar-capillary membrane. Steroids have been shown to reduce mucosal edema and to blunt changes in endothelial capillary permeability.[121] They stabilize cellular membranes and lysosomes and in theory may prevent propagation of tissue destruction.[22] Corticosteroids may also inhibit the chemotactic actions of the complement system.[80,122]

The potential side-effects and deleterious consequences associated with steroid use, however, have been shown to outweigh their theoretical benefits. Investigators have documented reduced lung bacterial clearance and increased mortality after steroid administration in animal models.[122] Stone et al found a two-fold increase in mortality after rats were exposed to smoke and then treated with steroids.[120] Positive blood cultures were twice as frequent in the steroid-treated group. Other animal studies have demonstrated an improved outcome with steroid administration. However, these studies limited the evaluation of outcome to the first 48 to 72 hours after the inhalation insult.[121,123]

The most frequently quoted clinical studies are from Moylan et al[124] and Stone et al.[120] Both investigators demonstrated increased mortality and morbidity as a consequence of pulmonary sepsis in patients who received steroids. In groups of patients matched for the presence of an inhalation injury and cutaneous burn, Moylan reported a 53% mortality (9/17) in a steroid-treated group (methylprednisolone for 48 hours) and only 13% (2/16) in the untreated group. There

was also a three-fold increase in infectious complications (bacteremia or pneumonia).[124] Stone et al noted that the only benefit of steroid therapy was its ability to interrupt severe bronchospasm when refractory to conventional bronchodilators.[120]

Clearly, steroids are contraindicated in the presence of a cutaneous thermal burn of any magnitude accompanying an inhalation injury, except to alleviate severe bronchospasm. Available data does not mitigate against steroid use in the patient that has an isolated inhalation injury. However, human studies have not demonstrated improvement or a difference in outcome in patients given steroids.[70,71]

In summary, antibiotic therapy should be instituted for documented infection based on the overall clinical picture, chest x-ray and documented cultures. Other sources of infection must be ruled out including the burn wound, indwelling catheters and remote sources—urosepsis acalculous cholecystitis, etc. Our recommended treatment protocol is shown in Table 3.

Ventilator Management Strategies

The ideal ventilator management strategy minimizes barotrauma and oxygen toxicity, while maximizing oxygen delivery to peripheral tissues. Increasingly complex strategies have evolved in an attempt to reduce ventilator-associated parenchymal injury while at the same time facilitate the healing process. It is important to point out that patients suffering from an inhalation injury may exhibit a different pathophysiologic response than other pulmonary insults that produce respiratory failure. Cioffi has postulated that, as the inhalation insult is acute and self-limited, the inhalation-injured lung should go on to heal within 10 to 21 days under most circumstances.[125]

Positive End-Expiratory Pressure. The beneficial effect of positive end-expiratory pressure (PEEP) in reducing the alveolar-arterial oxygen difference (intrapulmonary shunt) and improving arterial oxygen saturation (PaO$_2$) is well documented and remains an integral component of conventional management in

Minimize risks of infection
- Strict adherence to sterile techniques
- Early mobilization and ambulation
- Aggressive debridement of devitalized tissues
- Aggressive pulmonary toilet
  - Tracheobronchial suctioning as required
  - Frequent chest physiotherapy
  - Liberal use of bronchoscopy
- Humidification of inspired air and oxygen
- Thorough decontamination of respiratory equipment (ventilators etc)

Document infection
- Evaluate the respiratory system
  - Identify changes in sputum
  - Identify chest radiographic changes
    - Bronchoscopic evaluation with brushings for culture
- Serial blood cultures
- Rule out other sources of infection
  - Evaluate intravenous sites
  - Change indwelling catheters and culture
  - Evaluate all cutaneous burn sites
    - Maintain high index of suspicion for remote sites

Antibiotic therapy
- Directed use for documented infection only
- Regimen guided by organism sensitivities and institutional epidemiology

Table 3. Treatment protocol for inhalation injury.

patients with respiratory failure.[126,127] Proper utilization of PEEP facilitates a decreased FiO_2 requirement and minimizes O_2 toxicity. The observed improvement in arterial oxygen saturation is a result of an increased functional residual capacity (FRC) due to alveolar recruitment.[126]

It must be pointed out, however, that PEEP has not been shown to improve outcome in patients that have suffered an acute lung injury. Furthermore, one must remain cognizant of adverse effects at higher levels of PEEP. These have included barotrauma[108] and reduction of cardiac output (secondary to decreased venous return).[128] Investigations have also demonstrated that PEEP can accelerate interstitial lung water formation and

subsequent pulmonary edema.[129] However, increasing the level of PEEP is often the initial and appropriate step taken to achieve adequate oxygen saturation in the patient that has sustained pulmonary injury.

Inverse Ratio Ventilation. Inverse ratio ventilation (IRV) differs from conventional ventilation modes in that the inspiratory phase is prolonged such that the I:E ratio is <1. IRV is thought to improve oxygenation by way of an "auto-PEEP" phenomenon that leads to increased FRC by initiating alveolar recruitment.[130] The advantage of IRV over PEEP is that mean airway pressures can be increased without a concomitant elevation in peak pressures. This translates, at least theoretically, into less barotraumata.[131]

Pressure controlled ventilation (PCV) is commonly utilized in combination with IRV. PCV delivers an inspired gas flow at a constant pressure for a predetermined portion of the respiratory cycle. The resulting tidal volume is determined by the preset pressure, the I:E ratio and the inherent compliance of the pulmonary tree. Early investigations have revealed that PCV, when compared with conventional volume-controlled ventilation, significantly lowers peak airway pressure while at the same time producing a similar minute ventilation and maintaining equal gas exchange ($PaCO_2$ and PaO_2). While mean airway pressures are elevated in PCV, there appear to be no adverse hemodynamic effects, e.g., no alteration in cardiac index, pulmonary artery pressure or oxygen delivery.[132]

Studies have suggested that PC-IRV improves PaO_2 in settings where conventional modes failed to achieve acceptable oxygenation.[132,133] Tharrat et al evaluated 31 patients with severe respiratory failure (of which two had suffered severe burn and inhalation injury) and compared ventilatory parameters for each patient during conventional ventilation (SIMV) and PC-IRV. During PC-IRV, the peak inspiratory pressures were reduced an average of 24 cm of H_2O (from 66 to 42 cm H_2O), the mean airway pressures increased from 30-35 cm H_2O and the average PaO_2 improved from 69 to 80 mmHg.[133] It is tempting to speculate that the decreased barotrauma, lower potential for oxygen toxicity, and higher

PaO_2 achieved with PC-IRV would facilitate earlier restoration of the damaged alveolar-capillary membrane, but this has yet to be demonstrated. There are, as yet, no studies that have demonstrated an improved overall outcome when PC-IRV was used. However, PC-IRV has become the first line salvage strategy in these patients that fail to achieve adequate oxygenation by conventional methods.

High Frequency Ventilation. High frequency ventilation (HFV) has been demonstrated to be effective in improving arterial saturation in several clinical trials[134] and has recently been evaluated in a small population of patients that sustained an inhalation injury as their primary pulmonary insult.[125] The major characteristics of HFV include a ventilatory cycle of greater than 60 breaths/min, utilization of lower peak airway pressures than in conventional ventilation modes, demonstrated lower transpulmonary pressures (and less hemodynamic compromise) than conventional ventilators and an increased FRC with more efficient intrapulmonary gas distribution than conventional ventilators.[134] In addition, HFV has been reported to improve clearance of bronchial secretions, an important adjunct in the inhalation injured patient.[135]

Cioffi et al reported their early experience with HFV in 15 patients that sustained moderate to severe inhalation injury (documented by xenon scan and bronchoscopy). The incidence of intrapulmonary sepsis (20%) and barotrauma (10%) was significantly less than that predicted by an historical cohort of patients from this institution. It is significant that in 10 patients who received HFV within 24 hours of diagnosis there were no deaths (predicted mortality of 40%).[125] These early results are quite encouraging and clearly must be more extensively studied in prospective, randomized trials.

Extracorporeal Techniques. The basis of extracorporeal techniques lie in the hypothesis that, in resting the injured respiratory system, one might "buy time" for the healing process to occurr.[136] Extracorporeal techniques encompassing both oxygen delivery and/or CO_2 removal have not been evaluated in patients suffering inhalation injuries per se. If,

however, as has been suggested, the inhalation insult is a self-limiting process with expected restoration of alveolar-capillary integrity, extracorporeal techniques could potentially be of some utility in select patients. The merits and pitfalls of ECMO techniques are discussed briefly within the context of salvage therapy in patients suffering severe respiratory failure and ARDS.

Zapol and colleagues, in a randomized prospective multicenter trial, reported their results with ECMO as salvage therapy in patients with severe respiratory failure and compared this to conventilation ventilation. Partial venoarterial bypass was instituted and demonstrated to temporarily correct the hypoxemia and hypercapnea associated with severe lung injury. Furthermore, ECMO facilitated delivery of lower ventilatory pressures and lower inspired oxygen concentrations. However, of 90 patients enrolled in both arms of this study, there were only four survivors in each group, and there was no difference in survival at two weeks (9.5% and 8.3%, respectively).[137]

Utilizing a variant in extracorporeal techniques, Gattinoni et al have attempted venovenous bypass to remove CO_2 while maintaining adequate oxygenation with apneic respiration of the lungs with 3-5 "sigh" breaths/min. Preliminary results were reported in an uncontrolled study of 43 patients, and this technique in their hands yielded a survival of 49% (21/43) in a group of patients with a historical mortality of greater than 90%. Their efforts were impressive, and the complications common to ECMO (bleeding and sepsis) were minimized.[136] However, their results have not been duplicated, or reevaluated in a prospective controlled study.

There is a philosophical appeal to the extracorporeal approach, but the complexity of continuous prolonged bypass, the manpower required and the potential difficulties that may arise in establishing bypass conduits in patients with concomitant burn injury will limit its usefulness in patients with an inhalation injury. Furthermore, current data demonstrate no survival advantage in patients with severe respiratory failure.

CURRENT PROBLEMS AND FUTURE DIRECTIONS OF INVESTIGATION

A problem in efforts to understand the inhalation injury remains our inability to accurately quantify the degree of this insult. For this reason it is difficult to compare patient groups and treatment regimens. While demonstration of an upper airway injury by endoscopic evaluation may influence initial therapy,[138] studies have demonstrated no correlation between lower airway endoscopic findings and survival, length of ventilator dependence or the degree of ventilator support required.[139,140] Radionuclide (xenon) scanning remains an important adjunct in the diagnosis of inhalation injury and is readily available at most institutions. It has recently been suggested that such studies add little in the way of prognostic or diagnostic information.[4] However, it currently remains the most objective study presently available to quantify lower airway injury. As such, it should remain an important adjunct in the initial evaluation of the patient with an inhalation injury as it may allow for stratification of patients and evaluation of our interventions.

In spite of advances in the understanding of the inhalation insult and the pathophysiologic events that culminate in pulmonary parenchymal injury, management remains centered around supportive care. As aggressive as our current interventions may appear, we remain unable to interrupt the events that often culminate in respiratory failure. For some patients the initial insult is simply too severe to overcome. However, it is clear that others succumb to septic insults and pathophysiologic processes that we are unable to arrest. Herein lies not only the major problem, but the primary challenge to clinicians and researchers alike. Early work in animal models has demonstrated that we are indeed capable of interrupting the pathways that produce pulmonary and other end-organ injury.[141-143] These studies are to be applauded but should serve only as a doorstep to further investigation.

Clearly, the appropriate endpoint is a demonstration of improved outcome (survival) in this patient population. Septic complications continue to plague the patients that have sustained inhalation injuries, and mortality rates remain effectively unchanged over the last 20years. It can only be hoped that as we continue to unravel the immune response to injury and begin to understand the mechanisms of the systemic inflammatory response our treatment interventions will truly become meaningful.

REFERENCES

1. Cark WR, Nieman OF. Smoke inhalation. Burns 1988; 14:473-494.
2. Thompson PB, Herndon DN, Traber DL et al. Effect on mortality of inhalation injury. J Trauma 1986; 26:163-165.
3. Tredget EE, Shankowsky HA, Taerum TV et al. The role of inhalation injury in burn trauma: A Canadian experience. Ann Surg 1990; 212:720-727.
4. Shirani KZ, Pruitt BA, Mason AD. The influence of inhalation injury and pneumonia on burn mortality. Ann Surg 1987; 205:82-87.
5. Kinsella J. Smoke inhalation. Burns 1988; 14:269-279.
6. Haponik EF, Crapo RO, Herndon DN. Smoke inhalation. Am Rev Resp Dis 1988; 138:1060-1063.
7. Aub JC, Pittman H, Brues AM. The pulmonary implications: A clinical description. Ann Surg 1943; 117:834-840.
8. Stone HH. Pulmonary injuryassociated with thermal burns. Surg Gynecol Obstet 1969; 129:1242-1246.
9. Moylan JA. Smoke inhalation and burn injury. Surg Clin North Am 1980; 60:1533-1540.
10. Chu C. New concepts of pulmonary burn injury. J Trauma 1981; 21:958-961.
11. Prien T, Traber DL. Toxic smoke compounds and inhalation injury: A review. Burns 1988; 14:451-460.
12. Heimback DM, Waeckerle JF. Inhalation injuries. Ann Emerg Med 1988; 17:1316-1320.
13. Dyer RF, Esch VH. Polyvinyl chloride toxicity in fires. JAMA 1976; 235:393-397.
14. Markowitz JS, Gutterman EM, Schwartz S et al. Acute health effects among firefighters exposed to polyvinyl chloride fire. Am J Epidemiol 1989; 129:1023-1031.
15. Davies JWL. Chemicals versus lung tissue: An aspect of inhalation injury revisited. J Burn Care Rehab 1986; 7:213-222.
16. Terril JB, Montgomery RR, Reinhardt CF. Toxic gases from fires. Science 1978; 200:1343-1347.
17. Beretic T. The challenge of fire effluents. Br Med J 1990; 300:696-698.
18. Demling RH, LaLonde C. Airway and pulmonary

abnormalities. In: Demling RH, ed. Burn Trauma. New York: Thieme, 1989: 3-18.

19. Robinson L, Miller RH. Smoke inhalation injuries. Am J Otolaryngol 1986; 7:375-380.

20. Strongin J, Hales CA. Pulmonary disorders in the burn patient. In: Martyn JA, eds. Acute managementofthe Burned Patient. Philadelphia: WB Saunders, 1990: 25-45.

21. Desai MH, Rutan RL, Herndon DN. Managing smoke inhalation injuries. Postgrad Med 1989; 86;69-76.

22. Trunkey DD. Inhalation injury. Surg Clin North Am 1978;58:1133-1140.

23. Demling RH. Postgraduate course: Respiratory injury part III: Pulmonary dysfunction in the burn patient. J Burn Care Rehab 1986; 7:277-284.

24. Pruitt BA, Erickson DR, Morrison A. Progressive puilmonary insufficiency and other pulmonary complications of thermal injury. J Trauma 1975; 15:369-379.

25. Moritz AR, Henriques FC, McClean R. The effects of inhaled heat on the air passages and lungs. Am J Pathol 1945; 21:311-331.

26. Peters WJ. Inhalation injury caused by the products of combustion. Can Med Assoc J 1981; 125:249-252.

27. Dressler DP, Hozid JL, Nathan P. Smoke inhalation. In: Thermal Injury. St. Louis: CV Mosby, 1988: 152-171.

28. Herndon DN, Thompson PB, Linares, HA et al Postgraduate course: Respiratory injury part I Incidence, mortality, pathogenesis and treatment of pulmonary injury. J Burn Care Rehab 1986; 7: 184-191.

29. Herndon DN, Langer F, Thompson P. Pulmonary injury in burned patients. Surg Clin North Am 1987; 67:32-46.

30. Till GO, Johnson KJ, Kunkel R et al. Intravascular activation of complement and acute lung injury. J Clin Invest 1982; 69:1126-l135.

31. Stein MD, Herndon DN, Stevens JM. Production of chemotactic factors and lung cell changes following smoke inhalation in a sheep model. J Burn Care Rehab 1986; 7:117-l21.

32. Traber DL, Linares HA, Herndon DN. The pathophysiology of inhalation injury: A review. Burns 1988; 14:357-364.

33. Traber DL, Herndon DN, Stein MD. The pulmonary lesion of smoke inhalation in an ovine model. Circ Shock 1986; 18:311-323.

34. Molteni A, Clark WR, Traber DL et al. The endocrine response of the lung to thermal injury. In: Dolecek R, eds. Endocrinology of Thermal Trauma. Philadelphia: Lea and Feibiger, 1990: 174-215.

35. Fein A, Leff A, Hopewell PL. Pathophysiology and management of the complications resulting from fire and the inhaled products of combustion: A review of the literature. Crit Care Med 1980; 8:94-98.

36. Norris JC, Moore SJ, Home AS. Synergistic lethality induced by the combination of carbon monoxide and cyanide. Toxicology 1986;40:121-129.

37. Goldblum LR, Ramirez RG, Absalon KB. What is the mechanism of carbon monoxide toxicity? Aviat Space Environ Med 1975; 46:1289-l291.

38. Thorn SR. Smoke inhalation. Emerg Med Clin North Amer 1989; 7:371-387.

39. Demling RH. Smoke inhalation injury. Postgrad Med 1987; 82:63-68.

40. Silverman SH, Purdue GF, Hunt JL. Cyanide toxicity in burned patients. J Trauma 1988; 28:171-176.

41. Astry CL, Jakab GJ. The effects of acrolein exposure on pulmonary antibacterial defenses. Toxicol Appl Pharmacol 1983; 67:49-54.

42. Grundfest CC, Chang J, Newcombe D. Acrolein: A potent modulator of lung macrophage arachadonic acid metabolism. Biochem Biophys Acta 1982; 713:149-159.

43. Hales CA, Barkin PW, Jung W et al. Synthetic smoke with acrolein but not HCl produces pulmonary edema. J Appl Physiol 1988; 64:1121-1133.

44. Regan RH. Review of clinical experience in handling phosgene exposure gases. Toxicol Ind Health 1985; 1:69-71.

45. Summer W, Haponik E. Inhalation of irritant gases. Clin Chest Med 1981; 2:273-287.

46. Purser DA, Buckley P. Lung irritants and inflammation during and after exposures to thermal decomposition products from polymeric materials. Med Sci Law 1983; 23:142-150.

47. Flury KE, Dines DE, Rodarte JR et al. Airway obstruction due to inhalation of ammonia. Mayo Clin Proc 1983; 58:389-393.

48. Montague TJ, Macneil AR. Mass ammonia inhalation. Chest 1980; 77:496-498.

49. Dowell AR, Kilburn KH, Pratt PC. Short term exposure to nitrogen dioxide. Arch Intern Med 1971; 128:74-80.

50. Charan NB, Meyers CG, Lakshminarayan S. Pulmonary injuries associated with acute sulfur dioxide inhalation. Am Rev Resp Dis 1979; 119:555-559.

51. Deitch EA, Gelder F and McDonald JC. Sequential prospective analysis of the nonspecific host defense systems after thermal injury. Arch Surg 1984; 119:83-98.

52. Alexander JW, Ogle CK, Stinnet JE et al. A sequential prospective analysis of immunologic abnormalities and infection following severe thermal injury. Ann Surg 1978; 188:809-816.

53. Sharma VK, Agarwal DS, Satyanand et al. Profile of complement components in patients with severe burns. J Trauma 1980; 20:976-978.

54. Deitch EA. Infection in the compromised host. Surg Clin North Am 1988; 68:181-97.

55. Pruitt BA, Erickson DR, Morris A. Progressive pulmonary insufficiency and other pulmonary complications of thermal injury. J Trauma 1975; 15:369-379.

56. Achauer BM, Allyn PA, Furnas DW et al. Pulmonary complications of burns. Ann Surg 1973; 177:311-319.

57. Demling RH, Lalonde C. In: Demling RH, ed. Burn

Trauma. New York: Thieme Medical Publishers, 1989:149-167.

58. Chernock EL, Meehan JJ. Postburn respiratory injuries in children. Pediat Clin North Am 1986; 27:661-676.

59. Cohen MA, Guzzardi LJ. Inhalation of products of combustion. Ann Emer Med 1983;12:628-632.

60. Hocking WG and Golde DW. The pulmonary alveolar macrophage. N Engl J Med 1979; 301:580-587.

61. Demarest GB, Hudson LD, Altman LC. Impaired macrophage chemotaxis in patients with acute smoke inhalation. Am Rev Resp Dis 1979; 119:279-286.

62. Loose LD, Megirian R, Turinsky J. Biochemical and functional alterations in macrophages after thermal injury. Infect Immun 1984; 44:554-558.

63. Balis JU, Shelley SA. Quantitative evaluation of the surfactant system of the lung. Ann Clin Lab Sci 1972; 2:410-419.

64. Nieman GF, Clark WR, Wax SD et al. The effect of smoke inhalation on pulmonary surfactant. Ann Surg 1980; 191:171-181.

65. Jarstrand C: Role of surfactant in the pulmonary defense system. In: Robertson B, ed. Pulmonary Surfactant. New York: Elsevier, 1984:187-201.

66. Coonrod JD, Yoneda K. Detection and partial characterization of antibacterial factors in alveolar lining material of rats. J Clin Invest 1983; 71:129-141.

67. Shennib H, Molder DS, Chin RC. The effects of pulmonary atelectasis and re-expansion on lung cellular immune defenses. Arch Surg 1984; 119:274-277.

68. DiVincenti FC, Pruitt BA, Reckler JM. Inhalation injuries. J Trauma 1971; 11:109-117.

69. Stone HH. Pulmonary burns in children. J Pediat Surg 1979; 14:48-52.

70. Wroblewski DA, Bower GC. The significance of facial burns in acute smoke inhalation. Crit Care Med 1979; 7:335-338.

71. Levine BA, Petroff PA, Slade CL et al. Prospective trials of dexamethasone and aerosolized gentamicin in the treatment of inhalation injury in the burned patient. J Trauma 1978; 18:188-193.

72. Clark WR, Bonaventura M, Myers W. Smoke inhalation and airway management at a regional burn unit: 1974 -1983. J Burn Care Rehab 1989; 10:52-62.

73. Herndon DN, Barrow RE, Traber DL et al. Extra-vascular lung water changes following smoke inhalation and massive burn injury. Surgery 1987; 102:341-349.

74. Fowler AA, Hamman RF, Good JT et al. Adult respiratory distress syndrome: risk with common predispositions. Ann Intern Med 1983;98:593-597.

75. Herndon DM, Thompson PR, Brown M et al. Diagnosis, pathophysiology, and treatment of inhalation injury. In: Boswick JA, ed. The Art and Science of Burn Care. Rockville: Aspen Publishers, 1987.

76. Pepe PE, Potkin RT, Reus DH et al. Clinical predictors of the adult respiratory distress syndrome.

Am J Surg 1982; 144:124-130.

77. Ashbaugh DG, Bigelow DB, Petty TL et al. Acute respiratory distress in adults. Lancet 1967; 2:319-323.

78. Tale RM, Repine JE. Neutrophils and the adult respiratory distress syndrome. Am Rev Resp Dis 1983; 128:552-559.

79. Weiss SJ. Tissue destruction by neutrophils. N Engl J Med 1989; 320:365-376.

80. Stevens JH, Raffin TA. The adult respiratory distress syndrome. Postgrad Med Journal 1984; 60:505-513

81. Traber DL, Schlag G, Redl H et al. Pulmonary edema and compliance changes following smoke inhalation. J Burn Care Rehab 1985; 6:490-494.

82. Burns TR, Greenberg D, Cartwright J et al. Smoke inhalation: An ultra-structural study of reaction to injury in the human alveolar wall. Environ Research 1986; 41:447-457.

83. Till GO, Beauchamp L, Menapace D et al. O_2-radical dependent lung damage following thermal injury of rat skin. J Trauma 1983; 23:269-277.

84. Heffner JE, Sahn SA, Repine JE. The role of platelets in the adult respiratory distress syndrome: culprits of bystanders? Am Rev Resp Dis 1987; 135:482-492.

85. Fry DE, Perlstein L, Fulton RL et al. Multiple system organ failure: the role of uncontrolled infection. Arch Surg 1980; 115:136-140.

86. Montgomery AB, Stager MA, Carrico CJ et al. Cause of mortality in patients with the adult respiratory distress syndrome. Am Rev Resp Dis 1985;132:485-489.

87. Harlan JM, Harker LA, Reidy MA et al. Lipopolysaccharide-mediated bovine endothelial cell injury in vitro. Lab Invest 1983; 48: 269-274.

88. Brigham KL, Meyrick B. Endotoxin and lung injury. Am Rev Resp Dis 1986; 133: 913-927.

89. Haslett C, Worthen GS, Giclas PC et al. The pulmonary vascular sequestration of neutrophils in endotoxemia is initiated by an effect of endotoxin on the neutrophil in the rabbit. Am Rev Resp Dis 1987; 136: 9-18.

90. Rinaldo JE, Christman JW. Mechanisms and mediators of the adult respiratory distress syndrome. Clin Chest Med 1990; 11:621-632.

91. Deitch EA, Ma WJ, Ma L et al: Endotoxin induced bacterial translocation: a study in mechanism. Surgery 1989; 106:292-300.

92. Cerra FB. Hypermetabolism, organ failure, and metabolic support. Surgery 1987; 101:1-14,

93. Stephens KE, Ishizaka A, Larrick JW et al. Tumor necrosis factor causes increased pulmonary permeability and edema. Am Rev of Resp Dis 1988; 137:1364 -1370.

94. Tracer KJ, Lowry SF, Cerami A. Cachectin/TNF-alpha in septic shock and septic adult respiratory distress syndrome. Am Rev Resp Dis 1988; 138:1377-1379.

95. Solomkin JS, Costa LA, Satoh PS et al. Complement activation and clearance in acute illness and injury: evidence for C5a as a cell-directed mediator of ARDS in man. Surgery 1985; 97: 668-678.

96. Chenoweth ED, Cooper SW, Hugh TE et al. Complement activation during cardio-pulmonary bypass. N Engl J Med 1981; 304: 497-503.

97. Craddock PR, Fehr J, Brigham KL et al. Complement and leukocyte-mediated pulmonary dysfunction in hemodialysis. N Engl J Med 1977;296:767-774.

98. Seeger W, Hartmann R, Neuhoff H et al. Local complement activation, thromboxane-mediated vasoconstriction, and vascular leakage in isolated lungs. Am Rev Resp Dis 1989; 139:88-99.

99. Cochrane CG. The enhancement of inflammatory injury. Am Rev Resp Dis 1987; 136:1361-1362.

100. Voelkel NF, Stenmark KR, Westcott JY et al. Lung eicosanoid metabolism, Clin Chest Med 1989; 10:95-105.

101. Garcia JGN, Noonan TC, Jubiz W et al. Leukotrienes and the pulmonary microcirculation. Am Rev Respir Dis 1987; 136:161-169.

102. Flick MR. Mechanisms of acute lung injury. Crit Care Clin 1986; 2:455-470.

103. Kunkel SL, Spangler M, May MA et al. Prostaglandin E_2 regulates macrophage-derived tumor necrcosis factor gene expression. J Biol Chem 1988; 163:5380-5384.

104. Sittig K, Deitch EA. Effect of bacteremia on mortality after thermal injury. Arch Surg 1988; 123:1367-1370.

105. DeLos Santos R, Seidenfeld JJ, Anzueto A et al. One hundred percent oxygen lung injury in adult baboons. Am Rev Resp Dis 1987; 136: 657-661.

106. Fisher AB, Forman HJ, Glass M. Mechanisms of pulmonary oxygen toxicity. Lung 1984; 162: 255-259.

107. Summer WR. Adult respiratory distress syndrome. In: Haponik EF, eds. Respiratory Injury: Smoke Inhalation and Burns. New York: MacGraw-Hill Information Services Co., Health Professions Division, 1990:88.

108. Haake R, Schlichtig R, Ulstad DR et al. Barotrauma: pathophysiology, risk factors and prevention. Chest1987;91:608-613.

109. Woodring JH. Pulmonary interstitial emphysema in the adult respiratory distress syndrome. Crit Care Med 1985; 13: 786-791.

110. Navar PD, Saffle JR, Warden GD. The effect of inhalation injury on fluid resuscitation requirements after thermal injury. Am J Surg 1985; 150: 716-720.

111. Clark WR, Nieman GF, Goyette D et al. Effects of crystalloid on lung fluid balance after smoke inhalation. Ann Surj 1988; 208: 56-64.

112. Herndon DN, Traber DL, Traber LD. The effect of resuscitation on inhalation injury. Surgery 1986; 100: 248-251.

113. Loke J, Farmer W, Matthay RA et al. Acute and chronic effects of fire fighting on pulmonary function. Chest 1980; 77: 369-373.

114. Land T, Goodwin OW, McManus WF et al. Upper airway sequelae in burn patients requiring endotracheal intubation ortracheostomy. Ann Surg 1985; 201:374-382.

115. Slutzker AD, Kim R, Said SI. Bronchiectasis and progressive respiratory failure following smoke inhalation. Chest 1989; 95:1349-1350.

116. Perez-Guerra F, Walsh RE, Sagel SS. Bronchiolitis obliterans and tracheal stenosis: Late complications of inhalation burn. JAMA 1971; 218:1568-1570.

117. Adams C, Moison T, Chandrasekher AJ et al. Endobronchial polyposis secondary to thermal inhalation injury. Chest 1979;75:643-645.

118. Arturson G: Respiratory responses to burn injury. Burns 1975; 1: 254-26.

119. Johansen WG, Seidenfeld JJ, Gomez P et al. Bacteriologic diagnosis of nosocomial pneumonia following prolonged mechanical ventilation. Am Rev Resp Dis 1988; 137: 259-264.

120. Stone HH, Rhame DW, Corbitt JD et al. Respiratory burns: a correlation of clinical and laboratory results. Ann Surg 1967; 165: 157-168.

121. Dressler DP, Skornik MS, Kupersmith S. Corticosteroid treatment of experimental smoke inhalation. Ann Surg 1976; 183: 46 52.

122. Skornik WA, Dressler DP. The effect of short-term steroid therapy on lung bacterial clearance and survival in rats. Ann Surg 1974; 179:415-421.

123. Beeley JM. Mortality and lung histopathology after inhalation injury. Am Rev Resp Dis 1988; 133:191-196.

124. Moylan JA, Chan CK. Inhalation injury-an increasing problem. Surgery 1978; 188:34-37.

125. Cioffi WG, Graves TA, McManus WF et al. High-frequency Percussive ventilation in patients with inhalation injury. J Trauma 1989;29:350-354.

126. Petty TL. The use, abuse, and mystique of positive end-expiratory pressure. Am Rev Resp Dis 1988; 138:435-478.

127. Ashbaugh DG, Petty TL, Bigelow DB et al. Continuous positive pressure breathing(CPPB) in adult respiratory distress syndrome. J Thorac Cardiovasc Surg 1969; 57:31-41.

128. Eaton RJ, Taxman RM, Avioli LV. Cardiovascular evaluation of patients treated with PEEP. Arch Intern Med 1983; 143:1958-61.

129. Nieman GF, Bredenberg CE, and Paskanik AM. Positive end-expiratory pressure accelerates lung water accumulation in high surface tension edema. Surgery 1990; 107:156-162.

130. Cole AGH, Welter SF, Sikes MK. Inverse ratio ventilation compared with PEEP in adult respiratory failure. Intens Care Med 1984; 10:227-232.

131. Gurevitch MJ, Van Dyke J, Young ES et al. Improved oxygenation and lower peak airway pressure in severe ARDS: Treatment with inverse ration ventilation. Chest 1986; 89:211-217.

132. Lain DC, DiBenedetto R, Morris SL et al. Pressure control inverse ratio ventilation as a method to reduce peak inspiratory pressure and provide adequate ventilation and oxygenation. Chest 1989; 95:1081-1088.

133. Tharrat RS, Allen RR, Albertson TE. Pressure controlled inverse ratio ventilation in severe adult respiratory failure. Chest 1988; 94:755-762.

134. Hurst JM, Branson RD, Davis K et al. Comparison

of conventional mechanical ventilation and high-frequency ventilation. Ann Surg 1990; 211:486-491.

135. Thangathuria D, Holm AP, Mikhail M et al. HFV in management of a patient with severe bronchorrhea. Resp Management, 1988.

136. Gattinoni L, Pesente A, Maschioni D et al. Low frequency positive pressure ventilation with extra - corporeal CO_2 removal in severe acute respiratory failure. JAMA 1986; 256:881-886.

137. Zapol, WM, Snider MT, Hill JD et al. Extracorporeal membrane oxygenation in severe acute respiratory failure. JAMA 1979; 242:2193-2196.

138. Haponik EF, Meyers DA, Monster AM et al. Acute upper airway injury in burn patients: Serial changes of flow volume curves and upper airway nasopharyngoscopy. Am Rev Resp Dis 1987; 135:360-366.

139. Head JM. Inhalation injury in burns. Am J Surg 1980; 139:508-512.

140. Bingham HG, Gallagher TJ, Powell MD. Early bronchoscopy as a predictor of ventilatory support for burned patients. J Trauma 1987; 27:1286.

141. Priest PB, Brinson DN, Schroeder DA et al Treatment of experimental gram-negative sepsis with marine monoclonal antibodies directed against lipopolysaocharide. Surgery 1989; 106:147-155.

142. Dunn DL, Priest PB, Condie RM et al. Protective capacity of polyclonal and monoclonal antibodies directed against endotoxin during experimental sepsis. Arch Surg 1988; 123:1389-1393.

143. Mathison JC, Wolfson E, Ulevitch RJ. Participation of TNF in the mediation of gram-negative bacterial lipopolysaccharide-induced injury in rabbits. J Clin Inves 1988; 81:1925-1938.

CHAPTER 7

THE IMMUNE CONSEQUENCES OF TRAUMA: AN OVERVIEW

David J. Dries

INTRODUCTION

Trauma, as a whole, is the single greatest killer of the young adult population and the leading cause of loss of productive life span, far exceeding that due to neoplasia or atherosclerotic cardiovascular disease. Mortality following trauma proceeds in a three peak pattern with the first peak associated with immediate death due to critical injury. The second component of mortality following trauma is failure to recognize or treat life threatening problems within the initial "Golden Hour". The third component of mortality after injury is related to overwhelming infection which is the source of the majority of late deaths following traumatic injury.[1] This continues to be the case despite advances in critical care and antimicrobial therapy.

Numerous authors document alteration in cells of the immune response when severe injury or operative procedures have occurred. Risk of infection is increased in association with these changes, which result in a diminished host response to infecting microorganisms. Among the changes noted in multiply injured patients are depressed cell-mediated immunity with decreased HLA-DR receptor expression on monocytes and diminished production of cytokines including interleukin-1 (IL-1), interleukin-2 (IL-2), and interferon gamma.[2] In addition, the immunosuppressor prostaglandin PGE_2 is seen in increasing amounts. Polk, among others, have observed a decrease in monocyte HLA-DR expression in patients with severe injury and correlated this finding with poor clinical outcome. Monocyte HLA-DR expression is required for adequate antigen presentation to T-cells and is thought essential in the cell-mediated immunity needed for response to infectious agents in traumatized patients.[3]

Faist and associates have demonstrated that alteration in cell-mediated immunity following trauma is related to disruption of the monocyte T-cell interaction. A shift is noted in cell ratio in the compartments of the peripheral blood mononuclear cells, with an increase in prostaglandin E_2 production by macrophages and a simultaneous decrease of functionally competent $CD3^+$, and $CD4^+$ lymphocytes.[4] T-cell dysfunction in these states of stress is associated with impaired synthesis of crucial cytokines, including IL-2 and interferon gamma (IFN-γ). Reduction in IL-2 synthesis results in incomplete T-cell responses to antigenic stimuli while the IFN-γ deficit results in inefficient macrophage antigen presentation among other problems.

On the contrary, overstimulation or excessive response of the immune inflammatory system may cause multiple organ failure syndrome, the physiologic end point of late death in severely injured patients.[5] Cytokine administration or production in these patients may, therefore, be inappropriate or lead to excessive inflammatory cascade response with deleterious effects in a variety of physiologic and metabolic ways detrimental to host survival. The problem, which has yet to be resolved, is determination of appropriate time and dosage for immune stimulation or blockade of damaging substances produced in the immune response to optimize patient outcome.

Injury induced immune suppression appears reversible, and as its causes are better understood, hope has risen for control of immune response in favor of the patient. Unfortunately, the immune deficit associated with injury is unique and at times difficult to study, mainly because of the great variety in the extent and combination of injuries each of which may make a specific contribution to the immunological deficit. Most of the information now available is related to assessment of patients with thermal injury.

IMMUNE DEPRESSION IN THERMAL INJURY PATIENTS

Major thermal injuries create a significant multicentric immunological depression thought to predispose patients to subsequent infection. Impairment of immune response is universal in patients with injuries covering greater than 40% of the total body surface and particularly in the very young or very old. Ninnemann in several reviews has listed the immunological changes occurring in thermal injury patients:[6]

1. Loss of skin test reactivity and recall antigen response.

2. Release of endotoxin, other tissue degradation products, hormones, cytokines and lymphokines with immunosuppressive or inappropriate immunostimulatory proprieties.

3. Activation of the complement system using both the classical and alternative pathways with production of complement split products with immunoregulatory functions.

4. Reduced monocyte/macrophage function with increased suppressor macrophage function with production with immunosuppressive prostaglandin E_2 and reduced phagocytosis.

5. Transient depression in B-cell number and immunoglobulin production.

6. Depression of neutrophil function including chemotaxis, phagocytosis, intracellular killing and chemiluminescence.

7. Decreased serum opsonic activity and fibronectin production.

8. Diminished natural killer cell and lymphokine activated killer cell function.

9. Depression of T-lymphocyte response with increased suppressor cell activity.

10. Reversal of T-lymphocyte helper/suppressor cell ratios has also been reported.

The acute burn period is a time of diminished macrophage and lymphocyte function with vigorous suppressor T-cell activity and reduced immune response characterized by production of immunosuppressive mediators and the presence of leukopenia or lymphopenia. With respect to cytokine production, deficits in IL-2 production with associated T-cell activation have been noted.

The chief clinical interventions for reversing burn induced immune response deficits: removal of dead or injured tissue and restoration of the skin barrier to wound colonization, are critical to controlling the immunological perturbations which persist. Closure of the burn wound leads to restoration of immune competence and frequently, full recovery of the injured individual. The timing of restoration of immune competence is associated with the rate at which burn wound control can be achieved.

Many workers believe that burns represent a model by which immunological changes occurring following other types of traumatic injury, and following major surgery, can be better understood. Many of the changes which occur in burn patients also appear to follow blunt or penetrating trauma. However, few attempts have been made to study patients with other types of injuries due to the difficulty in grouping patients for study and establishing a correlation between type and severity of injury and the development of immune depression. The threshold of injury which results in loss of immune competence has not been evaluated in traumatized individuals to the degree that this has been possible in the burn patient.

As with the burn patient, the most important clinical evidence of immune depression is the dramatic increase in septic complications accompanying major injury. Baker and associates, in a review of accidental deaths in San Francisco, found that 78% of late mortality was due to sepsis. Polk et al noted a similar incidence for septic death (75%) in patients with major thermal injury.[7,8]

As most of the trauma patients in the study of Baker dying from sepsis had multiple injuries, it was hypothesized that many of these deaths could have been prevented by more extensive early debridement. This procedure has been shown to enhance immune competence in thermal injury.

Patients with major trauma are frequently anergic. Christou and Yurt found that lack of skin test reactivity (anergy), detected on patient admission was indicative of frequent sepsis and later patient death. A decrease in neutrophil function has been noted to accompany anergy following blunt trauma. In a subsequent study of blunt trauma victims, these workers found that patients with normal skin test reactivity at admission sustained no mortality or significant infectious complications while individuals with skin test anergy have a 20% rate of sepsis and a 16% mortality rate. Deficits in neutrophil function and adherence were detectable within hours of injury and appeared related to anergy and circulating immunosuppressive factors in the blood.

Patients undergoing major surgical procedures are also prone to develop immune response depression. Ninnemann reports an early study in this area carried out by Slade and associates measuring in vivo and in vitro immune function following nephrectomy in normal renal transplant donors. These individuals had normal immune response prior to surgery, but postoperatively sustained a fall in total lymphocyte, B-cell and T-cell numbers. Mitogen and mixed lymphocyte responses also decreased upon induction of anesthesia and after operation. While these patients sustained no clinically significant problems with infection, other data suggests that immune depression in surgical patients may have adverse clinical outcomes. Using standard skin testing, Christou and associates in a prospective evaluation of over 500 skin test positive surgical patients found that 6.4% of these individuals developed longlasting anergy in the postoperative period. This group had a 41% rate of significant infection and 22% mortality rate, compared to an infection rate of 5% and a mortality rate of 3% in the patients who were not anergic. While major surgical procedures appear to result in anergy, the extent of operation required to produce immune depression and anergy was not determined. Later work suggests that procedures of smaller scope may also be associated with suppression of T-lymphocyte function.

Subsequent studies by other workers evaluated leukocyte function in association with operative trauma. When Christou and Meakins reported a series of patients with anergy and depressed neutrophil chemotactic response, they concluded that the worst combination for the individual involved was cutaneous anergy coupled with decreased neutrophil chemotaxis. If both deficits occurred together, a high rate of sepsis and frequent mortality was predicted. Christou and Meakins pointed out that the serum of anergic patients contained mediators which appeared responsible for depressed neutrophil response. Lymphocyte response, particularly that of T-cells, is also depressed by surgery. This effect may be mediated by suppressor cell activation.

Cytokines and the Septic Syndrome

As recently reviewed by Filkins, an advance in understanding the immune response to trauma and other forms of injury of the past 20 years has been identification of a cell system centered on the mononuclear phagocyte or macrophage and substances, known as cytokines, at the base of a pathogenic chain of events resulting in sepsis and injury states.[9] Cytokines, whether lymphokines as derived from lymphocytes, monokines if obtained from mononuclear phagocytes, or generically related molecules from other immunocytes are defined as nonantibody regulatory proteins secreted by activated immunocytes mediating both local and systemic response to injury secondary to infection, trauma, inflammation, burns and hemorrhage.

The cytokines now include 13 interleukins; tumor necrosis factor (TNF) alpha and beta; interferons (IFN)—alpha, beta and gamma; colony stimulating factors (CSF) for granulocytes, monocytes, or both; chemotactic factors such as neutrophil activating proteins and macrophage inflammatory proteins; and a variety of growth and differentiation factors such as, transforming growth factor (TGF) platelet derived growth factor (PDGF) or fibroblast growth factor (FGF).

Filkins has modified Koch's postulates for proof that proposed agents are the cause of particular disease states to identify the role of cytokines in sepsis. These postulates can be summarized in three statements:

1. When the sepsis syndrome and septic shock are elicited, then cytokines must be elevated systemically.

2. When purified cytokines are injected into susceptible animal species, then the sepsis syndrome and septic shock must result.

3. When the specific antibody to the cytokine is injected therapeutically, then the sepsis syndrome and septic shock must be alleviated.

Recent human and animal evidence suggests that cytokines including TNF alpha, IL-1 beta and IL-6 can be demonstrated to be present and blocked with control of the septic state. Early human studies by Michie and associates demonstrated the association of TNF alpha production and endocrine and metabolic changes consistent with sepsis following administration of endotoxin to healthy volunteers.[10] Subsequent clinical studies permitted identification of IL-1 and IL-6 in similar circumstances. In addition, a combination of human and animal work demonstrates that administration of TNF alpha, IL-1 beta, and IL-6 produce sepsis syndrome in animal models and limited human studies. Finally, the recent development of monoclonal antibody therapy has led to evaluation of anti-TNF monoclonal antibody therapy in the clinical arena along with IL-1 receptor antagonist protein. Monoclonal antibodies to IL-6 have at this point seen only experimental application.

Role of Prostaglandins

Numerous authors have suggested that alteration of cell-mediated immunity following trauma is due to disruption of intact monocyte and T-cell interaction. Within this scenario, some report a shift in cell ratios in the compartment of peripheral blood mononuclear cells and increase in production of PGE_2 by stimulated macrophages.[11] This is temporally associated with decrease in CD3+ and CD4+ lymphocytes. This T-cell dysfunction in states of stress is associated with impaired synthesis of two cytokines: interleukin-2 (IL-2), and interferon-gamma (IFN-γ). Inability to produce adequate amounts of IL-2 results in incomplete T-cell proliferation while lack of interferon gamma results in inefficient macrophage antigen presentation. These functional deficits are thought critical to depressed cell-mediated immunity following trauma with subsequent infectious complications.[2,4]

Given the above, substances likely to provide immunoprotection and immune restoration are nonsteroidal antiinflammatory drugs blocking production of immunoreactive PGE_2, a common link near the end of the chain of macrophage/T-cell interactive dysfunction and synthetic stimulants, such as interferon gamma and thymopentin which result in T-cell activation, improved function and enhanced macrophage antigen processing.

Prostaglandin E_2 (PGE_2) may decrease T-cell activation by inhibiting production of IL-2. PGE_2 may inhibit IL-2 production through activation of a suppressor T-cell, though this mechanism has never clearly been demonstrated. PGE_2 may also act on T-lymphocytes by stimulation of adenylate cyclase activity with increased intracellular cyclic adenosine monophosphate concentration, a negative signal for T-cell activation. In burn patients, increased amounts of PGE_2 have been found in the wound, serum and adjacent lymphatics. Increased PGE_2 production by monocytes of burn patients has also been reported. Faist and coworkers have demonstrated increased monocyte production of PGE_2 in patients sustaining major trauma. A variety of investigators have administered cyclooxgenase inhibitors (particularly indomethacin) and evaluated outcome in patients and animals sustaining major surgical or traumatic stress. Restoration of interleukin-2 synthesis with improved outcome has been noted in both clinical and laboratory models. Thus, control of PGE_2 synthesis appears central to restoration of immune competence following various types of injury.

IMMUNE STIMULATION

Faist and coworkers have investigated immune stimulation in the setting of surgical or traumatic stress. Recent work suggests that administration of a cyclooxygenase inhibitor and a thymomimetic drug can prevent trauma-induced depression or breakdown of cell mediated immunity normally occurring after major operative or other forms of injury.[4] These workers note that administration of immune stimulant therapy was associated with consistent increase in levels of interferon gamma and recovery of IL-2 production. Similar findings have been reported in animal models with a variety of infectious and traumatic insults treated with exogenous administration of recombinant interferon gamma.

Faist and associates have investigated the immune restoration potential of combination therapy using thymopentin and indomethacin in 60 patients undergoing cardiac surgery utilizing cardiopulmonary bypass.[4] These patients also received perioperative immunologic screening with delayed type hypersensitivity skin test response and phenotyping for peripheral blood mononuclear cell specific and nonspecific induction of lymphoproliferative response. IL-2 synthesis was assessed in vitro.

Serum concentration of D-erythro-neopterin and gamma interferon were also assessed. These patients were evaluated in three groups containing 20 individuals each: one group received indomethacin for the first five postoperative days, while the second received thymopentin along with indomethacin for the first five postoperative days. The third group served as control. In the group receiving thymopentin and indomethacin therapy, delayed type hypersensitivity scores and proliferative responses in cell cultures were not depressed after operation in comparison to control patients. Cell surface expression for CD3, CD4 and IL-2 receptor positive subpopulations of lymphocytes was depressed in control patients following surgery while in patients receiving combination therapy with thymopentin and indomethacin protection with particular regard to CD4 and IL-2 receptor positive cell populations was noted. IL-2 production assessed in vitro was also protected in patients receiving indomethacin and thymopentin therapy. Thus, it appears that therapy combining agents blocking prostaglandin E_2 production as a mediator of immunosuppression along with provision of therapy to stimulate depressed cellular immune function in the initial postoperative period may provide improved immunologic outcome following major surgical or other traumatic insults. It should be noted however, that clinical efficacy was not demonstrated in this study. A total of seven infections were noted on clinical assessment with two patients dying with multiple organ failure. One death occurred in one of the treatment groups while the second occurred among the control patients.

Polk and associates have championed the role of gamma interferon treatment following trauma and various forms of infectious challenge. These workers have investigated interferon gamma treatment in animal models of subcutaneous and intraabdominal infection and initiated clinical studies utilizing this cytokine in patients sustaining multiple injuries. Interferon gamma is a T-cell product which stimulates macrophage activation as indicated by HLA-DR antigen expression. After initial work in which interferon gamma was efficacious in treating wound infection in a mouse model, these workers extended their animal work to include intraperitoneal infection with *Escherichia coli* followed by laparotomy and a second remote intramuscular infection with *Klebsiella pneumoniae*.[12] Interferon gamma was effective in improving outcome in survival studies with this dual infection model and was not associated with any adverse interaction with antibiotics administered as a part of this study. In addition, peripheral blood mononuclear cell Ia antigen expression was monitored, a parameter analogous to human monocyte HLA-DR antigen expression.

Ia antigen may play a crucial role in monitoring of antigen presentation and macrophage activation. In the animal model of Polk and associates, laparotomy resulted in subnormal levels of Ia antigen on mononuclear blood cells for three days after surgery. Laparotomy combined with infection resulted in a subnormal level of Ia antigen for five days following laparotomy. Low levels of Ia antigen, possibly coinciding with deficient antigen presentation and macrophage activation, could account for increased susceptibility of affected animals to infection. Interferon gamma therapy prevented decline in levels of Ia antigen expression. While interferon gamma has multiple immunoregulatory proprieties, it is possible that restoration of peripheral mononuclear cell Ia antigen levels could contribute to therapeutic effects and provide a marker for appropriate cytokine administration in animal and clinical studies.

Administration of cytokines and other immune stimulants is not without risk. Overstimulation or excessive response of the immunoinflammatory system is thought to cause multiple organ failure syndrome, the ultimate cause of death in many patients with severe infection. Thus, a potential adverse consequence of interferon gamma enhancement of the immune system may be inappropriate or excessive inflammatory cascade response to an otherwise minor inflammatory stimulus. Such a response may have adverse consequences on a variety of physiologic and metabolic functions and thus be detrimental to host survival.[13]

Jurkovich and associates have investigated some of the adverse consequences of interferon gamma therapy when given in combination with endotoxin administration.[5] In a study utilizing normal rabbits, these authors set up four treatment groups which were prepared for measurement of cardiac output, arterial pressure, arterial oxygen tension and white blood count. Animals receiving interferon gamma therapy coincident with endotoxin administration had significant decline in cardiac output, arterial oxygen tension and white blood count along with increased capillary permeability as indicated by pulmonary lavage fluid to plasma ratio of I^{125} labeled albumin when compared to other treatment groups. The doses of endotoxin and interferon gamma alone which were employed in this study had no effect on the measured variables when administered individually. Thus, it appears in animals without significant immune compromise, interferon gamma treatment may increase pathophysiologic response to endotoxin administration.

B-Cell Dysfunction

While many investigators have studied the impact of T-cell dysfunction in association with various forms of injury, alteration in antibody production by B-cells resulting in decreased opsonization and killing of bacteria may also be critical in permitting the increased incidence of sepsis and multiple organ dysfunction seen after injury.[14] B-cell function is directly affected by cytokine production (IL-1, IL-2, IL-5), the macrophage, and T-cells. B-cell function is also governed by interaction with T-cell subsets. Irregularity in any of the many steps in B-cell activation, including ingestion and presentation of bacterial antigen to the macrophage along with T- and B-cell interaction, could culminate in reduced B-cell response and ultimately require correction by therapeutic intervention.

Several workers have demonstrated that hemorrhage and thermal injury result in decreased serum immunoglobulin levels as well as decreased numbers of B-cells producing antibody. A change in B-cell function hierarchy also appears to occur such that following hemorrhage there are reduced bacterial antigen specific B-cell colony precursors, both in the spleen and in the intestine. These precursors are capable of activation to become plasma cells producing antibody necessary for direction against bacterial antigens. Other interactions requiring investigation in this area are unidentified immunosuppressive factors in the serum felt to be present after hemorrhage, accidental trauma and burns. These factors may act on B-cells directly or through functionally active T-cells subsets, particularly CD8 positive cells. Cytokines including IL-4 and IL-6 may ultimately be valuable in overcoming T-cell mediated suppression of B-cell function as they stimulate B-cell differentiation.

Nohr, Meakins and associates have investigated antibody production and response to tetanus toxoid immunization in patients receiving skin testing to determine delayed type hypersensitivity response.[15] These workers demonstrated a correlation between antibody production in response to immunization and delayed type hypersensitivity response as indicated by skin testing. Insufficiency or complete lack of antibody production in response to immunization corresponded to an increased risk of infection and ultimate septic mortality in the patients studied, coinciding with previously reported data from delayed type hypersensitivity as assessed by skin testing.

Monoclonal Antibody Therapy

Clinical use of monoclonal antibody therapy began with development of immunotherapy using polyclonal human antiserum directed against endotoxin core determinants in an attempt to reduce mortality in patients with gram negative bacteremia and protect high risk patients from septic shock.[16] The antiserum in these early trials was developed by immunization of volunteers with heat inactivated cells of mutant *E. coli* inducing an immune response to the core region of the endotoxin, the lipopolysaccharide component of the cell wall triggering many adverse systemic reactions and sequelae in patients with sepsis due to gram negative bacteremia. The

polyclonal antiserum is not commercially available due to toxicity associated with vaccination of serum donors and the recent recognition of the potential for transmission of infection with pooled human blood products. The more recent development of monoclonal antibody technique circumvents the problems of human donors and allows production of large quantities of antibody with known isotype specificity. In addition, human monoclonal antibodies offer the theoretical advantage of better function than antibodies derived from other species.

HA-1A is a human monoclonal IgM antibody binding to the lipid domain of endotoxin produced by a heteromyeloma cell line using the same heat inactivated *E. coli* J-5 vaccine used in production of the original polyclonal human J-5 antiserum. This monoclonal antibody and a similar product, E-5, have been employed in prospective multicenter randomized double blind placebo controlled clinical trials in patients with the sepsis syndrome and presumed diagnosis of gram negative infection. Among patients treated with these monoclonal antibodies in recent trials, the outcome was improved in patients with gram negative bacteremia extending in some cases to patients with multiple organ manifestations of the gram negative sepsis syndrome. No benefit of monoclonal antibody therapy was demonstrated in patients with sepsis which was not associated with gram negative bacteremia.

Given the results of this study, it is estimated that appropriately 400,000 patients developing sepsis annually in the United States may be candidates for treatment with monoclonal antibody to endotoxin. As noted previously, this agent is not effective for sepsis with gram positive bacteria or for nonbacteremic gram negative infections. If treatment criteria proposed in the original study were followed, 36% of patients with sepsis would be expected to benefit from therapy. If patients with gram negative bacteremia could be identified, it would be possible to reduce the cost of this therapy by approximately two-thirds without reducing effectiveness.[17] In current clinical practice, however, such identification is not feasible until blood culture results are available, which is frequently 48 hours after obtaining the specimens. This delay may make the use of currently available tests impractical for identifying appropriate candidates for antiendotoxin antibody therapy and decrease the effectiveness of the use of this drug. Schulman and associates[17] examined cost effectiveness using data obtained from the recent clinical study of monoclonal antiendotoxin antibody, HA-1A. Given two realistic strategies for application for this technology, annual cost of care using monoclonal antiendotoxin antibody were estimated between 1.3 and 2.3 billion dollars. Clearly, the economic and societal impact of these therapies must be closely examined as introduction to the clinical arena as anticipated.

In addition to cost considerations, the spectrum of coverage provided by monoclonal antibodies effective only against gram negative organisms must be weighed against the value of monoclonal antibodies to tumor necrosis factor, IL-1 and IL-6, directed at the common pathway of cytokine initiation for both gram positive and gram negative insults. These additional monoclonal antibody agents are rapidly moving toward clinical trials and may soon be evaluated in combination with each other and other existing therapies. We continue to lack appropriate indications to up regulate and down regulate immune response using these agents. Improved recognition of immunologic markers will significantly improve the efficiency and effectiveness of both monoclonal antibody cytokine and other immune response altering therapies in the critically ill.

Heat Shock Protein Genes

Adaptation to stress is essential to survival. Successful adaptation requires interaction between synergistic stress response systems. Various forms of stress induce expression of a group of genes known as heat shock protein genes.[18] Originally named on the basis of expression after heat stimulation, these genes are known to be induced in response to a variety of environmental and metabolic forms of stress including hypoxia, heavy metal exposure, sodium arsenite and localized trauma. Four major families of heat shock protein genes are recognized containing multiple genes in each (HSP-27, HSP-70, HSP-90, HSP-110). Heat shock proteins are among the most highly conserved proteins in existence and are thought to play a key role in protecting cells from adverse consequences of various forms of stress. These proteins appear to interact with various intracellular proteins and assist in assembly, disassembly, stability and intracellular transport. Current knowledge of heat shock protein regulation and function was initially obtained from cultured cells lines. Initial work in animals confirms induction of these proteins in a variety of tissues. Among tissues noted to have heat shock protein mRNA expression were brain, pituitary, thyroid, adrenal, heart, aorta, lung, kidney, liver, spleen, small bowel and skeletal muscle.

A number of laboratories are evaluating the role of heat shock protein genes in the molecular response to surgical stress.[19] Understanding the heat shock protein response to stress offers additional insight into the intrinsic mechanisms of cellular survival. The impact of various resuscitation protocols and medication therapies may ultimately be evaluated in terms of conservation or loss of heat shock protein expression as a key ingredient of cellular survival.

Gene Transfer as Immunotherapy

As the molecular response to stress and injury is better understood, transfer of genetic material which confers adaptive advantages may be desirable. Initial application of gene transfer technology to human gene therapy was approved in principal by the National Institutes of Health in January 1989. This decision allowed infusion into patients with advanced melanoma of lymphocytes subjected to retrovirus mediated gene transfer.[20] In the gene transfer experiments, an antibiotic resistance gene was introduced into the lymphocyte genome by retroviral infection thus allowing study of lymphocyte traffic and survival in vivo. This initial experiment constituted an exercise in gene marking, rather than therapy.

Results were encouraging as small numbers of transduced cells were noted in the circulation of patients tested for at least three weeks and in two patients for two months. Transduced cells were recovered from tumor deposits in three of five patients six days to two months after administration. No ill effects of gene transduction were noted in short-term studies and all safety studies were negative.

A wide range of inherited human disorders and possibly response to some acquired disorders may be treated by introduction of new genetic material into the proper type of cell. The principal requirement for somatic gene therapy is availability of a highly efficient and safe system for transferring the gene into the appropriate cell type. Ideally, the modified cell should be long in life resulting in long-term correction of the disorder. Modifying stem cells is, therefore, an attractive target for gene therapy. This early gene transfer experience in humans provides valuable information and constitutes critical progress toward development of gene therapy. We await other clinical trials intended to correct inherited or acquired disorders. If this technology rewards the initial promise shown, optimizing the genetic material of injured patients, possibly through gene transfer to critical stem cells of hematopoietic lineage, may prove attractive.

System Interaction

We are only beginning to investigate the interaction of various forms of immune therapy with other body systems. For example, septicemia is commonly associated with disturbance of hemostatic balance. Disseminated intravascular coagulation with widespread deposition of fibrin in the microvasculature is commonly found in septic shock and linked to development of multiple organ failure. As the role of tumor necrosis factor became more obvious in initiation of the septic syndrome, van der Poll and associates evaluated in vivo coagulation response to tumor necrosis factor in healthy volunteers.[21] These authors noted that a single injection of tumor necrosis factor was sufficient to create a rapid and sus-

tained activation of the common pathway of coagulation, probably induced through the extrinsic route. Thus, tumor necrosis factor may play an important part in activation of the hemostatic mechanism seen in septicemia. In addition, therapy with this cytokine or other cytokines, which may elicit release of tumor necrosis factor as a part of their actions, may result in undesirable activation of blood coagulation. Further studies in this and a myriad of additional areas are essential to better understanding of the impact of administration of pharmacologic doses of substances having a wide range of physiologic actions.

Conclusion

We now witness a knowledge explosion with regard to immune mechanisms and dysfunction associated with various forms of trauma and surgical stress. Research to date, both in terms of therapy and diagnosis, has been piecemeal. It seems apparent that combination therapy utilizing appropriately timed stimulants and blocking agents will be essential to appropriate control of the systemic response to various forms of surgical stress. Basic work describing the efficacy and toxicity associated with use of a myriad of new agents is nonexistent as are readily available markers allowing identification of specific interventions needed and their efficacy. Finally, the relationship of these powerful new mediators of the immune and metabolic response to trauma await incorporation into the vast knowledge base already available describing the neurohumoral and metabolic response to injury.

References

1. Trunkey DD. Trauma. Scientific American 1983; 249:28-35.
2. Faist E, Mewes A, Strasser T et al. Alteration of monocyte function following major injury. Arch Surg 1988; 123:287-292.
3. Hershman MJ, Cheadle WJ, Kuftinec D, Polk HC, Jr. An outcome predictive score for sepsis and death following injury. Injury 1988; 19:263-266.
4. Faist E, Markewitz A, Fuchs D et al. Immunomodulatory therapy with thymopentin and indomethacin. Ann Surg 1991; 214:264-275.
5. Jurkovich GJ, Mileski WJ, Maier RV et al. Interferon gamma increases sensitivity to endotoxin. J Surg Res

1991; 51:197-203.

6. Ninnemann JL. The immune consequences of trauma: An overview. In: Faist E, Ninnemann J, Green D, eds. Immune Consequences of Trauma, Shock and Sepsis. Berlin: Springer-Verlag, 1989:1-8.

7. Baker CC, Oppenheimer L, Stephens B et al. Epidemiology of trauma deaths. Am J Surg 1980; 140:144.

8. Polk HC. Consensus summary on infection. J Trauma 1979; 19:894-896.

9. Filkins JP. Cytokines: Mediators of the septic syndrome and septic shock. In: Critical Care: State of the Art (v12), Fullerton: Society of Critical Care Medicine, 1991:351-371.

10. Michie HR, Manogue KR, Spriggs DR et al. Detection of circulating tumor necrosis factor after endotoxin administration. N Engl J Med 1988; 318:481-486.

11. Miller-Graziano CL, Fink M, Wu JY et al. Mechanisms of altered monocyte prostaglandin E_2 production in severely injured patients. Arch Surg 1988; 123:293-299.

12. Hershman MJ, Polk HC, Jr, Pietsch JD et al. Modulation of infection by gamma interferon treatment following trauma. Infec Immun 1988; 56:2412-2416.

13. Redmond HP, Chavin KD, Bromberg JS, Daly JM. Inhibition of macrophage-activating cytokines is beneficial in the acute septic response. Ann Surg 1991; 214:502-509.

14. Abraham E. Host defense abnormalities after hemorrhage, trauma and shock. Intens Critic Care Dig 1990; 9:25-28.

15. Meakins JL, Nohr CW, Christou NV. Immunological response, infection and the surgical patient. In: Clowes GHA, ed. Trauma, Sepsis, and Shock: The Physiological Basis Therapy. New York: Marcel Dekker Inc., 1988:359-370.

16. Zeigler EJ, Fisher CJ, Sprung CL et al. Treatment of gram negative bacteremia and septic shock with HA-1A human monoclonal antibody against endotoxin. N Engl J Med 1991; 324:429-436.

17. Schulman KA, Glick HA, Rubin H, Eisenberg JM. Cost-effectiveness of HA-1A monoclonal antibody for gram-negative sepsis. JAMA 1991; 266:3466-3471.

18. Udelsman R, Blake MJ, Holbrook NJ. Molecular response to surgical stress: Specific and simultaneous heat shock protein induction in the adrenal cortex, aorta, and vena cava. Surgery 1991; 110:1125-1131.

19. Buchman TG, Cabin DE, Porter JM, Bulkley GB. Change in hepatic gene expression after shock/resuscitation. Surgery 1989; 106:283-291.

20. Rosenberg SA, Aebersold P, Cornetta K et al. Gene transfer into humans—immunotherapy of patients with advanced melanoma using tumor-infiltrating lymphocytes modified by retroviral gene transduction. N Engl J Med 1990; 323:570-578.

21. van der Poll T, Bulter HR, ten Cute H et al. Activation of coagulation after administration of tumor necrosis factor to normal subjects. N Engl J Med 1990; 322:1622-1627.

CHAPTER 8

EFFECTS OF TRAUMA ON T- AND B-CELL FUNCTION

Edward Abraham

Sepsis leading to multiple organ system failure (MOSF) remains the most important cause of late deaths after severe trauma. In several studies as many as 88% of the deaths occurring after admission of severely injured patients to the intensive care unit were due to infection. Although some of these infectious episodes are related to the nature of the patient's injury, such as bowel perforation and resultant peritonitis, most are due to nosocomial pneumonia and other secondary infections and are not clearly a result of the patient's underlying injury. This increased incidence of nosocomial infections in critically ill, injured patients suggested that trauma and blood loss in some way produced an immunocompromised state making these patients more susceptible to microbial colonization which then would lead to septic episodes. Accumulating evidence indicates that marked abnormalities in lymphocyte function affecting both T- and B-cells occurs after hemorrhage and injury and that these alterations in host defense function contribute in a significant and important manner to the increased susceptibility to infection following trauma.

T- AND B-CELL INTERACTIONS IN RESISTANCE TO INFECTION

Most nosocomial infections in critically ill patients involve extracellular gram negative bacteria, although the frequency of infection due to gram positive organisms, particularly coagulase negative *Staphylococcus,* is rising, probably secondary to the increased numbers of vascular catheters being used in the intensive care setting. Although the majority of nosocomial infections originate at the pulmonary mucosal surface, there also is evidence to suggest that the intestine may serve as an important source of nosocomial infection through translocation of bacteria from the gut lumen to mesenteric lymph nodes and then to the portal circulation, particularly in patients with conditions leading to mucosal ischemia.

Resistance to extracellular infection is primarily mediated by B-cells which produce antibodies able to attach to the surface of the bacteria. These antibacterial antibodies result in bacterial killing both by fixing complement and by enhancing the uptake and destruction of bacteria by phagocytic cells such as macrophages and neutrophils. For bacteria colonizing mucosal surfaces such as the lungs the most important class of immunoglobulin is IgA secreted by plasma cells residing in mucosal tissues. Mucosally based B- and T-cells, aside from being involved in the production of secretory IgA (sIgA), also show phenotypic and functional characteristics distinguishing them as a separate population distinct from systemic B- and T-cells primarily found in the blood, spleen and lymph nodes.

Resting B-cells have immunoglobulin on their surfaces able to recognize antigens with high specificity. These surface antibodies can bind bacterial antigens and then "present" the antigen to a T-cell. The antigen activated T-cell modulates the extent and degree of the antibody response to that antigen. Polysaccharides on the surface of bacteria are important bacterial antigens, and antibodies to bacterial polysaccharides have an important role in protection against infection due to the bacteria from which these polysaccharides are derived.

The role of B-cells as "antigen-presenting" cells is particularly important for bacterial polysaccharides which are able to activate antigen-specific T-cells only through this mechanism. In contrast, bacterial protein antigens often pass through intracellular processing pathways before being presented to T-cells and can be presented by many classes of cells including B-cells, macrophages and, most importantly, dendritic cells residing in the connective tissue stroma of lymph nodes, mucosal sites and other anatomic sites associated with lymphoid activity.

The nature and function of antigen presenting cells is particularly important when one is considering antibacterial defense mechanisms, because appropriate corrections of abnormalities in host defense functions requires identification of the components responsible for these alterations. An example of what may be misplaced emphasis on a particular cell type is the recent interest on alterations in macrophage antigen presenting functions following hemorrhage and trauma. For most bacterial antigens, which are polysaccharides, the macrophage does not have a major role in antigen presentation, and even for protein antigens, other cell types, particularly dendritic cells, are much more important than macrophages. Therefore, although it is pos-

sible that macrophage antigen presenting function contributes to the host defense abnormalities following injury, it is unlikely to play a central role in producing these alterations in immune function. In contrast, other macrophage associated activities—particularly cytokine generation—may be much more important in affecting immune response in the injured patient.

Following presentation of antigen to T-cells, the activated T-cell is able to modulate B-cell functionthrough helper/inducer or suppressor functions. In general, but not always, subpopulations of $CD4^+$ T-cells are responsible for helper/inducer functions, and subsets of $CD8^+$ T-cells for suppressor activity. However, it is important to remember that the antibody response to a number of important bacterial antigens—particularly polysaccharides—can be T-cell independent as shown by the generation of antigen-specific antibodies following immunization with these antigens in mice without T-cells. However, even in the case of these "T independent" polysaccharide antigens, in normal animals T-cells appear to be capable of modulating the magnitude of the antibody response after exposure to polysaccharide.

In response to a bacterial infection, there are a series of interactions between B- and T-cells leading to an antibody response to antigens born on the bacterial surface. Alterations in B- or T-cell function can affect the antibody response, and host resistance to the invading bacteria. For example, because B-cells are "committed" cells from the time that they leave the bone marrow, able to produce antibody to a single antigen, inadequate numbers of antigen-specific resting B-cells, able to be activated to become antibody secreting plasma cells, will result in an inadequate antibody response, even if all components of the T- and B-cell interaction are functioning perfectly. This issue of adequacy of numbers of B-cell clonal precursors able to produce bacterial antigen-specific antibodies is of particular concern after hemorrhage and trauma. We have found that in the spleen, lung and intestines there is a profound and longlasting depression of bacterial antigen-specific B-cell numbers occurring within three days of hemorrhage and lasting for more than three weeks following experimental hemorrhage, even with resuscitation.

Even if adequate numbers of bacterial antigen-specific B-cell clonal precursors are present in mucosal and systemic sites following injury, there still may be problems in recruitment of these B-cells from their resting state into an activated form where they become antibody secreting plasma cells. This inadequacy of activation of resting B-cells may result from inadequate T-cell "help" due to inadequate cytokine production or membrane signaling by CD4+ T-cells or to overactive T-cell "suppression" primarily due to CD8+ T-cells. Both of these mechanisms have been shown to be operative following hemorrhage and trauma. Several studies have shown that CD8+ T-cells isolated after hemorrhage and trauma are capable both of inhibiting T-cell proliferation and of altering bacterial antigen-specific B-cell function when injected into normal animals. There also is evidence that CD4+ T-cells are affected by injury and are less able to promote T-cell activation in this setting.

The role of macrophages in bacterial defense mechanisms, as mentioned above, depends to a great extent on the nature of the bacterial infection. Ingestion of bacteria by macrophages allowing antigens to be liberated in a setting where they can be captured by B-cells or dendritic cells may be important in initiating an adequate antibody response to the invading bacteria. Similarly, for intracellular bacteria, macrophages are important because they can process and present protein antigens derived from these microorganisms. It is important to remember though, that intracellular infections are relatively uncommon in the critically ill, injured patient and that normally the most important T-cell type in dealing with intracellular organisms is the CD8+ cytotoxic T-cell and not the antibody producing plasma cell.

Cytokines produced by macrophages may be important in modulating B- and T-cell responses to extracellular bacterial infection. For example, interleukin-1, produced by macrophages, has important functions in activating T-cells. Interleukin-6, also a mac-

rophage product, enhances antibody production by plasma cells. Similarly, the generation of other cytokines, particularly interleukins 2, 4 and 5, by activated CD4+ T-cells is important in enhancing the progression of resting B-cells to become antibody producing plasma cells. In contrast, activated CD4+ T-cells, particularly of the TH1 subset, also produce interferon gamma, a potent suppressor of antibody production by B-cells. Therefore, it is not only the rate of production of these cytokines which is important in modulating T-B interactions, B-cell function, and antibody production but also the relative balance between levels of the cytokines in the milieu where the immune response is taking place.

B-Cell Alterations Induced by Hemorrhage and Trauma and Potential Mechanisms for their Correction

As mentioned previously, hemorrhage results in greater than ten-fold decreases in the number of bacterial antigen-specific B-cell clonal precursors in mucosal, i.e., lungs and intestine, and systemic sites. The decreases in bacterial antigen-specific B-cell numbers are apparent within one day of hemorrhage but become most profound three days following blood loss. Return to normal numbers of antigen-specific clonal precursors is not seen until more than three weeks following hemorrhage in resuscitated mice. Interestingly, the numbers of B-cell clonal precursors committed to the production of antibodies against nonbacterial antigens do not appear to be diminished by hemorrhage or trauma. The functional significance of this hemorrhage induced disappearance of bacterial antigen-specific B-cell clonal precursors is shown by the almost total lack of an antibody response when animals are immunized with bacterial antigens three days following hemorrhage. The depression in bacteria antigen-specific antibody response is most profound at mucosal sites, particularly the lungs, where immunization between three days and three weeks of hemorrhage results in essentially no increase in the numbers of mucosally associated plasma cells producing antibody to that antigen nor in antigen-specific secretory antibody titers at mucosal sites. The lack of a bacterial antigen-specific mucosal immune response following hemorrhage translates into a marked increase in susceptibility to infection at these sites. For example, whereas more than 8×10^7 organisms of *Pseudomonas aeruginosa* are required to produce *any* mortality from pneumonia in normal, unhemorrhaged mice, less than *one quarter* of this number of bacteria will produce 100% mortality when injected into the lungs of mice four days following hemorrhage.

There are important lessons with major therapeutic implications to be learned from the experiments which examined bacterial antigen-specific B-cell repertoires following hemorrhage. In particular, these studies demonstrated that within the first 24 hours of hemorrhage there is little change in the numbers of bacterial antigen-specific B-cells in either systemic or mucosal sites. These findings imply that immunization within this "time window" after hemorrhage and injury might result in a near normal antibody response which would be protective against infection. However, because systemic and mucosal B-cells function in largely separate manners, with little transfer of circulating antibodies to mucosal surfaces, systemic immunization, although resulting in increased serum levels of antibodies, produces little or no enhancement of antigen-specific secretory antibodies at mucosal surfaces. Similarly, immunization at mucosal surfaces results in enhanced levels of antigen-specific secretory IgA but little change in titers of circulating antigen-specific antibodies.

Therefore, if one wished to protect the injured patient from nosocomial pneumonia, the most frequent initial infection in this patient population, it then would be necessary to immunize at a mucosal site in order to obtain increased titers of secretory immunoglobulin, particularly IgA, in the lungs. One advantage of this approach is that immunization at one mucosal surface, such as the intestines or nasal mucosa, results in generalization of that secretory antibody response to other mucosal sites, such as the lungs since mucosally associated B- and T-cells migrate

from one mucosal site to another. Theoretically then, in the injured patient increased resistance to nosocomial pneumonia could be accomplished by immunization with relevant bacterial antigens applied to any mucosal surface as long as the immunization was performed within the first 24 hours following injury, before the numbers of bacterial antigen-specific B-cells becomes too small to generate an adequate antigen-specific antibody response.

Several experiments have demonstrated that vaccination shortly after injury does result in increased resistance to pulmonary infections. For example, oral immunization with *Pseudomonas aeruginosa* polysaccharide co-administered with a potent mucosal adjuvant (cholera toxin) immediately following hemorrhage resulted in significant improvement in mortality from *Pseudomonas aeruginosa* pneumonia. Similarly, intranasal immunization of hemorrhaged mice with liposomes containing *Pseudomonas aeruginosa* polysaccharide also produced significant decreases in mortality due to *Pseudomonas aeruginosa* pneumonia.

Although these experimental results are promising and suggest that mucosal "vaccination" shortly after injury can decrease the incidence of infection and probably morbidity and mortality following injury, there remain major issues which must be resolved before this approach will be clinically applicable. It is clear that immunization against all possible infections, which might occur postinjury, is impossible. However, a polyvalent vaccine containing antigens from the most likely organisms could be envisaged. This vaccine would be similar to the present systemic vaccine against pneumococcus where the vaccine contains 23 polysaccharides from the most prevalent pneumococcal strains.

In a practical sense, the route of immunization after trauma may be quite important. Injured patients often have an ileus and are unable to tolerate oral administration of medications. Therefore, the fact that intranasal administration of bacterial antigens encapsulated in polysaccharides *after* hemorrhage results in enhanced resistance to infection suggests that this may be a very powerful and clinically useful technique in decreasing the incidence of infection and thereby improving the survival of critically ill injured patients. However, as mentioned above, it will be important to develop polyvalent liposomal vaccines able to protect against a wide range of organisms likely to cause nosocomial pneumonia and other infection following injury. Polysaccharide antigens are available for many of the clinically important *Pseudomonas aeruginosa* , *Escherichia coli* and *Klebsiella pneumoniae* strains and could be used in liposomal vaccine formulations. Unfortunately, bacterial polysaccharides by themselves are often poorly immunogenic. While encapsulation in liposomes can improve the immune response to these polysaccharide antigens, the increases in antigen-specific antibody titers, as well as the improvement in survival from *Pseudomonas aeruginosa* pneumonia, able to be achieved following intranasal immunization with these liposomal vaccines are relatively modest. Additional work is required, using clinically safe and effective adjuvants able to be included in the liposomal membrane or interior, in order to further enhance the bacterial antigen-specific mucosal immune response and resistance to infection.

T-cell Alterations Induced by Injury and Possible Approaches to their Correction

A major effect of trauma on immune function involves the activation of CD8$^+$ T-cells which are not only able to suppress the proliferation of other T-cells but more importantly to affect bacterial antigen-specific B-cell function. Modulation of the activities of these CR8$^+$ cells would be expected to reverse at least some of the suppression in antibacterial antibody responses found after injury. Two possible approaches to affecting T-cell function are available: either one can eliminate the cellular population which is producing the unwanted immunologic activity or the suppressive activities of that T-cell population can be reversed, by blocking excessive production of suppressive products or by increasing the activity of counter-regulatory cell

population in order to reverse suppressive effects of CD8$^+$ cells. Unfortunately, both of these approaches are associated with significant difficulties and potentially adverse side effects, particularly in the clinical setting of trauma.

Although CD8$^+$ cells are known to be activated by injury, complete elimination of the CD8$^+$ population in the injured patient would be unlikely to result in an overall improvement of those patients' clinical condition and outcome. CD8$^+$ cells are important in resistance to intracellular organisms, such as viruses and fungi, and elimination of this cellular population would be expected to produce significant immunosuppression in the critically ill, injured patient. However, methodology is now becoming available to identify CD8$^+$ subpopulations, and if an injury activated CD8$^+$ subpopulation could be targeted with monoclonal antibodies for elimination such an approach might reverse some components of injury induced immunosuppression without producing widespread immunologic alterations deleterious to this patient population.

The mechanisms by which immunologic suppression is induced are now being characterized, and the balance between the effects of cytokines released by activated lymphocytes may account for the modulation of immune response produced by these cells. Interleukin-2 (IL-2) release is consistently diminished after hemorrhage and injury. However, there is little evidence to suggest that treatment with exogenous IL-2 will reverse trauma induced immunologic dysfunction. Trauma and hemorrhage are known to be associated with alterations in the production of other cytokines, including tumor necrosis factor (TNF-α), interferon gamma (IFN-γ) and interleukins 1, 3, 5, 6 and 8. It is likely that the generation of other cytokines also is affected by injury. Further, the generation or activity of cell surface molecules such as integrins and selectins required for efficient cell-cell interactions in the immune response may be affected by injury, and these alterations may significantly affect immune response. It will be important to better define the trauma induced alterations in cytokine generation, looking at as wide a spectrum as possible of cytokines as well as other immunologically important mediators such as the cell adhesion molecules in order to define the patterns of alterations induced by injury and to develop an integrated approach to these alterations. Because of the complexity of T-T, T-B and other cellular responses involving T-cells, it is unlikely that treatment with a single recombinant cytokine or blockade of a single cytokine with monoclonal antibodies will correct the profound and widespread abnormalities found after injury. Rather, a more complex but biologically more realistic approach involving the modulation of multiple cytokine levels will probably be required to enhance antibacterial immune response in these critically ill, injured patients.

Evidence suggests that activation of CD8$^+$ T-cells after trauma may be the result of circulating immunosuppressive peptides. Several of these peptides have been partially characterized and show unique amino acid sequences not homologous with known proteins or portions of known proteins. In at least one circumstance, brief exposure, i.e. less than 60 seconds, of T-cells from normal animals to a hemorrhage induced immunosuppressive peptide was shown to induce suppressive activity among the previously normal T-cell population.

In the near future, further characterization of trauma-induced peptides will allow confirmation of their sequence, cloning of their genes and production of monoclonal antibodies against both the immunosuppressive peptides and their receptors on CD8$^+$ cells. The antipeptide and antireceptor monoclonal antibodies may have important therapeutic applications since their use would be expected to reverse trauma-induced CD8$^+$ cell activation as well as the alterations in antibacterial B-cell function induced by these CD8$^+$ cells. In addition, characterization and cloning of the trauma induced immunosuppressive peptides also may have therapeutic implications since these naturally occurring immunosuppressive peptides may be useful in organ transplantation through decreasing episodes of transplant rejection.

CONCLUSIONS

Multiple abnormalities in T- and B-cell function occur following trauma and lead to increased susceptibility to infection. Further characterization of the mechanisms leading to activation of CD8$^+$ T-suppressor cells and definition of the nature of those cellular interactions allowing these CD8$^+$ cells to affect the function of other T-cell populations and to alter antibacterial B-cell repertoires will lead to the development of therapies which are able to reverse the effects of these trauma-activated CD8$^+$ cells. It is probable that these therapies will be multifactorial, using monoclonal antibodies as well as exogenous administration of cytokines and other immunomodulatory agents. The utilization of these therapies is still some distance in the future, both because the characterization of T-cell induced suppression is, at present, incomplete and because it remains difficult to affect a single population of T-cells without causing profound and often deleterious effects on immune response.

However, even with our present less than complete understanding of trauma-induced alterations in immune function, important therapeutic interventions can be envisaged in the near future. We now know that the disappearance of antibacterial B-cell numbers is somewhat delayed following hemorrhage and injury, allowing a "window of opportunity" when vaccination would be both feasible and potentially of great use in decreasing the incidence of infection, particularly those infections originating at mucosal surfaces, such as the lungs. Mucosal vaccines, able to increase titers of secretory IgA in the intestines and lungs, are presently being developed. A major issue in improving the efficacy of these mucosal vaccines is finding safe and clinically effective adjuvants which can be incorporated into the vaccine formulations.

Ultimately, the approach to trauma induced immunosuppression will clearly be multifactorial. Early immunization will help decrease the incidence of infection among critically ill, injured patients. Better understanding of the nature of the alterations in immune function produced by trauma will identify those patients with severely altered immune response and will permit reversal of these alterations in host defense function. Because of the real financial costs associated with monoclonal antibody and other immunomodulatory therapies, the diagnostic component, where severely immunosuppressed patients are identified prior to the initiation of therapy, will be important so that these future therapies able to reestablish adequate antimicrobial immune function and to reduce the unacceptably high incidence of late morbidity and mortality in severely injured patients can be utilized most effectively.

SELECTED READING

1. Abraham E, Chang Y-H. Hemorrhage in mice produces alterations in intestinal B-cell repertoires. Cell Immunol 1990; 128:165
2. Abraham E, Freitas AA, Coutinho AA. Hemorrhage in mice produces alterations in B-cell repertoires. Cell Immunol 1989; 122:208
3, Abraham E, Freitas AA, Jagels M, Chang Y-H. Transfer of T- or CD8+ cells from hemorrhaged mice produce alterations in bacterial antigen-specific B-cell repertoire in normal syngeneic recipients. Immunobiology 1990; 181:379
4. Abraham E, Robinson A. Oral immunization with bacterial polysaccharide and adjuvant enhances antigen-specific pulmonary secretory antibody response and resistance to pneumonia. Vaccine 1991; 9:757
5. Chaudry IH, Ayala A, Ertel W, Stephan RN. Hemorrhage and resuscitation: Immunologic aspects. Am J Physiol 1990; 259:R663
6, Gregoriadis G. Immunologic adjuvants: A role for liposomes. Immunol Today 1990; 11:89
7. Liu Y-J, Johnson GD, Cordon J, MacLennan ICM. Germinal centers in T-cell dependent antibody responses. Immunol Today 1992; 13:17
8. Mestecky J. The common mucosal immune system and current strategies for induction of immune responses in external secretions. J Clin Immunol 1987; 7:265
9. Reidy JJ, Ramsay G. Clinical trials of selective decontamination of the digestive tract: Review. Crit Care Med 1990; 18:1449
10. Robinson A, Abraham E. Hemorrhage in mice produces alterations in pulmonary B-cell repertoires. J Immunol 1990; 145:3734
11. Underdown BJ, Schiff JM. Immunoglobulin A: Strategic defense initiative at the mucosal surface. Ann Rev Immunol 1986; 4:389

CHAPTER 9

CYTOKINES AND POST-TRAUMATIC SEPSIS

James P. Filkins

INTRODUCTION

A most dreaded sequela of trauma—even when it is initially managed early, aggressively and successfully by the accepted current standards of resuscitative therapy and care—is the progressive development of sepsis, the sepsis syndrome, refractory septic shock with multiple system organ failure and eventually septic demise. Unfortunately, many aspects of the pathogenesis of posttraumatic septic morbidity and mortality are still shrouded in ignorance. Fortunately, one area of septic shock research involving gram-negative bacteria and their constituent endotoxins has recently undergone remarkable progress which is already paying dividends in current trauma management while also providing a sound rationale for future therapeutic development. Thus, it is now generally accepted that gram-negative septic shock is predominately a dysregulated systemic inflammatory response to endotoxin that is intimately related to an inappropriate activation of the mononuclear cells of the immune system such that inordinate levels of septic mediators occur—especially the key family of intercellular signaling peptides termed cytokines. The end-result is a progressive failure of host-defense homeostasis, i.e., immune dyshomeostasis, which culminates in organ system failure and death.

This chapter overviews the state of the art as to the role of cytokines in the pathogenesis of septic shock and presents the current status of investigations designed to intervene in the cytokine-driven progression of the septic state. A step-wise sequence of topics are related to the putative causal relations during in vivo septic states, i.e., the endotoxin-macrophage interaction, the cellular and molecular biology of the activation of macrophage cytokine synthesis and secretion, the circulatory actions of cytokines, the target tissues and actions of cytokines, and the organ dysfunction elicited by altered cytokine states. For each step in the pathogenetic sequence, examples of therapeutic interventions are stipulated. An overview of cytokines in their role in septic shock is presented initially.

Cytokines and the Pathogenesis of Septic Shock

The cytokines of the immune system are now recognized as equal in stature to the two traditional major classes of intercellular signaling molecules—the neurotransmitters of the nervous system and the hormones of the endocrine systems. While studies of the neural and endocrine mechanisms in trauma are extensive and longstanding, the key role of the cytokines in posttraumatic pathophysiology is a relatively recent developing area of intensive biomedical investigation. Furthermore, just as interactions of the nervous and endocrine systems underwrite the field of the neuroendocrinology of trauma, similar interactions between the immune system and nervous-endocrine systems are being revealed as the rapidly developing new hybrid research domains of neuroimmunology, immuno–endocrinology and even psychoneuro–immunoendocrinology. Thus while a focus on cytokines in trauma is in itself intensive and rewarding, there is a bevy of potential therapeutic implications in the interactive domains of the three major communication systems—nervous, hormonal and immune.

Although the cytokine domain is still growing, five major families—interferons, interleukins, tumor necrosis factors, colony stimulating factors and cell-tissue growth factors—and some 50 individual peptide-protein molecules have now been identified. Most prominent presently in the trauma-sepsis pathogenesis connection are four key inflammatory cytokines—interleukins (IL) -1, -6 and -8 and tumor necrosis factor (TNFα).

In order to ascribe a primary etiological role to any given cytokine in the pathogenesis of the posttraumatic septic syndrome, three types of experimental evidence must be present:

1. When the sepsis syndrome prevails, then cytokines are present.

2. When a purified cytokine is administered to a test subject, then the sepsis syndrome ensues.

3. When steps are taken to nullify the cytokine signal, then the sepsis syndrome is alleviated.

Over the past few years, experimental investigations in humans and animal models of sepsis have by and large applied the above three criteria to four cytokines—IL-1, IL-6, IL-8 and TNF-α. As reviewed recently,[5] data are indeed available to support their elevations systemically during sepsis, their intrinsic ability to directly or indirectly elicit the sepsis syndrome, and finally that their antagonism using a variety of anticytokine therapeutic approaches abrogates the septic state. Thus, while much still needs to be learned, cytokines are firmly established as key early mediators of the septic state. The remainder of this chapter will therefore focus on five potential therapeutic attack points in the pathobiology of cytokine production and actions in septic states.

Step 1: Endotoxin-Macrophage Interactions

Bacterial endotoxin is produced and released by the autolysis of gram-negative bacteria either at a site of infection or within the intestinal tract compromised by lack of gut wall integrity. Once released, endotoxin may either interact locally or gain access to the circulation and the mononuclear leukocytes within. In the circulation, endotoxin may initially interact with specific binding or carrier proteins. On the one hand, some proteins like BPI (bactericidal permeability increasing) proteins may bind and inactivate endotoxin. On the other hand, some proteins like LPB (lipopolysaccharide binding) proteins may actually ferry endotoxin and then dock with a reactive mononuclear phagocyte. Recent studies have indicated specific endotoxin receptors on monocytes and lymphocytes, e.g., the CD-14 system. Apparently, the endotoxin-LPB complex is recognized by the monocytes and so initiates a reaction pattern in the macrophages which includes eventual cytokine synthesis and secretion. This first step in cytokine genesis can be abrogated by therapeutic use of BPI to inactivate endotoxin directly or by preventing the LPB-endotoxin complex from binding to its receptor by the use of antireceptor antibodies, e.g., anti CD-14 monoclonals. It is also possible that custom designed endotoxins with select deletions in their active lipid A toxophore groups may bind to cell membrane receptors but not initiate cytokine production. In addition, if there is immunization or treatment with monoclonal antibodies to the endotoxin, then the initiation of the entire septic process is abrogated. Indeed the recent surge of interest in therapeutic approaches to gram negative sepsis using monoclonal antibodies is evidence for the potentially powerful strategy of blocking the entire reaction at its root cause—neutralization of the reactive endotoxin molecule.

STEP 2: THE CELLULAR AND MOLECULAR BIOLOGY OF MACROPHAGE CYTOKINE SYNTHESIS AND SECRETION

Once endotoxin activates the macrophage to its inherent secretory phenotype, the production and secretion of cytokines such as IL-1, IL-6 and IL-8 and TNF-α may proceed in a dysregulated fashion. Attempts to manipulate the signal transduction process mediating cytokine production from an endotoxic stimulus have suggested a number of intracellular signal processes ranging from calcium ions to protein kinases. While not currently a readily accessible attack point in the therapeutic schema, it is possible that selective inhibitors of specific protein kinases such as the C-isoform family may afford another approach to deactivating the macrophage cytokine production line.

Evidence exists that the endotoxic molecule may be modified by intracellular enzymes such as acyloxyacyl hydrolases (AOAH) and thus it is either partially inactivated or transformed into a form with altered cytokine eliciting ability. Thus manipulation of the AOAH system by selected enzyme inhibitors may alter the progression of endotoxic activation of macrophages to elicit cytokines.

Since cytokines are synthesized de novo in response to an endotoxin stimulus, obligatory gene activation sequences are required.

Another therapeutic attack point is to interfere with the normal molecular biology of cytokine gene production by the use of regulatory element manipulators, antisense mRNAs or translational control inhibition. Indeed recent studies with glucocorticoids have revealed that their major mode of cytokine regulation is at the genetic level.

Since cytokine synthesis is often inhibited by co-release of eicosanoids, the appropriate use of select prostaglandins may diminish cytokine production. Finally as the biology of the mysterious process of cytokine secretion is revealed, steps in the peptide translocation across the macrophage cell membrane may soon be modulated.

STEP 3: NEUTRALIZATION OF THE CIRCULATORY CYTOKINES

Once released by macrophages, cytokines are rapidly engaged in interactions with their target tissues, i.e., cells which bear the appropriate cytokine receptor. While in transit either in the circulation or in the local areas of the interstitial fluid and matrix, it is still possible to immunoneutralize specific cytokines. Indeed a powerful new approach uses monoclonal antibodies to cytokines alone or in combination with similar antiendotoxin antibodies. This combination regimen is analogous to both blocking the trigger and stopping the bullets simultaneously. Undoubtedly anticytokine therapy will have some mixed effects—beneficial in hypercytokinetic states but perhaps detrimental in normal states of cytokine physiology where their normal host protection roles are maximized.

STEP 4: CYTOKINE—TARGET TISSUE INTERACTIONS

Even if cytokines gain access to the neighborhood of their target tissues, it is possible to antagonize or impede their interactions. One approach is to use shed receptors from the cells to bind the cytokine and to neutralize the signal. A second approach is to use nature's own anticytokines such as the recently discovered interleukin-1 receptor antagonist protein. By blocking receptor inter-actions, the biologic effects of cytokines can be abrogated. Finally, it is possible to actively use one cytokine to antagonize another—indeed transforming growth factor (TGF)-B is a potent nullifier of many actions of IL-1 and TNF.

Step 5: Reduction of Cytokine-Induced Tissue and Organ Dysfunction

The area of signal transduction by cytokines in their respective target tissues is only beginning to be elucidated. Some targets such as endothelial cells respond by up-regulating some receptors of their own; thus it is possible to immunoneutralize these receptors and turn off the cytokine effector pathway. In particular the use of antibodies to leukocyte adhesion receptors can prevent neutrophils sticking and eventually damaging actions. Various drug categories such as radical scavenger, antiproteinases, steroids, NSAIDS, anticoagulants, PAF antagonists and NO blockers may also ameliorate cytokine target effects and reduce organ damage.

Summary

A most important issue in trauma care is the pathogenesis of secondary septic states and the use of new and developing strategies to deal with such. Within the last few years, an outpouring of significant research has firmly established that cytokines from activated macrophages and other cells of the immune-inflammatory system are key mediators of the septic state. A major benefit of the extensive research efforts into cytokine pathobiology has been the availability of new strategies to impact the pathogenetic steps in septic processes. The investigative tacts as summarized in this review article must be viewed as a contemporary menu and further research must aggressively pursue new dimensions of this field of investigation in order to eventually alleviate the dreaded life-threatening syndrome of posttraumatic septic shock.

Selected Reading

1. Aggarwal BB Pocsik E. Cytokines: From clone to clinic. Arch Biochem Biophys 1992; 292: 335-359.
2. Bone RC. Multiple system organ failure and the sepsis syndrome. Hospital Practice 1991; 26: 101-126.
3. Billau A,Vandekerckhove F. Cytokines and their interactions with other inflammatory mediators in the pathogensis of sepsis and septic shock. Eur J Clin Invest 1991; 21: 559-573.
4. Dinarello CA. The proinflammatory cytokines interleukin-1 and tumor necrosis factor and treatment of the septic shock syndrome. J Infect Dis 1991; 163: 1177-1184.
5. Filkins JP. Cytokines: mediators of the septic syndrome and septic shock. In: Critical Care. State of the Art 1991;12: 351-372.
6. Hinshaw, L.B. Pathophysiology of endotoxin action: An overview. In: Cellular and Molecular Aspects of Endotoxin Reactions Vol. 1 of the Endotoxin Research Series. 1990:419-426.
7. Michie HR, Wilmore DR. Sepsis, signals and surgical sequelae: A hypothesis. Arch Surg 1990; 125:531-536.
8. Rackow EC, Astiz ME. Pathophysiology and treatment of septic shock. JAMA 1991; 266:548-554.
9. Raetz CRH, Ulevitch RJ, Wright SD et al. Gram-negative endotoxin: an extraordinary lipid with profound effects on eukaryotic signal transduction. FASEB 1991; 5: 2652-2660.
10. Tracey KJ. The acute and chronic pathophysiologic effects of TNF: Mediation of septic shock and wasting cachexia.In: Beutler B, ed. Tumor Necrosis Factors: The Molecules and Their Emerging Role in Medicine. Raven Press Ltd, 1992: 16 255-283:

CHAPTER 10

NEUTROPHIL FUNCTION IN THE INFLAMMATORY DISEASES OF TRAUMA AND BURN INJURY

Joseph S. Solomkin
Robert C. Bass

INTRODUCTION

A variety of postinjury sequelae including capillary leak syndrome, noninfectious lung injury—Adult Respiratory Distress Syndrome (ARDS)—and multisystem organ failure are now the primary causes of late mortality following trauma and burns. We recognize these events as interrelated and unwanted consequences of phagocytic responses to proinflammatory stimuli. Over the last decade there has been enormous progress in understanding the biochemical bases for neutrophil function, the mechanisms of cell regulation during inflammatory events and the role of neutrophils in the homeostasis of inflammation. These advances have supported and clarified the relationship between injury, leukocyte abnormalities and subsequent clinical disease.

The starting point for this discussion is the recent notion that the function of neutrophils in a matrix environment is substantially different from that of suspension phase cells. It is now appropriate to consider neutrophil function in relation to intravascular events and, separately, in relation to tissue-based events. Importantly, it is now recognized that through its surface receptors, the neutrophil has a substantial role in the recognition, propagation and regulation of the inflammatory response. Elements of neutrophil function include cytokine/messenger production, peptide synthesis and release and uptake and deactivation of proinflammatory mediators. This information challenges the classical perception of the neutrophil as primarily a phagocytic cell. This material has led us away from the study of cell functions such as chemotaxis, phagocytosis and microbicidal activity, and towards characterization of cell signalling processes and the participation of neutrophils in the multicellular sequence leading to inflammation and its resolution.

Prior to the discovery of tumor necrosis factors (TNF) in 1985 and the subsequent identification through biochemical technology of myriad interleukins, colony stimulating factors, growth factors and interferons, neutrophil responses were analyzed in relation to plasma protein cascade systems which participated in inflammation. The coagulation, kinin and complement cascades were believed to play paramount roles in the whole organism response to tissue injury or contamination. Research into the role of cytokines in acute inflammation defined a previously unrecognized network for regulation of acute inflammation centered upon macrophage-like cells. The pluripotent and overlapping effects of the multiple mediators provided a direct explanation for the hallmarks of severe trauma, including induction of acute phase responses and the regulatory changes in the functioning of effector cells including neutrophils, lymphocytes, macrophages and a range of epithelial cell types. An integrated view of the induction of inflammation now meshes complement-mediated and cytokine-mediated events.

Established Roles for Neutrophils in Acute Trauma and Burn Injury: A Role for Complement in Intravascular Events

Investigation of alterations of neutrophil function in injured patients has been spurred by the recognition of the high incidence of infection in these patients with its attendant morbidity and mortality. Research has focused on burn patients because of the ability to quantify the extent of injury by burn size and depth and because physiologic reserve limits the rapidity of wound excision and grafting. This provides a prolonged interval with a relatively stable injury to allow characterization of abnormalities of inflammatory cell function.

Measurement of plasma levels of complement metabolites has confirmed the activation of complement early in the course of burn injury. A potential source of activated complement components in the injured patient has recently been clarified. Burn injury is associated with oxidative injury to erythrocytes, presumptively as part of an ischemia/reperfusion process occurring in the vasculature of injured tissue. Both neutrophils and xanthine oxidase cause oxidant production through well recognized pathways. These erythrocytes serve as platforms for complement activation through the classical pathway. In the immediate postinjury period granulocyte function is altered in a pattern consistent with cell exposure to intravascular complement activation products. Phagocytosis is noted to be increased in the first 10 days

after burn. Changes in oxidative activity are correlated with the degree of complement activation, and can be conferred on normal cells by the burned patient's serum. Multiple reports of neutrophil chemotaxis show a consistent pattern of suppressed spontaneous or random migration with continued directional responses to FMLP and a specific loss of migratory responsiveness to C5a and its metabolites.

The complement activation product C5a, at nanogram concentrations, is known to regulate several neutrophil functions in vitro including adherence, aggregation, chemotaxis, degranulation and oxide radical production. Each of these responses may be viewed as means of localizing neutrophils to areas of inflammation and priming the cells for responses needed to facilitate transendothelial migration and subsequent chemotaxis.

An important means of regulation of the chemotactic response involves the interplay between C5a and three serum proteins. Carboxypeptidase N rapidly converts C5a in plasma to its desArg derivative resulting in a ten- to twenty-fold reduction in chemotactic potency. However, a second agent, vitamin D binding protein, identical to group-specific component globulin functions as a binding platform for $C5a_{desArg}$ to alter its receptor interactions and enhance the chemoattractant activity of the complex. A third protein, chemotactic factor inactivator, previously believed to be a C5a peptidase, is now known to exert its effect by altering the interaction between $C5a/C5a_{desArg}$ and Gc globulin, particularly lessening the affinity of the C5a receptor for the complex. Thus an increase in chemotactic factor inactivator would serve to suppress neutrophil responsiveness to plasma $C5a_{desArg}$. It is not known whether any of these factors are acute phase reactants. This regulatory system is likely a model which may be useful for other neutrophil stimulants.

Priming of Neutrophils

The induction of a potentiated state for heightened oxidative and phagocytic responses to a second stimuli is another function amenable to regulation. Pretreatment of normal neutrophils with C5a or $C5a_{desArg}$ leads to enhanced activity of the NADPH oxidase through faster activation in response to second stimuli and a higher maximal rate of oxidant production.

Analysis of neutrophil priming in response to pretreatment with $C5a_{desArg}$ revealed the up regulation of many previously cryptic receptors including FMLP, CR3 and CR1 receptors and the integrin family of adherence proteins. The secondary granular component of the neutrophils acts as a repository for a variety of spare receptors. Priming of the cell with C5a results in degranulation of the cells, with release of granular enzymes such as lysozyme and vitamin B_{12} binding protein and the enhanced expression of FMLP, CR1, CR3, laminin, vitronectin and fibronectin receptors on the cell surface. More recently, receptor upregulation from granular pools has been shown to occur without enzyme release.

Activation of circulating (suspension-phase) neutrophils by C5a and other chemoattractants results in the enhanced expression of adherence receptors, termed integrins, composed of a CD18 molecule and a CD11 moiety. The CD11 components confer ligand specificity. C5a additionally results in expression of endothelial lectin-like adherence molecules termed ELAM-1 and ICAM-1 that facilitate neutrophil endothelial interactions. While endothelial pretreatment with TNF-α enhances neutrophil adherence, the mechanisms appear to be separable from those initiated by C5a and to result in more transient effects. Furthermore, the monokine IL-1 induces endothelial gene expression and production of IL-8, a molecule that inhibits neutrophil adherence to endothelium and also serves as a neutrophil chemoattractant.

This mechanism for upregulating both receptor number and subsequent cellular responses to oxidant-generating stimuli was found to be a common property of other classes of chemoattractant/secretagogues. Leukotrienes and PAF mimic many of the effects of C5a including chemotaxis, secretion by cytochalasin-pretreated cells of granular enzymes and various oxidants and enhanced adherence. The similar types of responses of neutrophils induced by multiple chemical classes of mediators suggest that this event is overdetermined and is fundamental to the inflammatory response to tissue injury.

Priming is routinely assayed using the neutrophil oxidative burst. This cell response is closely regulated with rapid on and off times for suspension phase cells. This is effected through rapid recycling of cytoplasmic cofactors for the membrane bound NADPH oxidase. This activity appears to serve to promote highly localized matrix destruction by oxidation of extracellular proteins and more rapid digestion by an array of neutrophil export enzymes such as elastase and collagenase. Such activity is limited to the leading front of the cell which is tightly adherent to the target; this reduces the activity of oxidant scavengers such as ceruloplasmin and enzyme inactivators such as α1 proteinase inhibitor. Oxidative burst activity and localized degranulation serve other regulatory functions including inactivation of cytokines and receptor loss from the neutrophil surface, both best studied in relation to TNF-α. This high level of regulation of oxidant production is not seen with matrix adherent cells stimulated with cytokines.

Neutrophil Responses in Tissue Matrices: Enter the Cytokines

The adult respiratory distress syndrome (ARDS) is useful as a paradigm for examining the effects of a matrix environment on neutrophil function and for examining the mechanisms of neutrophil mediated tissue damage. Aside from the clinical importance of this syndrome, pulmonary architecture can be assessed through x-ray and functional abnormalities are easily quantified by blood gas determinations. ARDS is characterized histologically by a neutrophil alveolitis with disruption of the alveolar-capillary interstitium and injury to both epithelial and endothelial cells. As this lesion evolves, fibrosis with thickening of the alveolar-capillary junction occurs. This fibrosis persists for several weeks and causes inelasticity and impaired gas exchange. These abnormalities in turn are responsible for the prolonged ventilator dependency and high morbidity and mortality rates associated with ARDS.

The mechanisms by which neutrophils could participate in this disease remained unclear until macrophage production of powerful neutrophil stimulants was recognized. Early theories based on massive intravascular complement activation were compromised by absence of identified chemoattractants that would move neutrophils into the alveolar interstitium. Animal studies involving activation or infusion of large quantities of C5a failed to produce interstitial injury.

A variety of cytokines relevant to the pathogenesis of ARDS have been identified. These include IL-8, a neutrophil chemoattractant secreted by alveolar macrophages following the initial burst of LTB_4 release and TNF-α.

It has been known for sometime that alveolar macrophages can secrete LTB_4, a potent neutrophil chemoattractant but a modest stimulant for superoxide production. Conversely, TNF-α causes hemorrhagic necrosis of lungs and other organs if infused in large quantities. C5a appears to serve as a necessary cofactor. Neutrophils undergo a large respiratory burst in response to small quantities of several cytokines, including TNF, G-CSF, and GM-CSF, but only when adherent to serum or plasma coated surfaces or extracellular matrix proteins. Traditional suspension phase assays of the effects of TNF-α upon neutrophils demonstrated modest oxidant production that continued for a prolonged period of time, neutrophil activation through enhanced FMLP receptor expression and enhanced oxidative responsiveness to subsequently encountered stimuli. However, if neutrophils are allowed to adhere to fibronectin-coated plates, a process greatly accelerated by C5a, and then stimulated with TNF-α, GM-CSF, G-CSF or interferon-γ at very low doses (10-100 ng/ml), superoxide is produced at rates near those maximally achieved with PAM. The time course for this response is considerably different from that for suspension phase cells triggered by stimuli such as FMLP. There is a prolonged lag phase of 15-30 minutes, and superoxide production continues for approximately 90 minutes. The elaborate on/off mechanisms for suppressing oxidant production clearly are bypassed.

More recently, neutrophils have been shown to make messenger RNA for NADPH oxidase and cytochrome b, a required cofactor for the enzyme. Additionally, neutrophils make mRNA for both IL-1α and TNF-α. The identification of these functions suggests that neutrophils in tissue may function more like macrophage lineage cells than previously thought and may regulate early events at a site of contamination. It is currently believed that neutrophil adherence actuates signal transduction pathways, altering the type, time course and magnitude of PMN responses.

In this scheme, macrophage activation through tissue injury or tissue contamination with microorganisms causes release of various molecules that affect neutrophil-endothelial interactions in the local microvasculature as described above and induce neutrophil chemotaxis into the interstitium (IL-8 and LTB_4). Upon entry of the neutrophil into the interstitium, adherence of the neutrophil to matrix components magnifies the exocytic responses induced by TNF-α, GM-CSF and perhaps other local macrophage secretion products. A speculative assumption is that the adherence process activates a transductional pathway for receptor-ligand interactions. The result of these processes is a near maximal release of oxidants and neutrophil enzymes into the interstitium, an effect not observed with neutrophils in suspension.

SURFACE RECEPTOR-MEDIATED EVENTS, SIGNAL TRANSDUCTION AND REGULATION

The alterations in neutrophil function as a result of trauma and the chain of events leading to neutrophil mediated tissue damage may be understood as the end result of alterations of cell surface receptors and of receptor coupling mechanisms. Surface receptors are the cell's primary avenue of communication with its environment and provide a high degree of specificity for cell responses to environmental stimuli. Surface receptor interactions with various cytokines, bacterial products, connective tissue and structural molecules mediate neutrophil chemotaxis, priming, degranulation, adherence and regulation.

Neutrophil chemoattractant, exocytic and phagocytic responses are mediated by spatial sensing and differential occupancy of specific receptors. Receptors serve to transduce signals through the membrane, and are then removed from the cell surface by endocytic processes. This internalization of the receptor-ligand complex provides a means of regulating the inflammatory response by removing proinflammatory mediators from the cell's milieu and preventing repeated stimulation of the cell by the same ligand. Recycling of receptors occurs in relation to the extracellular concentration of ligand. At low (chemotactic) doses, such recycling allows a continued response across a ligand gradient. Higher, degranulating concentrations, immobilize cells by not allowing recycling.

Tumor necrosis factor binds to neutrophils via a cell surface glycoprotein receptor. The neutrophil receptor for TNF is subject to down-regulation by previous exposure to cell activating stimuli such as C5a and down-regulation correlates well with inhibition of TNF-induced PMN function. The receptor has two extracellular domains that are released from the cells in soluble form when the cell is activated, and both are capable of binding TNF. These TNF binding proteins have been purified from human urine and have been demonstrated to protect cells from the toxic effects of TNF. Interleukin-1 has also been implicated as an important mediator of the septic response and acts synergistically with TNF to cause tissue damage. A natural monocyte protein that acts as an IL-1 receptor antagonist has been identified, cloned and shown to reduce endotoxin and IL-1 induced inflammation as well as mortality from endotoxic shock in animal models. These cytokine antagonists are now being evaluated in humans. They raise the hope that by utilizing recombinant binding proteins and/or receptor agonists against TNF, IL-1 or other cytokines the deleterious effects of the septic state may be ameliorated.

Another potential point of regulation of neutrophil function involves alterations in the cell's second messenger systems which include the guanine nucleotide binding proteins. These proteins exist in two forms, one inactive [GTP-bound] and one active [GTP-bound] and have an intrinsic GTPase activity which terminates their active state. There appear to be at least two classes of GTP nucleotide regulating proteins. The classical model for guanine nucleotide binding protein function is in relation to cell surface receptor coupling. Ligand-receptor interactions lead to binding of GTP to the active site (the α subunit of the $\alpha \beta \gamma$ trimer) at the cell surface. The α subunit binds to an activating site on adenylate cyclase, resulting in production of large numbers of cAMP second messengers. Other second messenger systems, particularly activation of a phosphoinositol phosphatase C resulting in production of diacylglycerol and Ca^{2+} and subsequent protein kinase C activation. Cytosolic guanine nucleotide binding proteins, which include the Ras, Ras related, and Rho proteins, fulfill a wide range of regulatory functions in all organisms.

Neutrophil activation with the bacterial chemotactic peptide FMLP is coupled to various effector functions via pertussis toxin-sensitive and insensitive pathways. Pertussis toxin ADP-ribosylates the GTP binding sites, blocking effector functioning. A 40 kDa G-protein has been purified from neutrophil membranes which is ADP-ribosylated in the presence of pertussis toxin.

This outline for the function of guanine nucleotide binding proteins as a transductional mechanism provides numerous points for intrasystem regulation and potential therapeutic intervention. It is probable that the cytosolic GTP binding proteins function to polymerize actin and then facilitate granule movement within the cell and to the cell surface. This area has only recently been defined and represents an important area for academic and therapeutic research.

NEUTROPHIL-ENDOTOXIN INTERACTIONS

Currently much work is focused on the elucidation of the components involved in the priming of neutrophils by endotoxin. Several receptors that bind specifically to endotoxin have been identified on the surface of neutrophils. These are the members of the CD11/CD18 family of receptors (integrins), CD14, and a distinct 80 kd protein. However whether these receptors are responsible for the neutrophil responses to endotoxin is still under active investigation. Prior exposure of macrophage to endotoxin is known to blunt the cell's subsequent production of TNF in response to repeated challenge with endotoxin. It is possible that a similar mechanism may exist in neutrophils and be important in the modulation of an inflammatory response. This leads to the notion that down regulation of surface receptors for LPS may occur, similar to that seen with C5a receptors.

There is considerable evidence that endotoxin plays a role in inducing the deleterious hyperfunction of the immune system that can accompany infection. Whether this is true in trauma and burn patients remains to be seen. Thus the consequences of blockade of endotoxin's effects presents a fruitful area of research. Monoclonal antibodies specific for the lipid A portion of endotoxin are undergoing clinical trials. The means by which these antibodies work is subject to conjecture. Binding of endotoxin, blockade of a receptor or an agonist-desensitizing effect are possibilities. Alternatively, they may shift the cellular response to endotoxin from the macrophage to the neutrophil with a resultant improved survival for the host. That the neutrophil may be the primary humoral element responsible for clearance of endotoxin is supported by the finding that current antiendotoxin antibodies only work in nonneutropenic patients.

The morbidity and mortality engendered by the marked inflammatory responses to injury, including increased susceptibility to infection and noninfectious inflammatory injury, have lead to a vigorous effort to understand and control these responses. As research into the cellular and molecular events of the inflammatory response leads to a clearer understanding of the process, points in the chain of events subject to intervention are being identified. The powerful techniques of molecular biology are being brought to bear on the study and treatment of the inflammatory processes that threaten the injured, stressed and septic patient. It is anticipated that as these studies yield insights into the cellular and molecular events of the inflammatory response, the means of altering and controlling it will be developed.

SELECTED READING

1. Senior RM, Campbell EJ. Neutral proteinases from human inflammatory cells: A critical review of their role in extracellular matrix degradation. Clin Lab Med 1983; 3:645-666.
2. Becker EL. The short and happy life of neutrophil activation. J Leukoc Biol 1990; 47:378-389.
3. Robbins RA, Hamel FG. Chemotactic factor inactivator interaction with Gc-Globulin (vitamin D-binding protein): A mechanism of modulating the chemotactic activity of C5a. J Immunol 1990; 144 (6):2371-2376.
4. Hannum CH, Wilcox CJ, Arend WP et al. Interleukin-l receptor antagonist activity of a human interleukin-1 inhibitor. Nature 1990; 343:336-340.
5. Nathan CF. Neutrophil activation on biological surfaces: Massive secretion of hydrogen peroxide in response to products of macrophages and lymphocytes. J Clin Invest 1987; 80:1550-1560.
6. Nathan C, Srimal S, Farber C et al. Cytokine-induced respiratory burst of human neutrophils: Dependence on extracellular matrix proteins and CDl1/CD18 integrins. J Cell Biol 1989; 109:1341-1349.
7. de la Harpe J, Nathan CF. Adenosine regulates the respiratory burst of cytokine-triggered human neutrophils adherent to biologic surfaces. J Immunol 1989; 143:596-602.
8. Dubravec DB, Spriggs DR, Mannick JA, Rodrick ML. Circulating human peripheral blood granulocytes synthesize and secrete tumor necrosis factor alpha. Proc Natl Acad Sci USA 1990; 87:6758-6761.
9. Lomax KJ, Leto TL, Nunoi H et al. Recombinant 47-kilodalton cytosol factor restores NADPH oxidase in chronic granulomatous disease. Science 1989; 245:409-412.
10. Akard LP, English D, Gabig TG. Rapid deactivation of NADPH oxidase in neutrophils: continuous replacement by newly activated enzyme sustains the respiratory burst. Blood 1988; 72:322-327.
11. Borregaard N, Heiple JM, Simons ER, Clark RA. Subcellular localization of the b-cytochrome component of the human neutrophil microbicidal oxidase: translocation during activation. J Cell Biol 1983; 97:52-61.
12. Porteu F, Nathan CF. Shedding of tumor necrosis factor receptors by activated human neutrophils. J Exp Med 1990; 172:599-607.
13. Gabig TG, Eklund EA, Potter GB, Dykes JR, III. A neutrophil GTP-binding protein that regulates cellfree NADPH oxidase activation is located in the cytosolic fraction. J Immunol 1990; 145:945-951.
14. Curnutte JT, Scott PJ, Mayo LA. Cytosolic components of the respiratory burst oxidase: resolution of four components, two of which are missing in complementing types of chronic granulomatous disease. Proc Natl Acad Sci USA 1989; 86:825.
15. Philips MR, Abramson SB, Kolasinski SL, Haines KA et al. Low molecular weight GTP-binding proteins in human neutrophil granule membranes. J Biol Chem 1991; 266:1289-1298.
16. Cockcroft S. G-proteins and exocytotic secretion in phagocytic cells. FEMS Microbiol Immunol 1990; 2:3-8.

CHAPTER 11

IMMUNE MODULATION

David L. Dunn

Although significant clinical advances over the last 20 years that consist of the development of new antimicrobial agents, the use of fluid resuscitation, metabolic support and aggressive nutritional supplementation have led to a reduction in mortality, even today the lethality of gram-negative bacteremia remains greater than 10% and exceeds 30% in immunocompromised patients. Thus, it has become increasingly evident that refinements in the use of currently available modalities may not be capable of providing additional decreases in mortality rates. This observation of the continued high mortality of gram-negative bacterial infections, sepsis and septic shock despite optimal treatment with current measures has provided an impetus for the development of new adjuvant therapies.

New immunomodulatory therapies, in particular those that are targeted both against microbial virulence factors and that are designed to interdict the deleterious systemic responses provoked by these microbial factors, therefore have been developed. These new therapies may exert a significant impact upon this lethal disease process. Because gram-negative bacteria possess the cell wall component lipopolysaccharide (endotoxin, LPS) that appears to be primarily responsible for the high morbidity and mortality associated with serious gram-negative bacterial infections, it may be possible to target therapy directly against this compound. Current evidence suggests that endotoxin may exert deleterious effects upon the host by direct toxicity, by the production of secondary monokine mediators, or both. Host monokines such as tumor necrosis factor (TNF), interleukin-l (IL-1) and interleukin-6 (IL-6) are secreted in response to gram-negative bacterial infection and following endotoxin challenge and are assuredly essential components of the host response to such infections. Unfortunately, endotoxin may not only initiate but may perpetuate the release of these monokines, and it has become obvious that excessive monokine production may in and of itself produce end organ damage, organ failure and death.

Thus, the host response to a septic insult may be equally, if not more important, than the direct toxicity caused by the infecting pathogen. Most probably, effective therapy for gram-negative bacterial sepsis requires not only the elimination of infection and neutralization of microbial virulence factors but also abrogation of the release of the secondary host mediators that occurs during such infection. This concept constitutes the basis for the use of antibodies directed against endotoxin and endotoxin-induced monokines as adjuvant treatment of gram-negative bacterial infections. These new therapies hopefully will serve to reduce the high mortality associated with clinical gram-negative bacterial sepsis that persists despite optimal therapy.

Structure of Endotoxin

LPS is composed of three distinct regions, each region possessing unique pathogenic and antigenic properties. These three regions are: 1) the outer polysaccharide (O-antigen), that is unique to and comprises the major antigenic determinants of each gram-negative bacterial strain; 2) core polysaccharide that links outer polysaccharide to lipid A and that is structurally similar among many bacterial genera; and 3) lipid A, the potent toxic moiety of endotoxins that is structurally homogeneous among most gram-negative organisms. The core polysaccharide region of LPS links O-antigen to lipid A and is composed of 10-12 saccharide residues. Colonies of organisms that display core polysaccharide on their surfaces are crinkled or rough in appearance, resulting in the name "rough" bacteria. The core region is itself composed of three regions: outer, intermediate and inner (deep) core. The outer region is composed of hexoses that are linked to hep–toses that constitute the primary constituents of the intermediate core. The deep core is composed of three residues of 2-keto-3deoxy-D-mannoctulosonic acid (KDO) that are linked to lipid A. A single core type is known for *Salmonella sp*, while five types have been identified for *E coli*. Lipid A is structurally the most highly conserved portion of LPS among different genera of gram-negative organisms, and forms the toxic moiety of endotoxin. Lipid A is linked to KDO through an ester linkage and the primary structure is composed of diphosphorylated diglucosamine residues containing ester- and amide-linked fatty acids.[1]

Host Response to Endotoxin

The mononuclear phagocyte (monocyte, macrophage) has emerged as the central effector cell in the host response to endotoxin. LPS-stimulated macrophages have been demonstrated to release TNF, IL-1, IL-6, arachidonic acid metabolites, toxic metabolites of oxygen, proteolytic enzymes, and procoagulant factors. In addition macrophage functional capacity is altered after binding of LPS: phago- cytosis, adherence, oxidative burst, protein synthesis and expression of Ia on the cell surface are all enhanced. The accumulated evidence supports the essential role of the macrophage in the generation of the septic response to endotoxin administration. This has been confirmed in studies of the C3H/HeJ endotoxin-unresponsive strain of mouse: adoptive transfer of bone marrow derived macrophages from C3H/HeN endotoxin-responsive mice into C3H/HeJ animals restores sensitivity to endotoxin.[2]

A growing awareness of those host responses that occur during gram-negative bacterial infection has made it increasingly clear that the vast majority of the systemic effects caused by endotoxin are related to the effects of the release of host mediators. A great deal of attention therefore has been focused upon endotoxin-induced cytokine production. These mediators appear to induce many, if not all of the systemic responses associated with morbidity and lethality. Endotoxin induces systemic and local production of diverse cytokines, in particular TNF, IL-1, IL-2, IL-6 and interferon γ. Within this array of host cytokines, particular attention has been focused on TNF, IL-1 and IL-6 because their presence has been most closely associated with the occurrence of morbid sequelae of gram-negative bacterial infections, sepsis and shock.

The role of TNF during sepsis has been extensively studied in experimental models of gram-negative bacterial infection, in clinical volunteers receiving endotoxin and during severe clinical infection. Using an analysis similar to that proposed by Koch to identify association of a microbe with disease, it has been possible to construct evidence that TNF is a critical component of the host response to gram-negative bacterial sepsis. Three lines of evidence are used: 1) the association of elevated TNF levels with lethal gram-negative bacterial and endotoxin challenges; 2) the lethality of direct administration of high doses of TNF to animals; and 3) the observation that anti-TNF antibodies reduce the lethality associated with both gram-negative bacterial and endotoxin challenges.[3-5]

TNF has been associated with the onset of sepsis after gram-negative bacterial challenge in mice and baboons. Serum TNF levels characteristically peak rapidly following bacterial challenge and decline to undetectable levels thereafter. The early peak in TNF characteristically occurs one to two hours after infection and rapidly decreases as levels of other cytokines rise and peak. The time course and degree of the TNF increase appears to be dependent on the nature of the challenge. In chronic sepsis models such as that induced by cecal ligation and perforation, no detectable increase in TNF is observed in mice. In contrast, after endotoxin challenge mice exhibit a marked increase in serum TNF levels. The differential host response to varying degrees of TNF secretion is likely to occur clinically as well, and these observations suggest that differential effects of TNF may occur depending on the absolute level in vivo.

The critical role of TNF during the host response to gram-negative bacterial or endotoxin challenge is further supported by experiments in which high doses of TNF are administered. TNF administration results in a dose dependent increase in tachypnea and hypotension, decline in arterial pH and increase in serum lactate. At necropsy, animals receiving lethal doses of TNF demonstrate hemorrhagic lung lesions, bowel necrosis and hemorrhage and hemorrhage into the kidneys, pancreas and adrenal glands. These pathophysiological and histological changes closely mimic those found when endotoxin is administered, implicating TNF as an essential mediator of endotoxin-induced systemic changes.

Additional evidence implicating TNF in the pathogenesis of gram-negative bacterial infections has been obtained by assessing the effects of TNF attenuation following septic challenge. For example, immunization with TNF reduces the mortality associated with endotoxin challenge. Similarly, when polyclonal or monoclonal antibodies (mAbs) directed against TNF are administered in experimental models, the morbidity and mortality associated with either TNF administration itself, or that caused by gram-negative bacterial or endotoxin challenges can be reduced. A recent clinical trial employing anti-TNF antibody for the treatment of sepsis has provided a preliminary indication that

this approach may be of benefit.

Another cytokine that has been implicated as an important inducer of endotoxin-related systemic changes is IL-1. IL-1 plays a critical role in many different immunological processes, foremost of which are inflammatory reactions to bacterial infection. Induction of fever during infection has been largely attributed to the direct and indirect actions of IL-1. In addition to inducing the febrile response associated with bacterial sepsis, IL-1 increases the production of acute phase proteins, induces hypotension and provokes a series of other proinflammatory effects associated with the onset of bacterial sepsis. A large body of evidence has implicated IL-1 as a critical mediator of the toxicity associated with gram-negative bacterial infections. In animal models of gram-negative infection, elevated levels of IL-1 have been observed several hours after infection is induced. Blockade of endotoxin or TNF by specific anti-LPS or anti-TNF antibodies reduced IL-1 levels and reduced mortality. When IL-1 was administered at high doses, IL-1 induced both fever and hypotension in rabbits. Blockade of the biological activity of IL-1 by infusion of an IL-1 receptor antagonist (IL-1ra) has recently been shown to reduce the mortality of gram-negative bacterial infection in several animal models, including rabbits, newborn rats and baboons. In rabbits, hypotension following gram-negative bacterial infection is attenuated by the administration of IL-1ra.

Similar to TNF and IL-1, IL-6 is an important mediator that may play a significant role in producing the systemic effects that occur during of gram-negative bacterial and endotoxin challenge. Elevated levels of IL-6 have been demonstrated in diverse types of infectious diseases including gram-negative and gram-positive bacterial infections. Of importance is the observation that IL-6 has been found to accumulate at the local site of inflammation in many different types of infections. IL-6 production that occurs early following a septic insult may primarily augment the host response to a septic insult by virtue of its effects on acute phase protein synthesis and its capacity to augment cellular immunity. Additional evidence for the role of

IL-6 as a mediator of sepsis comes from recent studies demonstrating that anti-IL-6 anti-bodies protect against either a lethal gram-negative bacterial or a TNF challenge.[6]

A series of elegant animal studies have provided compelling evidence that the host responses associated with gram-negative bacterial infections are mediated through the effects of endotoxin and endotoxin-induced cytokines. Because of important differences in special sensitivity to endotoxin and due to the practical difficulty in determining the onset of gram-negative bacterial sepsis in humans, similar demonstrations in septic patients have not been as evident. One means to study the role of endotoxin and endotoxin-induced cytokines in humans, however, has been to infuse these mediators into healthy human subjects. These studies have yielded compelling evidence implicating both endotoxin and the endotoxin-induced cytokines TNF, IL-1 and IL-6 as potent effectors of the host response that occurs during gram-negative bacterial infections in man.

Infusion of endotoxin into healthy volunteers produces a symptom complex that includes myalgias, chills, headache and nausea mimicking the symptoms associated with the early onset of gram-negative bacterial sepsis. A similar symptom complex is produced following TNF and IL-1 infusion. Following TNF infusion, the onset of symptoms is immediate while symptoms following endotoxin infusion begin 90 to 120 minutes after endotoxin infusion, a time interval corresponding with the peak of plasma TNF levels. In addition to producing symptoms characteristic of gram-negative bacterial infections, either endotoxin or TNF infusion induces hemodynamic changes that include tachycardia, increased cardiac output and a reduction in systemic vascular resistance. In contrast to the onset of symptoms, the peak tachycardia and fever responses induced by either endotoxin or TNF occur four hours after infusion. While these symptoms and hemodynamic alterations are nonspecific and associated with diverse infectious and noninfectious diseases, these observations are consistent with the hypothesis that TNF and IL-1 mediate many of the toxic effects associated with the presence of endotoxin in the bloodstream of humans.

Endotoxin-induced cytokine responses in man are also similar to those observed to occur in animals. The cytokine cascade in response to endotoxin stimulation in vitro is identical to that using murine derived cell lines and complements the similarities found between the two species in vivo. In human volunteers, endotoxin infusion is associated with a rapid increase in serum levels of both TNF and IL-6: TNF peaks within one to two hours while IL-6 peaks within two to four hours. Elucidating the pattern of cytokine responses that occurs in critically ill patients with documented gram-negative bacterial infections, however, has proved difficult. Similar to those observations regarding TNF, elevated plasma levels of IL-1 and IL-6 have been documented in some patients during episodes of gram-negative bacterial sepsis, but this has not been a consistent finding. While IL-1 levels have been found to be higher in patients dying from gram-negative bacterial sepsis, elevated IL-1 levels have not been uniformly found in these patients and did not correlate with outcome when other prognostic variables were analyzed via logistic regression analysis. Elevated IL-6 levels have also been observed in patients with septic shock.

ANTIBODY IMMUNOTHERAPY OF GRAM-NEGATIVE BACTERIAL SEPSIS

The morbidity and mortality associated with gram-negative bacterial infection have been reduced but by no means eliminated through the use of current therapeutic interventions. Fluid and nutritional support together with the administration of effective antibiotics mitigate but apparently cannot eliminate the toxicity that assuredly results from both the direct effects of endotoxin upon cells and tissues and the host response that is provoked by the endotoxin-stimulated release of secondary mediators. Immunotherapy employing anti-endotoxin antibodies represents a new type of therapy for gram-negative bacterial sepsis that may serve to decrease the morbidity and mortality of gram-negative sepsis through: 1) repletion or augmentation of host defenses; 2) neutralization of the toxicity of endotoxin; and 3) interdiction of the release of deleterious cytokines that may result in the clinical manifestations of sepsis.

In the initial years of research in this area, several intriguing lines of evidence suggested that anti-endotoxin antibodies might prove useful in the treatment of gram-negative bacterial sepsis: 1) the ability of active immunization with *Pseudomonas aeruginosa* to provide protection, albeit limited, against infection with the homologous organism in patients with malignancies; 2) correlation of high titers of naturally occurring anti-endotoxin antibodies with decreased frequency of shock and death in patients with gram-negative bacterial sepsis; and 3) the demonstration of protection against lethal endotoxemia after passive immunization of animals with hyperimmune serum. Subsequent fractionation of protective serum samples revealed that the protective component was in the antibody fraction. Based upon these findings, both polyclonal and monoclonal antibodies have been produced against different structural regions of gram-negative bacterial endotoxin over a 20-year period. Antibody preparations that display binding specificity against O-antigens (serotype-specific antibodies) or against deep core/lipid A structures (crossreactive antibodies) have been developed and some, but not all, have demonstrated protective capacity.

Serotype-specific antibodies appear to have limited utility since during clinical infection: 1) several days may elapse between onset of sepsis and the identification of a gram-negative bacterial organism, precluding the administration of the correct antibody during the critical early phase of sepsis; 2) the causative gram-negative pathogen may never be identified because the patient develops low grade culture negative bacteremia and concurrent endotoxemia; or 3) an antibody may not be available against the causative bacterial strain.

EXPERIMENTAL STUDIES

Early investigators first suggested that a toxic moiety common to many different types of endotoxin might exist and that administration of antibody directed against this "toxophore" might assist the reticuloendothelial system in its uptake and degradation. Through purification and differential extraction of bacterial endotoxins, the shared toxic moiety was localized to the deep core region of endotoxin and was identified as being associated with lipid A. Subsequently, the identification and use of mutant bacterial species that lack the O-antigens of endotoxin has permitted the development of a large number of antibodies against deep core/lipid A epitopes. These regions of LPS appear to be poor immunogens, and the use of whole bacteria and their derived endotoxin has greatly facilitated research in this area. The mutant organisms express these determinants extensively on their cell surface and thus represent both excellent immunogens and targets for antibody binding studies. Polyclonal anticore LPS antibody preparations have been examined in a large number of animal models. Although protective capacity has not been invariably demonstrated, a recent meta-analysis has indicated that the vast majority of these preparations provide protective capacity.[1,7-9]

In addition to inconsistent protective capacity, polyclonal antibody preparations have several important limitations: 1) production of the antibody depends on immunizing single animals or individuals to produce antibody which necessarily results in variable antibody reactivity and limits the supply of antibody; 2) immunization with mutant strains such as *E. coli* J5 may lead to the production of antibodies directed against antigenic determinants outside of the deep core and lipid A regions of LPS that may have no protective benefit; and 3) these antibody preparations are difficult to characterize with regard to binding specificity and protective capacity. In response to these problems, several groups of investigators have developed murine and human mAbs directed against various portions of LPS. The generation of hybridomas producing mAbs that bind LPS allows the production of large quantities of highly monospecific antibody directed against specific epitopes within the O-antigen or deep core/lipid A regions. Interestingly, however, only one study has directly compared protection after monoclonal and polyclonal antibody administration, and both preparations exhibited similarly protective capacity.

Several groups have developed mAbs directed against the O-antigen region of *E. coli* 0111:B4 LPS that are capable of providing extremely efficient protective capacity in experimental models of both bacterial infection and endotoxin challenge. Although serotype-specific mAbs demonstrate efficient protection in animal models of peritonitis, intravenous bacteremia or endotoxemia, protection is limited to the homologous organism, and crossprotection does not occur.[10,11] While the use of cocktails of mAbs in prophylaxis and treatment of gram-negative bacterial infections has been suggested, a more promising approach has been the development and isolation of crossreactive mAbs directed against the highly conserved core and lipid A regions of LPS.

Antideep core mAbs produced after immunization of mice with rough mutant organisms have demonstrated varying degrees of crossreactivity in vitro against diverse gram-negative bacterial species. In fact, even those that demonstrate extensive binding to lipid A and of broad crossreactivity in vitro are not invariably protective. The majority of mAbs generated against rough mutant gram-negative organisms have lacked reactivity against homologous wild-type smooth organisms or LPS derived from these organisms, heterologous organisms or LPS or lipid A.[12-19] There are several possible explanations for the apparent lack of crossreactivity of mAbs that include: 1) choice of binding target; 2) physical alteration of binding target by fixation; 3) inaccessibility of deep core/lipid A epitopes on intact bacteria and on LPS; and 4) occurrence and antigenicity of unique binding determinants within the deep core/lipid A region.

Thus although the protective capacity of passively transferred anticore/lipid A antibodies has been comprehensively examined, unequivocal demonstration of protective capacity has not yet been forthcoming. The mechanisms that determine antibody reactivity and protective capacity are only now being delineated and represent a complex series of interactions of anticore LPS antibodies with molecular, cellular and systemic components of host defenses. Many factors govern these interactions and may determine the degree of protective capacity in animal models and in clinical studies, including: 1) polyclonal or monoclonal nature of the antibody; 2) epitope specificity; 3) antibody subclass or fragment type utilized; 4) dose and dosing interval of antibody administration; and 5) interaction with other treatment modalities such as antibiotics. These factors need to be carefully examined and correlated with protective capacity in animal models and in clinical studies in order to develop new, broadly crossreactive antibodies that may provide clinical benefit.

CLINICAL TRIALS

Naturally occurring antibody directed against both *S. minnesota* Re, *E. coli* J5 and lipid A has been demonstrated in patients with gram-negative bacteremia, and the presence of these antibodies has been positively correlated with decreased morbidity and mortality. In addition, Pollack et al found that survival of patients with *Pseudomonas* sepsis was positively correlated with the presence of naturally occurring anti-*E. coli* J5 antibodies. The discovery of naturally occurring anti-endotoxin antibodies provided support for the concept that anti-endotoxin antibody immunotherapy might prove efficacious during the treatment of gram-negative bacterial sepsis and led to trials in which the effect of passive transfer of polyclonal anti-LPS antibody was studied.

Initial investigations of the efficacy of polyclonal anti-LPS antibody against gram-negative bacterial sepsis were instituted by Lachman et al who administered freeze-dried human plasma containing high titers of naturally occurring anti-LPS IgG to women in septic shock of gynecologic origin. A decrease in mortality from 47% to 7% was reported in patients receiving high-titer plasma of undetermined specificity compared to those who received normal plasma. In contrast, intramuscular administration of hyperimmune globulin known to contain high titers of anti-LPS antibody to patients who developed septic shock after surgical procedures resulted in no decrease in endotoxemia or mortality. Analysis of serum antibody titers from the donor population from which the hyperimmune globulin was prepared revealed a high proportion of serotype-specific antibody and it is therefore possible that the lack of protection resulted from the administration of antibody with inappropriate specificity.[20]

The development of polyclonal anticore antisera with broad crossreactivity in vitro led to performance of a randomized, double-blind trial of human polyclonal anti-*E. coli* J5 plasma. Ziegler et al assessed outcome in relation to death from gram-negative bacteremia in patients with presumed gram-negative bacterial sepsis and found a 17% decrease in mortality in those patients who received a single unit of antibody. The degree of protection was greater in those treated patients (44% vs 77%) with clinical evidence of shock, with or without positive blood cultures.[21] In a separate clinical trial, this same anti-*E. coli* J5 antiserum preparation or control serum was administered to a group of patients identified as being at high risk for, but without clinical signs of bacteremia. Anti-*E. coli* J5 antiserum failed to prevent localized gram-negative infections although the infections that occurred appeared less severe than those experienced by controls. The incidence of shock and death was reduced in those patients receiving anti-*E. coli* J5 antiserum providing support for the findings of the initial trial. In a subsequent human trial of anti-*E. coli* J5 antiserum prophylaxis, however, the administration of pre- and postimmune anti-*E. coli* J5 antisera to neutropenic patients resulted in no reduction in bacteremia, febrile episodes or mortality.

Two multicenter double-blinded, randomized clinical trials have been performed in which the effect of crossreactive anti-lipid A mAbs has been examined in populations of patients with a presumptive diagnosis of gram-negative bacterial sepsis. In both trials routine resuscitative and supportive measures including fluid, pressors and administration of appropriate antibiotics were implemented or continued, and patients were followed for 28 to 30 days or until death. In one trial, administration of a single 100 mg dose of human IgM mAb designated HA-1A was compared to placebo. In 196 patients with gram-negative bacteremia, 63% of patients receiving HA-1A survived 28 days compared to

48% of controls. A 42% reduction was observed when mortality was examined in those patients with septic shock. In a similar trial involving 486 patients, the effect of administration of two 2 mg/kg doses of a murine IgM mAb (E5) was compared to administration of placebo. Although survival was similar between the two groups, a subgroup of 137 E5 treated patients who were not in shock at the time of entry into the study were noted to exhibit enhanced survival. The results of these trials are extremely encouraging, and should serve to promote the continuance of further treatment and prophylaxis trials. [22,23]

MONOKINE ABROGATION

While anti-LPS antibodies are likely to be a useful adjunct to standard treatment modalities, their usefulness is limited to treating patients with gram-negative bacterial infections. A wide array of microorganisms, however, have been found to initiate the cytokine cascade associated with sepsis. Therefore, new therapies directed at the host response to microbial products may prove effective in patients with polymicrobial infections and in those patients without a particular infection source identified. The best characterized of these approaches is the use of antibodies to abrogate or block the biological activity of TNF. Based on substantial animal data demonstrating the protective effect of monoclonal and polyclonal antibodies directed against TNF, one study has described the use of anti-TNF mAbs in the treatment of septic patients. This preliminary study utilized a murine mAb directed against human TNF and reported no acute toxicity attributable to the antibody, and possible efficacy in three patients.

While IL-1ra and anti-IL-6 antibodies have shown promise in animal models of gram-negative bacterial infections, this mode of therapy is just in the process of being applied clinically. As with other immunomodulatory therapies, a cautious approach toward therapies that abrogate cytokine responses is warranted. Although substantial evidence implicates TNF, IL-1 and IL-6 as critical mediators of the toxicity associated with gram-negative bacterial infections, each has been shown to have some immunostimulatory functions that may provide beneficial effects. Inhibition of salutary effects such as local recruitment of host defenses at the local level could have disastrous consequences.

Controversies

Although there are substantial experimental data and compelling evidence from early clinical trials that has supported the clinical application of anti-endotoxin antibodies, important questions remain unanswered regarding the optimal antibody preparation to use, the patient populations most likely to benefit from anti-LPS antibodies and the mechanism of action of these antibodies. Perhaps most importantly, the optimal epitope against which to direct anti-endotoxin antibodies has not been defined. Although directing the antibody against lipid A or core determinants has demonstrated broad in vitro crossreactivity and crossprotection, the site of anti-LPS mAb binding that provides optimal protective capacity has not been precisely identified. The "cryptic" nature of this binding site has led some investigators to question the existence of a truly a crossreactive LPS binding site.

As noted above, antibodies used in early clinical trials have been IgM mAbs with reported reactivity against lipid A. E5 is a murine mAb while HA-1A was generated by the fusion between human spleen cells and mouse-human heteromyeloma cells. Purified HA-1A has been reported to have reactivity in vitro not only to lipid A but also to gram-positive bacterial antigens, fungal antigens and unrelated lipids. The affinity constant of HA-1A for isolated lipid A from two bacterial species is relatively low (10^4 M^{-1}) for lipid A derived *S. minnesota* Re595 and *P. aeruginosa* according to some investigators, although other investigators have reported an affinity constant of (10^7 M^{-1}) for *S. minnesota* RE595 lipid A. Detailed binding specificity of E5 has not yet been published. It should be obvious that precise delineation of the binding specificity and potential crossreactivity of these antibody preparations may be an essential component not only in selecting the most efficacious preparation but also in evaluating their clinical efficacy.

A second problem that has been evident during clinical trials using anti-endotoxin antibodies concerns the selection of the patient population that is most likely to benefit from this form of therapy. Because use of anti-endotoxin antibody is being considered as empiric therapy for patients with suspected gram-negative bacterial infections, it is clear that a significant proportion of these patients will assuredly be found later to have another cause for their sepsis. Consequently, these patients will receive anti-endotoxin antibody "unnecessarily." In one trial, no difference in mortality was noted when patients who developed clinical parameters of sepsis and received anti-endotoxin antibody were compared to those who received only placebo. One explanation for this finding may be that many of these patients did not benefit from anti-endotoxin antibody therapy because they did not have gram-negative bacteremia nor endotoxemia. Thus although the clinical data demonstrates the safety of anti-endotoxin antibodies, this form of therapy may lead to significant expenditures in a large group of patients without endotoxemia who will receive no benefit from the antibody. The anticipated cost of currently available antibody preparations has been estimated at $2,000-$3,000 per dose, and multiple dosing regimens are being considered.

Because as many as 400,000-800,000 patients might qualify as candidates for this therapy based on the presumptive diagnosis of gram-negative bacterial sepsis, this new therapy could represent an annual cost of up to $1.6 billion dollars each year in the U.S. Although the cost of anti-endotoxin antibody therapy may be offset by cost savings afforded by the benefits achieved, the most cost efficient way in which to administer these antibodies would be to identify patient populations most likely to respond to this therapy. As one would expect, preliminary clinical trials have indicated that patients with gram-negative bacteremia and endotoxemia are those subgroups that indeed will most likely benefit from this therapeutic modality.

Cultures remain the primary method by which to identify the presence of gram-negative infection and require more than 24 hours to process. Unfortunately, current endotoxin assay techniques still have significant limitations restricting their widespread clinical use. Rapid and accurate assays of gram-negative bacterial infection and endotoxemia are required not only for the identification of patients most likely to benefit from the antibody but are essential in evaluating the efficacy of this therapy. An accurate assessment of the impact of anti-endotoxin antibodies necessarily will require measurement of anti-lipid A antibody levels prior to passive immunization, obtaining serial blood cultures and serial plasma samples upon which endotoxin TNF, IL-1 and IL-6 determinations can be made. It is extremely important that such monitoring take place so that anti-endotoxin antibody therapy is used appropriately.

A final controversy that bears mention concerns the manner in which these antibodies function during human gram-negative bacterial sepsis. As has been previously discussed, animal models of gram-negative bacterial infection have provided important information regarding the ability of these antibodies to bind to intact bacterial organisms, enhance opsonophagocytosis and attenuate endotoxin-induced cytokine production. Animals studies, however, have several features that limit the extrapolation of the results obtained to human practice. Animal models used to study anti-LPS antibodies have generally consisted of those in which acute, monomicrobial bacterial infection or endotoxemia is induced. Although some instances of human gram-negative bacterial infections may be quite similar to these models, the majority of significant gram-negative bacterial infections in humans are characterized by a more indolent course. Human gram-negative bacterial sepsis may differ markedly from that observed in animal models of infection, and anti-endotoxin antibodies may act quite differently in the clinical and laboratory settings. In addition to measuring endotoxin levels and bacteremia, evaluation of anti-endotoxin antibody therapy in humans will require assessment of the effect of these antibodies on cytokine levels, hemodynamic parameters and other indices of sepsis. One study has attempted to correlate TNF before and after anti-endotoxin antibody therapy, and no significant correlation between TNF

levels and anti-endotoxin antibody treatment was observed. Further studies in this regard in the clinical setting may be essential in determining the mechanism of action of these antibodies during clinical infections.

Although anti-endotoxin antibodies have reached the level of clinical trials, several areas of investigation require pursuit in order to optimize the efficacy of this form of therapy. Many questions still remain regarding the optimal antibody class or subclass of these antibodies. It is well known that the biological activity of the immunoglobulin molecule is determined in part by the molecular composition of the heavy chain, and that differential biologic function is conferred by differences in this region which represent the basis for antibody class and subclass classification. For example, antibodies of the IgM class are potent activators of complement while antibodies of the IgG class are efficient opsonins by virtue of Fc portion of the immunoglobulin molecule that binds to specialized receptors on phagocytes. Since antibodies used in early clinical trials have exclusively been IgM antibodies, experimental investigation using anti-deep core/lipid A using class switch clones may have important clinical implications.

Another area that requires additional study is determining the optimal dosing requirements of patients receiving anti-endotoxin antibodies. Numerous experimental studies have demonstrated that anti-endotoxin antibodies are most efficacious when administered prior to initiation of gram-negative bacterial sepsis or endotoxemia. In most experimental models, the optimal time to administer antibody is several hours prior to infection, and administration of antibody several hours after infection is less effective or ineffective. Although the reason for this difference has not been directly studied, it may relate to a requirement for binding of the antibody to phagocytes prior to infection or to an inability of the antibody to protect against the larger bacterial inoculum that arises after the initiation of infection. Because the clinical features of gram-negative bacterial sepsis may appear only after infection has been established, this may represent a limitation of single dose treatment of septic patients. The efficacy of multiple doses of antibody and the optimal dosing regimen is an area that demands further study.

Another important area that requires additional study is the use of anti-endotoxin antibodies together with anti-cytokine antibodies. Combining these two modes of therapy is attractive in light of the intimate involvement of both endotoxin and cytokines in the pathobiology of gram-negative infections. When administered to septic patients, anti-endotoxin antibodies may prevent the continued activation of potentially deleterious host responses including cytokine release. Concomitant administration of anti-cytokine antibodies might serve to further abrogate those responses initiated by endotoxemia that occurred prior to the administration of anti-LPS antibody or that occurs because of lack of anti-LPS containment. Blockade of both the initiation and propagation of host response to infection may prove to be the most efficacious approach for the treatment of life-threatening gram-negative infection.

Acknowledgement

I would like to thank Ms. Lace Aase and Ms. Lora Esch for their assistance in preparing this manuscript.

References

1. Cody C, Dunn D. Endotoxins in septic shock. In: CRC Handbook on Mediators in Septic Shock. Neugebauer E, Holaday J, Eds. Boca Raton: CRC Press, In press.
2. Morrison D, Ulevitch R. The effects of bacterial endotoxins on host mediation systems. Amer J Pathol 1978; 93:527.
3. Tracey K, Teutler B, Lowry S, Merryweather J et al. Shock and tissue injury induced by recombinant human cachectin. Science 1986; 234:470.
4. Beutler B, Milsark I, Cerami A. Passive immunization against cachectin/tumor necrosis factor protects mice form lethal effect of endotoxin. Science 1985; 229:869.
5. Hesse D, Tracey K, Fong Y, Manogue K et al. Cytokine appearance in human endotoxemia and primate bacteremia. Surg Gynecol Obstet 1988; 166:147.
6. Starnes H, Pearce M, Tewari A, Yim J et al. Anti-IL-6 monoclonal antibodies protect against lethal Escherichia coli infection and lethal tumor necrosis factor: A challenge in mice. J Immunol 1990; 145:4185.
7. Dunn D, Ferguson R. Immunotherapy of gram-negative bacterial sepsis: Enhanced survival in a

guinea pig model by use of rabbit antiserum to *Escherichia coli* J5. Surgery 1982; 92:212.
8. Dunn D, Mach P, Cerra F. Monoclonal antibodies protect against lethal effects of gram-negative sepsis. Surg Forum 1983; 14:142.
9. Dunn D, Mach P, Condie R, Cerra F. Anticore endotoxin F(ab')₂ equine immunoblobulin fragments protect against lethal effects of gram-negative bacterial sepsis. Surgery 1984; 96:440.
10. Kirkland L, Ziegler E. An immunoprotective monoclonal antibody to lipopolysaccharide. J Immunol 1984; 132:2590.
11. Dunn D, Bogard W, Cerra F. Enhanced survival during murine gram-negative sepsis by use of a murine monoclonal antibody. Arch Surg 1985; 120:50.
12. Dunn DL, Mach PA, Cerra FB. Monoclonal antibodies protect against lethal effects of gram-negative bacterial sepsis. Surg Forum 1983; 34:142-144.
13. Dunn D, Bogard W, Cerra F. Efficacy of type-specific and crossreactive murine monoclonal antibodies directed against endotoxin during experimental sepsis. Surgery 1985; 98:283.
14. Teng N, Kaplan H, Herbert J, Moore C. Protection against gram-negative bacteremia and endotoxemia with human monoclonal IgM antibodies. Proc Natl Acad Sci 1985; 82:1790.
15. Dunn D, Priest B, Condie R. Protective capacity of polyclonal and monoclonal antibodies directed against endotoxin during experimental sepsis. Arch Surg 1988; 123:1389.
16. Dunn D. Antibody Immunotherapy of gram-negative bacterial sepsis in an immunosuppressed animal model. Transplantation 1988; 45:424.
17. Priest B, Brinson D, Schroeder D, Dunn D. Treatment of experimental gram-negative bacterial sepsis with murine monoclonal antibodies directed against lipopolysaccharide. Surgery 1989; 106:147.
18. Mayoral J, Schweich C, Dunn D. Decreased tumor necrosis factor production during the initial stages of infection correlates with survival during murine gram-negative sepsis. Arch Surg 1990; 125:24.
19. Mayoral J, Dunn D. Crossreactive murine monoclonal antibodies directed against the core/lipid A region of endotoxin inhibit production of tumor necrosis factor. J Surg Res 1990; 49:1.
20. Lachman E, Pitsoe S, Gaffin S. Anti-lipopolysaccharide immunotherapy in management of septic shock of obstetric and gynaecological origin. Lancet,1984; 1(8384):981.
21. Ziegler E, McCutchan J, Fierer J et al. Treatment of gram-negative bacteremia and shock with human antiserum to a mutant Escherichia coli. N Engl J Med 1982; 307:1225.
22. Ziegler E, Fisher C, Sprung C et al. Treatment of gram-negative bacteremia and septic shock with HA-1A human monoclonal antibody against endotoxin. N Engl J Med 1991; 324:429.
23. Greenman R, Schein R, Martin M et al. A controlled clinical trial of E5 murine monoclonal IgM antibody to endotoxin in the treatment of gram-negative sepsis. JAMA 1991; 266:1097.

CHAPTER 12

BIOLOGICAL RESPONSE MODIFICATION:
An Emerging Therapy in Critical Illness

Timothy G. Buchman

It has always seemed a little unfair to me that the privilege of looking back at the past and speculating about the future falls to those seniors who are about to become spectators. "Surgery," Dr. George Block once remarked, "is not an armchair sport." This chapter—an exercise of player's privilege—is a young surgeon's reflection on several past events, present trends and hazards several predictions as well.

Throw a pebble into a pond and you will see how surgery advances. The first anesthetic under the "ether dome" created a small splash—the real advances came as the ripple of anesthesia traversed all types of operative care. Penicillin was a life-saver for servicemen injured in World War II—but its true impact can best be seen in our current formulary of drugs which can arrest the growth of the most exotic microorganisms. Laparoscopy, once a "toy" reserved for gynecologic surgeons, has married high resolution video imaging—their offspring of minimally invasive techniques can now be found in virtually every surgical discipline, every operating room. Yet each of these advances—analgesia, antibiosis, operative imaging—will probably be dwarfed by an even greater advance in our midst today.

To understand this advance, it is necessary to return across oceans and go back in time to the "Voyage of the Beagle," to join Charles Darwin as he wandered about the Galapagos Islands. Among the species previously unseen by man, among the predators and prey, Darwin made his greatest observation. Darwin recognized in his subjects the occurrence of random mutations and recognized that the forces of natural selection would perpetuate only those mutations which favored survival in a hostile environment. Darwin substituted "evolution" for "God" in accounting for the natural self-restorative powers possessed by all living organisms. He would have agreed with the father of physiology, Claude Bernard, that much human pathology is a failure of homeostasis and that the goal of therapy should be to support the restorative homeostatic mechanisms naturally selected over the eons. Through the first half of this century, these tenets held: Restore the natural balance. Remove the cancer. Set the stage for healing. Drain the pus. "Mother nature" in her wisdom will do the rest. And so on.

Although natural selection ensured that humans were well-equipped to cope with natural challenges to our physiologic integrity, these pioneer biologists—Darwin and Bernard—could not foresee the *unnatural* challenges our patients face today.

Of surgery's great pursuits—ablation and restoration—the latter seems by far the nobler. An entire discipline, transplantation surgery, is single-mindedly devoted to restoring the infirm with healthy tissues donated by others. This therapy—allogeneic organ transplantation—created the challenge of overcoming the naturally protective immune response, and created for surgery a new class of challenges.

For the Galapagos tortoise, the cave man and even modern man, an immune response is a resource to be treasured. For the recipient of a cadaver kidney, it threatens the graft's (and thus the recipient's) survival. Here, then, is the first expression of what I believe to be surgery's transcendent idea, the idea which will shape trauma and critical care for decades to come:

"The advances of medicine in general and surgery in particular have so far outpaced the forces of natural selection that those hard-worn homeostatic responses must not be assumed to be salutary. The goal of surgical care can no longer be limited to merely setting the stage for healing because our stage—the ICU—bears little relationship to the stage on which homeostatic responses evolved. Rather, the approach to therapy must extend into understanding, manipulating and in some cases even extinguishing in our individual patients those homeostatic mechanisms which otherwise have ensured our survival as a species."

The operation of renal transplantation is elegant yet simple enough that today it is readily performed by a mid-level surgical resident. It is amazing in retrospect that so many patients survived the early transplants given the relatively indiscriminate immunosuppressive agents—prednisone and azathioprine—available at the time. It is even more amazing that the heresy of the therapy—the idea that a seemingly protective response might be more dangerous to the organism than the event which provoked it—also survived.

The early experiences in clinical trans-

plantation biology were important from another aspect as well. Although cancer specialists of that era recognized and were trying to take advantage of the fact that malignant cells grew with profoundly different kinetics than normal cells, the clinical transplanters were among the first to exploit the fact that expanding clones of lymphocytes had kinetics sufficiently distinct from other cells such that drugs which interfered with selected aspects of the cell cycle could be administered and have differential effects on the different cell populations. In other words, the early transplanters recognized the importance of cell targeting—that to modify a biological response, it was important to target therapy to that specific cell population responsible for the response.

Until the mid-1970s researchers relied heavily on such cell cycle strategies to experimentally (and therapeutically) distinguish among populations of cells. Two important advances occurred. First, it became apparent that cell surfaces, and in particular the proteins embedded in the plasma membrane, are distinct with respect to cell type. These proteins were recognized as receptors—for small molecular ligands such as epinephrine, for viruses and for larger proteins such as insulin. Second, Kohler and Milstein demonstrated a technique which made it possible to biosynthesize large quantities of "antibodies" which would specifically bind to any particular protein. For their discoveries related to biosynthesis of monoclonal antibodies, they were subsequently awarded the Nobel prize. This advance was rapidly applied to clinical transplantation immunology: one of the first monoclonal antibodies to come into clinical use, OKT3, recognizes a protein found only on the surface to T-lymphocytes. OKT3 is now a mainstay of immunosuppression, since administration of this monoclonal antibody to a patient rejecting a solid organ inactivates the entire T cell population, thereby attenuating the rejection episode. Yet until the early 1980s, antibody-based modification of biological responses seemed to be a clinical strategy largely confined to clinical immunology.

While the transplanters were busy trying to suppress unfavorable immunological responses, the infectious disease specialists were grappling with problems related to inadequate immunological responses. Despite the initial success of penicillin which came into wide clinical use in the Second World War and the subsequent success of several mechanistically distinct antibiotics, patients still seemed to succumb to the effects of septicemia if not to the infection itself. A turning point in this chapter of the story occurred in 1964 when Kass and co-workers, writing in the *New England Journal of Medicine*,[1] reported on a series of patients with documented gram negative sepsis who had been successfully treated with antibiotics, i.e., their subsequent cultures were negative, but who nevertheless died. These unfortunate victims of otherwise successful therapy were noted to have remarkably high endotoxin levels in their bloodstream. Those authors had the brilliant insight to suggest that endotoxin—then a poorly defined constituent of bacterial cell walls—or even "unrecognized toxic substances released into the blood as a consequence of endotoxemia," might be responsible for the poor outcomes. More than two decades would elapse before the groups at Rockefeller University led by Cerami and Tufts by Dinarello would identify tumor necrosis factor and interleukin-1 as those unrecognized toxic substances.

By the late 1970s, a group of visionaries including Abraham Braude and Elizabeth Ziegler had designed a clinical trial of immunotherapy against endotoxin in humans. They recognized that although endotoxins are nearly as unique to bacteria as fingerprints are to humans, at least one portion of the molecule—the Lipid A fragment—was common to all and, moreover, seemingly responsible for much of the pathophysiology. They obtained a mutant *E. coli* J5 whose endotoxin consisted only of Lipid A and a bit of the adjacent core portion of the molecule, killed the *E. coli* and used that material to immunize volunteer military recruits. The antisera crossreacted with endotoxins of virtually all gram-negative organisms. Antisera to J5 and (as control) to irrelevant antigens were then used to treat septic patients. In her landmark 1982 report in the *New England Journal of Medicine*, Dr. Ziegler demonstrated that immuno-

therapy could not only modify the biological response to endotoxin but also improved outcome in sepsis.[2] Despite this success, such immunotherapy did not explode immediately upon the clinical scene. Volunteer recruits (for immunization) were in limited supply; titers among immunized volunteers were quite variable; and the emergence of the human immunodeficiency virus rapidly diminished interest in blood products derived from pooled plasma.

Here, the basic science breakthrough could be brought to bear on a clinical problem. Kohler and Milstein's technique of producing an antibody specific for any antigen was exploited by Teng[3] who, collaborating with Braude and others, constructed a cell line which could be expanded in culture to provide an essentially limitless supply of a monoclonal antiendotoxin reagent. Years of animal experimentation just last year culminated in pivotal trials of two such antiendotoxin monoclonal antibodies. These studies showed that absorption of endotoxin by passive immunization with monoclonal antibodies could ameliorate the biological respone to gram-negative sepsis and thereby improve outcome.[4,5] The significance of this breakthrough for septic patients must not be minimized, but the real importance of this breakthrough, I think, is that it validates the earlier generalization: genetically programmed homeostatic responses (in this case, release of TNF and IL-1 in response to endotoxemia) which are beneficial to humans in the wild can be detrimental to humans treated in the modern hospital environment.

Perhaps the most important part of the endotoxin story was written by Beutler[6] and Tracey.[7] Working in Cerami's lab, these investigators purified and cloned TNF, and administered it to experimental animals. Fulfilling a modern version of Koch's postulates, they showed that endotoxemic animals secreted TNF; that exogenous administration of this naturally occurring substance caused the sepsis syndrome; and that passive immunization with an anti-TNF antibody could prevent the lethal effects of endotoxin. To be sure, bacterial endotoxin is a trigger of the sepsis syndrome—but it is the endogenous response that kills our patients. To paraphrase Walt Kelly's Pogo, "We have met the enemy, and they is us." Ohlsson[8] subsequently showed that interleukin-1 fulfilled Koch's postulates as an endogenous mediator of endotoxin-triggered sepsis syndrome, substituting an antagonist for the interleukin-1 receptor for an antibody directed against that messenger ligand. *This clinical challenge is already upon us: we must now learn which of these biologic response modifiers to administer; in what measure; at what time and in what combination so as to modify the autodestructive component of sepsis while preserving the favorable aspects of the immune response.*

At first glance, the current focus of biological response modification on cell proliferation and growth factors seems to be a recycling of the oncologists' interest in chemical strategies for limiting tumor growth. Although correct in part, such analysis is incomplete. The discovery of growth factors—extracellular macromolecules which can accelerate or retard cell cycling, division and expansion—provided valuable insights into the mechanisms by which such events are limited in normal tissues. But the identification, cloning and synthesis of dozens of such growth factors has made also available to surgeons a new set of tools with which to attack an old problem: poor healing of wounds.

All surgery involves the management of wounds. Healing is satisfactory in most cases, retarded in others, absent in a few—but in every case never fast enough nor strong enough for either surgeon or patient. Indeed, perhaps the greatest spur to the development of laparoscopic surgery was the desire to limit the size of iatrogenic wounds. Hunt and many others are presently applying combinations of synthetic growth factors to poorly healing wounds. In so doing, these investigators have gone beyond merely setting the stage for healing to manipulating multiple cell populations and their programs of gene expression in order to accelerate the synthesis and remodelling of repair molecules such a collagen. Here, even minor successes will have a substantial impact; consider the enormous economic effect of shortening by even a few percent the current recuperative period presently required after major operative surgery.

What lies ahead? Studies in our own laboratory are aimed at unravelling the cellular events which follow shock and resuscitation. Building on the startling observation that at least part of what we learned as ischemic injury actually does not occur until reperfusion,[9] we have observed that cells have a limited repertoire of responses to a wide variety of physiologic and environmental stresses. Moreover, we have observed that modern resuscitation from deep shock triggers several programs of gene expression which appear to be independently salutary but in combination are quite detrimental to cells and the tissues which they constitute.[10,11] Again, the eons of evolution could not have anticipated the restorative effects of hollow needles and intravenous fluids. Until quite recently, patients sustained such overwhelming stimuli for multiple programs of stress gene expression only as a preterminal event.

Is there a risk in all of this meddling? Yes, but it is probably minuscule. As long as we restrict our interventions to small numbers of humans who are unlikely to reproduce after their life-threatening process has been reversed, there should be no significant effect on the population as a whole. But as biological response modification becomes a common therapeutic strategy, surgeons in general and pediatric surgeons in particular could well be challenged to evaluate the long-term population effects of saving critically ill patients who will subsequently reproduce, and possibly perpetuate adverse mutations which otherwise would be lost from the gene pool. I do not mean to suggest that care should be withheld from any individual who might benefit, but rather that surgeons consider the potential effects of that care from a population perspective which many find unfamiliar.

Where are we going? Back, I think, to the pathology laboratory. The next ten years will see that discipline recast by the tools of molecular biology from a largely descriptive science to a mechanistic one. In a very real sense, we are going back to Darwin. This time, however, our goal will be to study not the successes but rather the failures of natural selection. Scientists are defining most inherited diseases in molecular terms. Intensivists—

clinical pathophysiologists—are coming to understand the notion that acquired molecular pathology—for example, the failure of anemic patients to synthesize erythropoietin—can be treated by molecular replacement.

As intensivists we are redefining our patients in terms of the biological response to injury, thinking more about the systemic effects of trauma than about the injuries themselves. And we will begin to manipulate those effects. We will manipulate skeletal and hepatic metabolism with targeted reagents which will be able to modulate intermediary metabolism and even reprogram gene expression in selected cell populations. Nutritional support will give way to a more global concept of metabolic intervention. Patients will benefit from current wound healing studies. We will apply the advances in prevention of sepsis syndrome to our at risk population.

Ten years ago Horace Judson summarized the advances in molecular biology in a book entitled, *The Eighth Day of Creation*. His history was accurate, but his visionary title was perhaps a little short-sighted. We are no longer as concerned with creating new forms of life as we are concerned with re-creating ourselves, cell by cell, response by response, tissue by tissue. Fifty years go, replacing whole organs was a dream. Today, French Anderson and other pioneers at the NIH are using gene replacement therapy to manage human disease.[12] Clinical reprogramming of genetically based events is now a reality.

For those of us at the front lines, in the trauma rooms and in the ICU, the potential of biological response modification as a therapeutic modality is great. Whether we will learn to apply this therapy wisely, effectively, economically and safely remains to be seen.

REFERENCES

1. Porter PJ, Spievach AR, Kass EH. Endotoxin-like activity of serum from patients with severe localized infections. New Engl J Med 1964; 271:445-447.
2. Ziegler EJ, McCutchan A, Fierer J et al. Treatment of gram-negative bacteremia and shock with human antiserum to a mutant Escherichia coli. N Engl J Med 1982; 307:1225-1230.
3. Teng NNH, Kaplan HS, Hebert JM et al. Protection against gram-negative bacteremia and endotoxemia with human monoclonal IgM antibodies. Proc Natl Acad Sci USA 1985; 82:1790-1794.
4. Ziegler EJ, Fisher CJ et al. Treatment of gram-negative bacteremia and septic shock with HA-1A human monoclonal antibodies. N Engl J Med 1991; 324:429-436.
5. Greenman RL, Schein RMH et al. A controlled clinical trial of ES murine monoclonal IgM antibody to endotoxin in the treatment of gram-negative sepsis. JAMA 1991; 266 (8):1097-1102.
6. Beutler B, Krochin N, Milsark IW et al. Control of cachectin (tumor necrosis factor) synthesis: Mechanisms of endotoxin resistance. Science 1986; 232:977.
7. Tracey KJ, Fang Y et al. Anticachectin/TNF monoclonal antibodies prevent septic shock during lethal bacteremia. Nature 1987; 330:662-664.
8. Ohlsson K, Bjork P et al. Interleukin-1 receptor antagonist reduces mortality from endotoxin shock. Nature 1990; 348:550-552.
9. Granger DN, McCord JM et al. Superoxide radicals in feline intestinal ischemia. Gastroenterology 1981; 81:22.
10. Buchman TG, Cabin DE, Vickers S et al. Molecular biology of circulatory shock: II. Expression of four groups of hepatic genes is enhanced following resuscitation from cardiogenic shock. Surgery 1990; 108:559-566.
11. Buchman TG, Cabin DE. Molecular biology of circulatory shock: III. HepG2 cells demonstrate two patterns of shock-induced gene expression which are independent, exclusive and prioritized. Surgery 1990; 108:902-911.
12. Culver K, Cornetta K, Morgan R et al. Lymphocytes as cellular vehicles for gene therapy in mouse and man. Proc Natl Acad Sci USA 1991; 88 (18):3155-3159.

CHAPTER 13

NUTRITIONAL SUPPORT OF THE INJURED PATIENT

Robert C. Morris

Nutritional or metabolic support of the injured patient encompasses a number of patient groups. The response to stress, that is, trauma with soft tissue or bony injury, significant thermal burns, or even infection is generally similar. These patients can be considered at various points along the spectrum of response that correlates change in metabolic activity with disease process.[2] However, when a specific disease process is considered, such as trauma, the correlation of metabolic activity and degree of injury may not be so clear, as one group showed no correlation between the injury severity score (ISS) and the degree of metabolic activity.[1]

Nutritional support of the injured patient is important because of the hypermetabolic response. The response to stress leads to a condition of increased energy expenditure. If this process is allowed to go unsupported, the consequences can be life threatening as a result of the obligatory body wasting that occurs.

THE METABOLIC RESPONSE TO INJURY

Historically, one of the earliest descriptions of the response to injury was reported by Cuthbertson. He showed that in patients who sustained long bone injuries a hypercatabolic state was produced and that excretion of N, S and P increased in proportion to amounts charactristics of cellular tissue.[3] It was Cuthbertson who initially described the "ebb" and "flow" phase of this response. As the "ebb" phase corresponds to the period immediately after injury it is generally short-lived and is due to hypovolemia and increased sympathetic activity. In mild degrees of stress, there may be no 'ebb' phase. The flow phase is prolonged and is characterized by negative nitrogen balance." The mediators of this response are both hormonal and inflammatory. In the early phase, as mentioned above, catecholamine stimulation with increased secretion of epinephrine and norepinephrine occurs. This is generally short lived and is complete within the first 24 hours. Also, during this early phase, certain hormonal responses occur which are characterized by increased secretion of glucagon and cortisol. The fact that these hormones are important has been validated by the infusion of cortisol, glucagon and adrenaline in normal volunteers. The infusion resulted in a raised basal metabolic rate, hyperglycemia, hyperinsulinemia and negative nitrogen

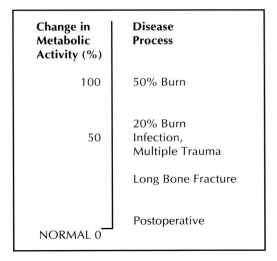

Change in Metabolic Activity (%)	Disease Process
100	50% Burn
50	20% Burn Infection, Multiple Trauma
	Long Bone Fracture
	Postoperative
NORMAL 0	

Fig.1. Adapted from Rombeau J L, Rolandelli RH, Wilmore D W. Nutritional Support. In: Care of the Surgical Patient.. New York: Scientific American Medicine 1991: Chapter 10

balance. Also, interleukin-1 and other cytokines have been implicated in the response as well. The known effects of cytokines are fever, granulopoesis, synthesis of acute-phase proteins and hyperinsulinemia. These effects are probably mediated by prostaglandins.

SUBSTRATE METABOLISM

As the hypermetabolic response is characterized by nitrogen loss and hyperglycemia, it is useful to examine fuel utilization. Control of gluconeogenesis comes under the hormonal influences of glucagon, epinephrine and cortisol. Insulin inhibits the process as well as plasma glucose under normal conditions. The central nervous system and red blood cells are dependent on glucose for energy and have a relatively constant rate of uptake and oxidation of glucose. In starvation, the brain adapts to the use of ketones; but in stress, ketogenesis is suppressed. Under normal circumstances, insulin inhibits the rate of hepatic glucose production and stimulates glucose uptake in muscle and adipose tissue, primarily. The threshold for the action of insulin on peripheral uptake is higher than the threshold for the effect of insulin on

hepatic production. During stress associated with injury and/or infection the effects of both insulin and glucose to suppress hepatic production of glucose are decreased. Glucose production in stress is mediated by hormonal stimulation at the liver where the hormones involved are glucagon and cortisol. The liver's capacity for glucose production is suppressed somewhat by the effects of glucose and insulin but not to the effects expected because of glucagon and cortisol action. If sepsis is an additive factor, there seems to be an inhibitory factor active that counterbalances the effects of glucagon and cortisol.

The brain cannot use fatty acids as they cannot cross the blood brain barrier, and RBCs depend on ATP production by glycolysis as there are no mitochondria. In addition, glucose uptake is increased by the presence of actively metabolizing wound tissue. During stress then, these tissues are obligatory users of glucose and uptake occurs independently of insulin action. Only at high rates of glucose infusion or ingestion do changes in clearance mediated by insulin become important, and euglycemia generally cannot be maintained with glucose infusion that is markedly higher that the endogenous rate of glucose production.

Where plasma glucose is sufficiently high to elicit an insulin response in normal patients, this is blunted in the critically ill patient. That is, the muscle and adipose tissue response is decreased to the action of endogenous insulin though glucose levels are elevated. In one experiment, despite high rates of exogenous insulin, the maximum rate of glucose uptake achieved was 6 mg/kg/min.

Gluconeogenesis involves lactate as the most important precursor and since much of the lactate is derived form plasma glucose via glycolysis, the resynthesis of glucose from lactate is a cyclic reaction. The energy to resynthesize glucose comes from fat oxidation in the liver. Glycerol is another precursor, and can account for as much as 20% of total glucose production in a long fast or stress situation. Alanine is the major amino acid precursor for gluconeogenesis.[5]

In the stressed patient, there is an increase in fat mobilization and an increase in

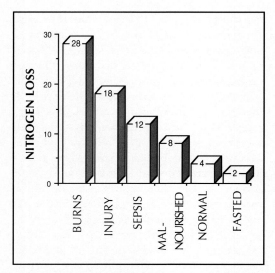

Fig. 2. Adapted from Goldstein SA, Elwyn DH. The effects of injury and sepsis on fuel utilization. Ann Rev Nutr 1989; 9:445-473.

fat oxidation. Ketone production is decreased. While lipolysis is increased, release of free fatty acids is reduced. This is described as futile cycling. Free fatty acid oxidation occurs at sites close to triglyceride hydrolysis, as free fatty acid levels are not elevated in plasma. In the liver, glucagon stimulates free fatty acid oxidation, whereas insulin stimulates lipogenesis by way of free fatty acid esterification.

In hypermetabolic patients, there is net fat oxidation or decreased lipogenesis or both. When glucose is provided in amounts of 1.2-1.5 REE, RQ rises but does not exceed 1.0, though an increase in CO_2 production occurs. In stress, there is a relative insensitivity of lipolysis to insulin, leading to increased free fatty acid turnover. Glucose oxidation is inhibited as a result of increased free fatty acid uptake and oxidation. When glucose intake is increased, lipogenesis does occur but not enough to result in an RQ greater than 1.0. Decreased lipogenesis together with inhibition of glucose oxidation results in the accumulation of glycogen in the liver and in the accumulation of triglyceride in the liver by lipogenesis, though at a reduced rate. Fat accumulates because of FAA reesterification, as the metabolic fate of glucose is either oxidation, glycogen deposition, or fat synthesis. Ketogenesis is suppressed by the effects of insulin.[6]

Skeletal muscle is the major site of nitro-

gen storage and nitrogen loss. In the stressed patient, there is an obligatory requirement for glucose by the brain since the adaptive response of brain utilization of ketone bodies does not occur as ketogenesis is suppressed. Brain oxidation is higher than normal, and this increase is quantitively the most important factor requiring increased muscle proteolysis. Normal daily requirement by the brain is 120 g glucose and would require 200 g protein (32 g N). Other processes require amino acids including protein synthesis in the wound, synthesis in liver for acute phase proteins and protein synthesis in inflammatory cells. Net catabolism of body protein occurs with the amount dependent on severity and type of injury. (Fig. 2) This was a study where N excretion was measured during 5% dextrose infusion. The numbers represent grams of N per 70 kg of body weight. Nitrogen balance (lessening of net N or protein loss) can be improved in response to N and energy intake.[3]

As described previously, catabolism of muscle protein provides substrate for hepatic and wound protein synthesis, and for gluconeogenesis. The mediators of this response appear to be glucagon and interleukin-1, with a lesser contribution by glucocorticoids.

A summary of the metabolic response to stress is shown in Fig. 3.[7]

Nutritional Support

Nutritional support of the injured patient should attempt to ameliorate the nitrogen loss that occurs as a result of the hypermetabolic response and to minimize any further problem with hyperglycemia. The strategies of providing nutritional support will be discussed.

Patients who are injured and starved have an accelerated loss of tissue in comparison to pure starvation. Patient selection is dictated by several factors: whether the patient was malnourished before injury, whether intolerance to feeding exists or is expected and whether the patient will require frequent trips to the operating room. When to feed the patient is generally a matter of clinical judgment. The enteral route of feeding is preferred as there is evidence of gut function early and feeding provides some protective effect from nonuse. The feasibility of early feeding has been demonstrated with no adverse consequences. In one study, it was shown that enteral feeding can be done early in injured patients with slowing of nitrogen loss and decrease in infectious complications.[8] In a second study, it was shown that because nitrogen loss was lessened or eliminated equally between groups and infectious complications were similar,[9] enteral feeding was as good as provision of nutrients parenterally.

When parenteral nutrition is required, multiple strategies are available for providing nutritional support both peripherally and centrally. One report suggests beginning patients on a peripheral regimen when there is a question of patient tolerance or of timing of enteral feeding. A standardized solution is given which has a volume of approximately 3000 ml and contains 100 grams of fat, 60 grams of amino acids and 240 grams of glucose. The solution can be given safely over 24 hours without risk of metabolic complications.[10]

ESTIMATION OF ENERGY EXPENDITURE

Before discussing estimation of energy expenditure, it is useful to define the components that are frequently described. Basal metabolic rate (BMR) is defined as the energy expenditure of a subject lying down and resting in a thermoneutral environment, having fasted for the previous 12 hours. Resting energy expenditure (REE) is the metabolic rate calculated from measurements made during rest in patients receiving continuous nutrition. REE is 110% of BMR, as this includes the specific dynamic action of foods or what is known as diet induced thermogenesis.

Measurement of energy expenditure is not readily performed, and estimating energy expenditure can be done using a number of

Hormones	Starvation Early	Starvation Prolonged	Stress
Epinephrine	↑	↓	↑↑
Cortisol	↑	↑	↑↑
Glucagon	↑↑	↑	↑
Insulin	↓	↓	↑
Metabolism			
Rate	No Change	↓	↑↑
RQ	No Change	↓	↑
Energy Substrate			
Glycerol	↑↑	↑↑	↑
Fatty Acids	↑↑	↑↑	↑
Glucose	↓	↓	↑↑
Ketones	↑↑	↑↑	↑
Lactate	↑	↑	↑↑
Alanine	↓	↓	↑
Fuel Utilization			
Fatty Acids	↑	↑	↓
Glucose	↑	↑	↓
Amino Acids	↑	↑	↑↑

Figure 3. Adapted from Deppe S.A. Metabolism in starvation, illness and injury. Problems in Critical Care. 1988; 2:547-555.

equations. The most common method reported of estimating energy expenditure is use of the Harris-Benedict equations. An estimate of resting energy expenditure can be done with the height, weight and age of the patient. One of the limitations using the Harris-Benedict equations is that they were derived from measurement made in normal subjects. What is felt to be a better estimate of energy expenditure is the use of indirect calorimetry performed by the gas exchange method. However, there are also limitations in methodology. These include high inspired fraction of oxygen, especially in mechanically ventilated patients, and problems determining oxygen consumption and carbon dioxide production due to leaks in the system, unstable gas analyzers and inaccurate volume measurements. Despite this, the use of indirect calorimetry can provide important information as measured vs. predicted REE may vary with a range of 70% to 140%. Reasons include fluid status, spontaneous vs. mechanically assisted ventilation, body temperature, drugs such as narcotics that may alter metabolic rate, state of illness or use of neuromuscular blocking agents.[11] Two recent reports of the utility of the metabolic cart are summarized. In a group of critically ill patients, the metabolic cart was used to determine REE. Fifteen percent of studies showed patients to be hypometabolic and 62% to be hypermetabolic. Use of the Harris-Benedict equation underestimated needs, but addition of an activity factor overestimated needs. Only 32% of patients were fed appropriately, 41% were underfed and 27% were overfed.[12] In a second group of head injured patients, indirect calorimetry was employed to measure REE. REE was an average of 160% of that predicted by the Harris-Benedict equation with no value less than 112%.[13]

It must be remembered that an estimation of energy expenditure is just somewhat of an educated guess. The patient that needs more intensive study of energy expenditure is the one in which there is significant nitrogen catabolism and sustained stress beyond two to three weeks. Knowledge of the limitations and the appropriate clinical setting should dictate the technique that is chosen.

NUTRIENT COMPOSITION

Once energy expenditure has been determined, the components can be assembled based upon a patient's particular needs. Protein requirements depend on the nutritional state of the patient. As most injured patients are well nourished or mildly malnourished prior to injury the strategy should be directed toward minimizing the loss of body cell mass. In this patient group nitrogen intake at 100-400 mg/kg/day should be provided. This is equivalent to ~1.0-2.5 grams of protein or amino acids/kg/day. This amount of nitrogen should limit loss to 3-4 grams per day. Nitrogen balance can be monitored by determining nitrogen loss in the urine. This can be done by a 24 hour urine collection and determining urine urea nitrogen. A constant is then added to approximate losses via skin and stool. Nitrogen intake can then be adjusted accordingly.

At least 100-150 grams/day of carbohydrate should be provided as glucose. Glucose should never be given in excess of 6 mg/kg/day or ~600 grams/day for the patient of normal body weight. At this level glucose uptake is saturated despite use of exogenous insulin. As fat oxidation does occur, fat can be provided as half of the nonprotein calories. Calorie provision with a mixed fuel source potentially limits the risk of hyperglycemia, respiratory failure and fatty acid deficiency. Electrolytes and minerals should be added to prevent hyponatremia, hypokalemia, hypomagnesemia, hypophosphatemia, vitamin and trace mineral deficiency. An algorithm is described (Fig. 4) where metabolic support is initiated with frequent monitoring of results and adjustment of the dose of nutrient components.[14]

Newer nutrients are being postulated as having a potential beneficial role in improving overall nutritional status or improving immune function. These include nucleic acids, omega-3 fatty acids, arginine, parenteral analogs of glutamine and branched chained enriched formulations of amino acids. The role of these have not been defined as the benefits versus conventional formulations have not been clearly demonstrated.

```
┌─────────────────────────────────────┐
│      Metabolic Support in the ICU    │
└─────────────────────────────────────┘
                  ▄
┌─────────────────────────────────────┐
│  Initiation                          │
│      fat:1.0 gm/kg/d                 │
│      glucose:4-5 gm/kg/d             │
│      amino acids:2.0 gm/kg/d         │
└─────────────────────────────────────┘
                  ▄
┌─────────────────────────────────────┐
│  Monitoring                          │
│      nitrogen balance                │
│      BUN                             │
│      RQ                              │
│      acute phase proteins            │
│      lytes, LFT's                    │
└─────────────────────────────────────┘
                  ▄
┌─────────────────────────────────────┐
│  Adjust Dosing                       │
│      positive nitrogen balance       │
│      R/Q ~ 0.9                       │
│      BUN<100 mg%                     │
│      rising prealbumin or transferrin│
│      ✓ lytes, Mg, Zn, Ca PO4         │
└─────────────────────────────────────┘
```

Fig. 4. Adapted from Cerra FB. Nutrient modulation of inflammatory and immune function. Amer J Surg 1991; 161:30-34.

Summary

Appropriate timing of feeding is not the total answer to control the hypermetabolic state, as feeding does not seem to blunt the early response to injury.[15] Metabolic support is important to lessen the effects of the obligatory nitrogen loss that occurs.

The metabolic response to injury is probably adaptive.[3] Fasting without injury elicits a protein sparing and fat consuming economy. With injury superimposed, the wound adds obligate glucose and amino acid consumption, with fat consumption continuing, but providing a lesser fraction of total energy expenditure and protein providing a greater portion. Hyperglycemia provides a glucose concentration gradient to the relatively ischemic wound and provides a continual source of fuel to insulin-independent tissue. Increased substrate cycles involving glucose, lipid, and protein are obligatory and contrib-

ute to energy expenditure. Compared to normal, fasted individuals, more carbohydrate is needed to reduce gluconeogenesis and more protein is required to reduce muscle catabolism. Metabolic, and hence dietary therapy should be provided to support the altered pattern of fuel utilization, that is, maintenance of the adaptive response while preventing undue body wasting.

References

1. Shaw JHF, Wolfe RR. An integrated analysis of glucose, fat and protein metabolism in severely traumatized patients. Ann Surg 1989; 209:63-72.
2. Rombeau JL, Rolandelli RH, Wilmore DW. Nutritional Support. In: Care of the Surgical Patient. New York: Scientific American, Inc, 1991:Ch. 10.
3. Goldstein SA, Elwyn OH. The effects of injury and sepsis on fuel utilization. Ann Rev Nutr 1989; 9:445-473.
4. Douglas RG, Shaw JHF.: Metabolic response to sepsis and trauma. Br J Surg 1989; 76:115-122.
5. Wolfe RR. Carbohydrate metabolism in the critically ill patient. Crit Care Clin 1987; 3: 11-25.
6. Wiener M, Rothkopf MM, Rothkopf G et al. Fat metabolism in injury and stress. Crit Care Clin 1987; 3:25-55,1987.
7. Deppe SA. Metabolism in starvation, illness and injury. Prob Crit Care 1988; 2:547-555.
8. Moore EE, Jones TN. Benefits of immediate jejunostomy feeding after major abdominal trauma: A prospective, randomized study. J Trauma 1986; 26:874-881.
9. Adams S, Dellinger EP, Wertz MJ et al. Enteral versus parenteral nutritional support following laparotomy for trauma: A randomized prospective trial. J Trauma 1986; 26:882-891.
10. VanWay CW. Nutritional support in the injured patient. Surg Clin N Amer 1991; 71:537-548.
11. Damask MC, Schwarz Y, Wiessman C. Energy measurements and requirements of criticaily ill patients. Crit Care Clin 1987; 3:71-96.
12. Makk LJK, McClave SA, Creech PW et al. Clinical application of the metabolic cart to the delivery of total parenteral nutrition. Crit Care Med 1990; 18:1320-1327.
13. Moore R, Najarian MP, Konvolinka CW. Measured energy expenditure in severe head trauma. J Trauma 1989; 29:1633-1636.
14. Cerra FB. Nutrient modulation of inflammatory and immune function. Amer J Surg 1991; 161:230-234.
15. Poret HA, Kudsk KA, Croce MA et al. The effect of enteral feeding on catecholamine response following trauma. Surg Forum 1991; 42:11-13.

CHAPTER 14

BACTERIAL TRANSLOCATION AND GUT BARRIER FAILURE

Mark R. Mainous
Edwin A. Deitch

INTRODUCTION

Multiple organ failure (MOF) continues to be a leading cause of death in critically ill patients. Although MOF has been the subject of extensive laboratory and clinical investigation over the past two decades, the precise mechanisms responsible for its onset and progression remain unknown. It appears clear, however, that MOF is a systemic process mediated by various endogenous and exogenous factors which results in the sequential failure of organ systems distant from the site of injury or primary disease, usually with a lag period of days to weeks between the initial insult and the development of MOF.

It has been suggested that MOF is the external expression of a septic syndrome secondary to the presence of uncontrolled infection.[1-3] This concept was widely accepted in the late 1970s and prompted several authorities to advocate empiric laparotomy for any patient who developed MOF in the absence of a clinically identifiable source of infection.[3,4]

Unfortunately, as more and more patients dying of MOF were subjected to abdominal exploration in search of an occult septic focus, it became clear that in a large proportion of these patients a source of infection could not be identified either clinically or at autopsy.[5-9]

Over the past decade, increasing clinical and laboratory evidence has accumulated supporting the concept that gut barrier failure may play a major role in the etiology of MOF. It is hypothesized that failure of the gut mucosal barrier may allow bacteria and endotoxin normally contained within the gastrointestinal tract to enter the portal circulation or gut lymphatics and to subsequently initiate a septic process leading to the development of MOF. The term "gut septic states" has been used by Border and coworkers to describe this phenomenon, [10] and Meakins has described the gut as the "motor" of MOF.[9]

Investigators working in Fine's laboratory in the 1950s and 1960s were the first to demonstrate that bacteria and endotoxin could escape from the gut and overwhelm the reticuloendothelial system resulting in sepsis and irreversible shock.[11-15] Wolochow, in 1966, coined the term "bacterial translocation" (BT) to describe the passage of bacteria across the intestinal wall.[16] This early work on BT was largely ignored for nearly 20 years, until several epidemiological studies were published documenting that the gastrointestinal tract is a clinically important reservoir for bacteria and fungi capable of causing life-threatening systemic infections in bone marrow recipients [17] and in granulocytopenic patients with hematologic malignancies.[18,19] Despite strong clinical evidence implicating the gastrointestinal tract as a reservoir of potential pathogens capable of causing systemic infection, the underlying mechanisms of how bacteria translocate across the gut mucosal barrier were poorly understood. The focus of our laboratory over the past decade has been to investigate potential mechanisms responsible for failure of the gut mucosal barrier as well as the relationships between the intestinal microflora, trauma, host defenses and MOF. In this review, experimental and clinical evidence supporting the concept of BT will be presented.

BIOLOGY OF INTESTINAL BARRIER FUNCTION

The gut lumen contains extremely high concentrations of bacteria and endotoxin; nevertheless, healthy individuals are remarkably resistant to BT. In order for BT to take place, a bacterium must first adhere to the epithelial cell surface, after which it must pass through or between the enterocytes to reach the lamina propria.[20] Unless the translocating bacteria or their products are able to invade the lymphatics or bloodstream and then spread systemically, the process will be of no clinical significance. Multiple defense mechanisms have evolved which function together to prevent this process from occurring. These defense mechanisms include the stabilizing influence of the indigenous intestinal microflora, mechanical defenses and immunological defenses.

One major defense against BT is the indigenous intestinal microflora itself. Van der Waaij coined the term "colonization resistance" to describe the protective role of the indigenous gut microflora in preventing the overgrowth of potential pathogens.[21] He demonstrated that by altering the ecology of the indigenous gut microflora using antibiotics, the resistance of the gut to the colonization of pathogens could be decreased.[21-23] It is now evident that the obligate anaerobic bacteria are responsible for colonization resistance. They outnumber the enteric gram-negative and aerobic gram-positive bacteria by 1000- to 10,000-fold and associate closely with the intestinal epithelium, forming, in effect, a barrier limiting the direct attachment of potential translocating bacteria to the epithelial cells. This anaerobic barrier is lost when broad spectrum antibiotics are administered because the obligate anaerobes are more sensitive to antibiotic suppression than is the remainder of the gut flora.[24] Loss of the anaerobic barrier then allows for the direct attachment of potential pathogens to the intestinal epithelium.

A second line of defense against BT is provided by the mechanical defenses of the gut. The intestinal mucus layer appears to be important in preventing bacterial adherence to the intestinal epithelium. Elimination of the mucus layer has been shown to result in increased numbers of bacteria adhering directly to the enterocytes.[25] In addition, small intestinal peristalsis prevents prolonged stasis of bacteria in close proximity to the intestinal mucosa and thereby reduces the chance that bacteria may have adequate time to penetrate the mucus layer and adhere directly to the epithelium. If peristalsis is impaired, as occurs with bowel obstruction or ileus, bacterial stasis will result, providing the bacteria with an increased opportunity to penetrate the mucus layer and adhere to the intestinal epithelium.[26,27]

The intestinal immune system, known as the gut-associated lymphoid tissue (GALT), regulates the local immune response to soluble and particulate antigens within the gastrointestinal tract. The exact role of the GALT in preventing bacterial adherence and translocation is unclear; however, it appears that secretory IgA produced by antigen-primed B lymphocytes lining the mucosal surface prevents mucosal invasion by binding to bacteria and blocking their attachment to epithelial cells without activating other arms of the immune system.[28,29] The importance of secretory IgA in preventing BT is unclear, however, since patients with selective IgA deficiencies are not at increased risk for developing gut-origin sepsis. Nevertheless, they do compensate for their IgA deficiency by producing increased amounts of secretory IgM.[30] Bile appears to be an important factor in preventing the escape of endotoxin from the gut. Bile salts are thought to prevent endotoxemia by binding to intraluminal endotoxin and forming detergent-like complexes that are poorly absorbed by the gut.[31,32] Although low levels of portal endotoxemia may occur normally, the reticuloendothelial cells of the liver are very efficient in clearing endotoxin from the portal blood. Systemic endotoxemia does not occur unless the reticuloendothelial function of the liver is impaired.[33]

Each of these defense mechanisms may be impaired in critically ill patients at risk of developing MOF. Many of these patients receive broad-spectrum antibiotics which disrupt the normal ecology of the gut microflora thereby leading to the overgrowth of potential pathogens. Alkalinization of the stomach for prophylaxis against stress bleeding may result in the colonization of the stomach with ingested bacteria. The presence of ileus may result in small intestinal stasis and bacterial overgrowth. The use of vasoactive drugs may cause a decrease in splanchnic blood flow, resulting in ischemic injury to the gut epithelium. Hyperosmolar enteral feedings or parenteral feedings may disrupt the ecology of the indigenous gut microflora as well as impair the mechanical defenses of the gut. Intestinal edema secondary to hypoalbuminemia and capillary leak syndrome may impair peristalsis and result in bacterial stasis, bacterial overgrowth and altered gut permeability. Furthermore, hepatic failure or obstructive jaundice may allow endotoxin to reach the systemic circulation, where it may induce a septic-like state. Thus, these and other conditions commonly seen in critically ill patients may promote failure of the gut mucosal barrier to bacteria and endotoxin.

EXPERIMENTAL EVIDENCE OF BACTERIAL TRANSLOCATION

There now exists a large body of evidence to suggest that BT may occur in critically ill patients and may contribute to the septic response and to the development of MOF. The focus of our laboratory investigations has been to study the various mechanisms by which BT may occur using several in vivo rodent models which mimic clinical situations commonly seen in critically ill patients. In these models, the animals are subjected to an actual or sham insult, and then killed at various time intervals following the insult. Blood, peritoneal fluid, the mesenteric lymph node complex (MLN) and various organs are harvested and cultured for translocating bacteria. The MLN receives its lymphatic drainage from the small intestine, cecum and proximal colon, and is normally sterile. Therefore, the presence of viable bacteria within the MLN is a very sensitive marker of BT. Additionally, cecal bacterial population levels are quantitated to determine the effect of the specific insult on the ecology of the indigenous gut microflora. Sections of the ileum and cecum are also examined histologically to determine the extent, if any, to which the gut mucosa has been damaged.

Our studies demonstrate that certain conditions commonly encountered in critically ill patients may promote BT. Furthermore, it appears that at least one of three basic pathophysiologic factors must exist in order for BT to occur: 1) disruption of the ecologic balance of the gut microflora; 2) physical disruption or impairment of the gut mucosal barrier; and 3) impairment of host immune defenses. In addition, BT is not an all-or-none phenomenon. Disruption or impairment of a single major intestinal defense mechanism will result in the translocation of bacteria to the MLN and occasionally to the liver and spleen where they are usually locally contained and cleared as the animal recovers. In conditions that more closely mimic the true clinical situation in which the animal receives several simultaneous or sequential insults, systemic BT is the rule. In some of these combined injury models, the majority of animals survive, while in other models the animals ultimately die in a septic-like state.

A nonlethal burn injury model was chosen initially in order to examine the relationship between BT and trauma. By altering the size of the thermal injury, the effect of varying levels of trauma on gut barrier function could be assessed.[34-36] BT occurred only in those animals receiving at least a 40% burn and was limited to the MLN. No systemic spread of bacteria occurred, and in the animals receiving less than a 40% burn even the MLNs remained sterile. We conclude from these studies that in healthy animals with a normal gut flora, BT does not occur following trauma unless the magnitude of the injury is relatively severe. These findings have been supported using other nonlethal trauma models.[37]

Since disruption of the ecology of the normal gut flora is common in severely injured patients as well as in those receiving broad-spectrum antibiotics, the effect of thermal injury on BT was also tested on animals whose gut flora had been disrupted either by sterilization of the gut followed by mono-association with *Escherichia coli* or by the administration of oral antibiotics which selectively kill the obligate anaerobes. In both of these models, not only did BT occur in those animals with less severe burns, but it involved systemic organs as well as the MLN.[35,36] These results suggest that the combination of trauma and intestinal overgrowth with gram-negative enteric bacilli results in the synergistic spread of bacteria from the gut to systemic organs.

Because of the clinical association between shock, infection and the development of MOF, we tested whether limited periods of hypotension (up to 90 minutes) would induce BT in a rat model of hemorrhagic shock.[38] Hemorrhagic shock consistently resulted in systemic BT, with the magnitude of BT and the mortality rate directly related to the duration of shock. Additionally, the mechanism of BT appears to be related to injury to the gut mucosal barrier, since the severity of mucosal damage increased as the duration of shock increased. These results are consistent with those of Chiu[39] who documented a cor-

relation between the magnitude of the mucosal injury with the severity of intestinal ischemia. Furthermore, the histologic appearance of the ileal mucosa in the shocked rats was similar to that reported in humans who had experienced periods of hypotension.[40,41]

Protein malnutrition is a common problem in critically ill patients, who often receive nutritional support via parenteral or enteral elemental diets. Although we have been unable to demonstrate evidence of BT in enterally fed, protein malnourished animals,[42] we and others have documented that parenteral[43,44] and enteral[44,45] elemental diets may promote BT. In addition, in a rat model, we have demonstrated that administration of an enteral elemental diet not only promotes BT but is associated with in vitro and in vivo depression of T lymphocyte-mediated immune function, all of which may be reversed rapidly by reinstituting a normal diet.[46]

Endotoxemia is relatively common following thermal or mechanical trauma,[47-50] and is associated with various conditions leading to MOF.[9,51] In addition, endotoxin has been shown to impair host immune defenses[52] and to increase gut mucosal permeability.[53,54] We have demonstrated that in mice with a normal gut flora, nonlethal doses of endotoxin will promote BT in a dose-dependent fashion, although the translocating bacteria are limited to the MLN and do not spread systemically.[55] However, an otherwise nonlethal dose of endotoxin combined with either protein malnutrition[42] or thermal injury[56] will result in systemic BT and a lethal septic state.

Histologic examination of the ileum and cecum of endotoxin-challenged animals characteristically shows physical disruption of the gut mucosal barrier[57] with edema of the lamina propria and separation of the epithelium, especially at the villous tips, an appearance very similar to that seen following hemorrhagic shock.[38] The degree of mucosal injury and the magnitude of BT may be significantly reduced in both the endotoxin-challenged[57] and hemorrhagic shock-treated animals[58] by the inhibition (using allopurinol) or inactivation (using a molybdenum-free, tungsten-enriched diet) of xanthine oxidase activity, indicating that the mucosal injury in these two models is mediated, at least in part by xanthine oxidase-derived oxygen free radicals. This hypothesis has recently been supported by work from Herndon's laboratory using a sheep model.[59]

The exact routes by which translocating bacteria reach the MLN, blood and systemic organs are not known with certainty. It has been proposed by Wells and coworkers[60,61] that macrophages function to transport viable bacteria from the lamina propria of the gut to the MLN, at which point they escape the MLN and gain access to the systemic circulation via the thoracic duct. We have recently demonstrated, using a model of systemic inflammation, that bacteria are capable of exiting the gut via both the mesenteric lymphatics and the portal blood, and that, in the face of a major inflammatory insult, the portal blood may be the most important route for the systemic spread of bacteria from the gut.[62]

Human data on BT is quite limited. We have shown that MLNs obtained at laparotomy from patients undergoing elective surgery rarely contain bacteria (4%), in contrast to 59% of patients operated on for simple small bowel obstruction in the absence of necrotic bowel or positive peritoneal fluid cultures.[63] The results of this study were similar to those reported by Ambrose and colleagues,[64] who sampled ileal serosa and MLNs from patients with and without Crohn's disease. They found that only 5% of patients without Crohn's disease had viable bacteria in their MLNs as opposed to 33% of patients with Crohn's disease. Based on an anecdotal report by Krause and coworkers,[65] in which *Candida* was recovered from the blood and urine of a healthy volunteer who drank a large quantity of *Candida albicans*, it appears that *Candida* is also capable of translocating from the gut. Rush has documented the presence of bacteremia and endotoxemia in the absence of visceral perforation in trauma victims admitted to the emergency room in shock.[50]

In addition to these studies, there have been three clinical reports indicating that intestinal permeability may be increased during an infectious episode,[66] shortly after major thermal injury,[67] or in healthy human volunteers who receive a single dose of endotoxin.[68] In addition, Marshall and colleagues,[69] in a large series of critically ill patients, have demonstrated the upper gastrointestinal tract to be an occult reservoir for organisms responsible for intensive care unit acquired infections. Although limited, the existing clinical evidence supports the concept that BT does indeed occur in humans.

RELATIONSHIP OF BACTERIAL TRANSLOCATION TO MULTIPLE ORGAN FAILURE

The precise relationship between BT and MOF is not known. Nevertheless, considerable data now exists which supports the concept that gut barrier failure may play a significant role in the pathogenesis of MOF. In addition, the defense mechanisms which normally protect the integrity of the gut mucosal barrier are frequently impaired in critically ill patients. Many of these patients are in some way immunocompromised and commonly receive broad-spectrum antibiotic therapy with resultant overgrowth by potential pathogens. Alkalinization of the stomach for stress bleeding prophylaxis in intubated patients may result in colonization of the stomach with oral flora and predispose to pneumonias and other infectious complications.[69,70] Hypotension or the use of vasoactive drugs may result in splanchnic hypoperfusion and lead to damage to the gastric or intestinal mucosa. Other factors, such as ileus, intolerance of enteral feedings and nutritional deficiencies may further impair gut barrier function.

If gut barrier failure does occur, the integrity of the reticuloendothelial function of the liver may play a critical role in preventing systemic sepsis and distant organ injury. The clearance of bacteria and endotoxin from the portal blood is dependent on Kupffer cell phagocytic activity. There is evidence to suggest that low levels of portal vein endotoxin may play a physiologic role in helping maintain normal hepatic reticuloendothelial activity.[71] However, markedly increased levels of portal vein endotoxin may actually result in liver injury.[72] Conversely, in the face of liver injury, endotoxin clearance is impaired and systemic resistance to endotoxin is decreased.[73] It is thus conceivable that gut barrier failure may result in a vicious cycle in which the translocation of bacteria and endotoxin through the portal venous system may result in liver injury or further compromise an already failing liver. Impaired clearance of gut-derived bacteria and endotoxin may eventually lead to spillover of bacteria and endotoxin into the systemic circulation, which may result in increased gut permeability and further translocation of intestinal bacteria and endotoxin. The ensuing septic state may eventually lead to distant organ injury which may be exacerbated by the release of various cytokines and other mediator substances from Kupffer cells and activated macrophages.

POTENTIAL THERAPY

The best treatment for gut barrier failure unquestionably lies in its prevention. Border and colleagues[10] have demonstrated in trauma victims that a policy of early definitive surgery, including prompt repair of injuries, debridement of necrotic tissues, control of bacterial contamination and early fixation of fractures is associated with a significant reduction in the incidence of gut-derived sepsis and MOF.

In addition, infection must be recognized and controlled early in its course. Abscesses must be adequately drained and systemic antibiotics used judiciously. In order to minimize intestinal bacterial overgrowth, perioperative antibiotics should be discontinued shortly after surgery, and when treating an established infection, the antibiotic spectrum should be kept as narrow as possible and administered for the shortest acceptable period of time.

The use of selective antibiotic decontamination of the gut to maintain colonization resistance has been documented to decrease the incidence of systemic infections in several groups of patients. However, since it is not clear whether selective antibiotic decontamination of the gut will improve survival, more information is needed before this approach

can be recommended for all patients at risk of developing MOF.

It is now clear that attempts to alkalinize the stomach in an effort to prevent stress bleeding may result in colonization of the stomach with gram-negative bacteria which may predispose to nosocomial pneumonias in intubated patients. Sucralfate provides cytoprotection for the gastric mucosa without raising the gastric pH and has been shown to be as effective as antacids or H_2-blockers in preventing stress bleeding, while minimizing the risk of nosocomial pneumonias in intubated patients.[74] Therefore, sucralfate appears to be the drug of choice in preventing stress-induced gastric bleeding in intubated patients.

Since the starved gut loses mucosal mass, villous height, and becomes more permeable to intraluminal bacteria and endotoxin, early enteral feeding appears to be important in maintaining gut mucosal integrity. Kudsk and coworkers have shown that animals receiving enteral nutrition tolerate a septic insult far better than do animals fed an identical diet parenterally.[75,76] Wilmore has suggested that gut barrier failure may occur in critically ill patients due to the fact that current methods of parenteral support do not support gut mucosal structure or function.[77]

Enteral nutrition may have beneficial systemic metabolic effects as well. Mochizuki and coworkers[78] have documented in a guinea pig model that immediate enteral feeding following thermal injury prevents the hypermetabolic response by maintaining gut mucosal mass and preventing the excessive secretion of catabolic hormones. The exact reason why enteral feedings maintain gut mucosal mass better than parenteral feedings is not fully understood although it appears that the optimal maintenance of gut mucosal mass and integrity requires the intraluminal delivery of nutrients as well as the availability of specific nutrients and factors not present in the currently available parenteral diets, such as glutamine[77] or bulk.[44] Furthermore, the protein content of the enteral formula is also important since high protein enteral feedings have been shown conclusively to improve host defenses, decrease the incidence of systemic infection and improve survival in thermally injured children.[79]

Recent studies also suggest that specific growth factors, such as epidermal growth factor and human growth hormone, may have trophic effects on the intestinal mucosa.[77] Therefore, in the future, optimal nutritional support may include a combination of specific enterally administered nutrients and mucosal trophic factors.

Nonintestinal factors may also impair gut barrier function. Hypotension, hemodynamic instability and vasoactive drugs, all of which may cause decreased gut perfusion, may promote BT by increasing intestinal permeability. Systemic insults or drugs that decrease intestinal motility may also be deleterious since ileus is associated with bacterial stasis and overgrowth. Thus, attention should be paid to the systemic factors that may influence intestinal function as well as to the factors which directly affect the gut.

CONCLUSION

It is unclear at this point exactly what role, if any, BT plays in the development of MOF. It is conceivable, however, that gut barrier failure may contribute to MOF by allowing bacteria and endotoxin to escape from the gut and enter the portal and systemic circulations where they may help fuel the septic process. We have demonstrated that at least one of three basic pathophysiological factors must be present in order for BT to occur. These factors include loss of colonization resistance, disruption of the gut mucosal barrier and impaired host immune defenses. Furthermore, BT is not an all-or-none phenomenon in that the relationship between the host's defense mechanisms and the magnitude of the insult determine whether the translocating bacteria and endotoxin are cleared or will cause systemic illness and remote organ injury. The status of the reticuloendothelial function of the liver may be important in limiting the magnitude of BT. Whether MOF can be prevented by the maintenance of the gut mucosal barrier, and whether survival can be improved in patients with established MOF by restoration of nor-

mal gut barrier function is unknown. Nevertheless, a large body of laboratory and clinical data exists which supports the hypothesis that BT may play an important role in the etiology of MOF, especially in those patients without a clinically identifiable focus of infection.

REFERENCES

1. Fry DE, Pearlstein L, Fulton RL et al. Multiple system organ failure: the role of uncontrolled infection. Arch Surg 1980; 115:136-140.
2. Baue AE. Multiple, progressive, or sequential systems failure: a syndrome of the 1970s. Arch Surg 1975; 110:779-781.
3. Polk HC, Shields CL. Remote organ failure: a valid sign of occult intraabdominal infection. Surgery 1977; 81:310-313.
4. Ferraris VA. Exploratory laparotomy for potential abdominal sepsis in patients with multiple organ failure. Arch Surg 1983; 118:1130-1133.
5. Meakins JL, Wickland B, Forse RA et al. The surgical intensive care unit: current concepts in infection. Surg Clin North Am 1980; 60:117-132.
6. Norton LW. Does drainage of intra-abdominal pus reverse multiple organ failure? Am J Surg 1985; 149:347-350.
7. Goris RJA, Boekhorst TPA, Nuytinck JKS et al. Multiple organ failure: generalized autodestructive inflammation. Arch Surg 1985; 120:1109-1115.
8. Faist E, Baue AE, Dittmer H et al. Multiple organ failure in polytrauma patients. J Trauma 1983; 23:775-787.
9. Carrico CJ, Meakins JL, Marshall JC et al. Multiple organ failure syndrome. Arch Surg 1986; 121:196-208.
10. Border JR, Hassett J, LaDuca J et al. Gut origin septic states in blunt multiple trauma (ISS=40) in the ICU. Ann Surg 1987; 206:427-446.
11. Ravin Ha, Rowley D, Jenkins C et al. On the absorption of bacterial endotoxin from the gastrointestinal tract of the normal and shocked animal. J Exp Med 1960; 112:783-790.
12. Jacob S, Weizel H, Gordon E et al. Bacterial action in the development of irreversibility to transfusion in hemorrhagic shock in the dog. Am J Physiol 1954; 179:523-540.
13. Schweinburg FB, Serigman AM, Fine J. Transmural migration of intestinal bacteria:study based on the use of radioactive Escherichia coli. N Engl J Med 1950; 242:747-751.
14. Fine J. Current status of the problem of traumatic shock. Surg Gynecol Obstet 1965; 120:537-544.
15. Ravin HA, Fine J. Biological implications of intestinal endotoxins. Fed Proc 1962; 21:65-68.
16. Wolochow H, Hildebrand GJ, Lammanna C. Translocation of microorganisms across the intestinal wall in rats:effect of microbial size and concenration. J Infect Dis 1966; 116:523-528.
17. Wells CL, Podzorski RP, Peterson PK et al. Incidence

of trimethoprim-sulfamethoxazole resistant Enterobacteriaceae among transplant recipients. J Infect Dis 1984; 150:699-706.

18. Tancrede CH, Andremont AO. Bacterial translocation and gram-negative bacteremia in patients with hematologic malignancies. J Infect Dis 1985; 152:99-103.

19. Schimpff SC. Infection prevention during profound granulocytopenia. An Intern Med 1980; 93:358-361.

20. Wells CL, Maddaus MA, Simmons RL. Proposed mechanisms for the translocation of enteric bacteria. Rev Infect Dis 1988; 10:95-979.

21. van der Waaij D, Berghuis-deVries JM, Lekkerkerk-van der Wees JEC. Colonization resistance of the digestive tract in conventional and antibiotic treated mice. J Hygiene (Camb) 1971; 69:405-411.

22. van der Waaij D, Berghuis-deVries JM, Lekkerkerk-van der Wees JEC. Colonization resistance of the digestive tracts and the spread of bacteria to the lymphatic organs in mice. J Hygiene (Camb) 1972; 70:3350342.

23. van der Waaij D, Berghuis-deVries JM, Lekkerkerk-van der Wees JEC. Colonization resistance of the digestive tract of mice during systemic antibiotic treatment. J Hygiene (Camb) 1972; 70:605-609.

24. Berg RD. Promotion of the translocation of enteric bacteria from the gastrointestinal tracts of mice by oral treatment with penicillin, clindamycin, or metronidazole. Infect Immun 1981; 33:854-861.

25. Banwell JG, Howard R, Cooper D et al. Intestinal microbial flora after feeding phytohemagglutinin pectins (Phaseolus vulgaris) to rats. Appl Environ Microbiol 1985; 50:68-80.

26. Savage DC, Dubois RS, Schaedler RW. The gastrointestinal epithelium and its aurochthonous bacterial flora. J Exp Med 1968; 127:67-76.

27. Plaut AG, Gorbach SL, Nahas L et al. Studies of intestinal microflora III: the microbial flora of small intestinal mucosa in fluids. Gastroenterology 1967; 53:868-873.

28. Tomasi TB. Mechanisms of immune regulation at mucosal surfaces. Rev Infect Dis 1983; 5(suppl): S789-S792.

29. Klein J. Responses dominated by B-lymphocytes: biological role of IgA. In: Klein J, ed. Immunology: The Science of Self-Nonself Discrimination. New York: John Wiley, 1982:530-531.

30. Brown WR, Savage DC, DuBois RS et al. Intestinal microflora of immunoglobulin-deficient and normal human subjects. Gastroenterology 1972; 62:1143-1152.

31. Cahill CJ, Paine JA, Bailey ME. Bile salts, endotoxin, and renal function in obstructive jaundice. Surg Gynecol Obstet 1987; 165:519-522.

32. Bertok L. Physico-chemical defense of vertebrate organisms:the role of bile acids in defense against bacterial endotoxins. Perspect Biol Med 1977; 21:70-76.

33. McCuskey RS, McCuskey PA, Urbaschek R et al. Kupffer cell function in host defense. Rev Infect Dis 1987; 9(suppl 15):S616-S619.

34. Maejima K, Deitch EA, Berg RD. Bacterial translocation from the gastrointestinal tracts of rats receiving thermal injury. Infect Immun 1984; 43:6-10.

35. Maejima K, Deitch EA, Berg RD. Promotion by burn stress of the translocation of bacteria from the gastrointestinal tracts of mice. Arch Surg 1984; 119:166-172.

36. Deitch EA, Maejima K, Berg RD. Effect of oral antibiotics and bacterial overgrowth on the translocation of GI-tract microflora in burned rats. J Trauma 1985; 25:385-392

37. Deitch EA, Bridges RM. Effect of stress and trauma on bacterial translocation from the gut. J Surg Res 1987; 42:536-542.

38. Baker JW, Deitch EA, Li M et al. Hemorrhagic shock induces bacterial translocation from the gut. J Trauma 1988; 28:896-906.

39. Chiu CJ, McArdle A, Brown R et al. Intestinal mucosal lesions in low-flow states. Arch Surg 1970; 101:478-483.

40. Penner A, Bernheim AI. Acute postoperative enterocolitis. Arch Path 1939; 27:966-983.

41. Sorenson FH, Vetner M. Hemorrhagic mucosal necrosis of the gastrointestinal tract without vascular occlusion. Acta Chir Scand 1969; 135:439-448.

42. Deitch EA, Winterton J, Li M et al. The gut as a portal of entry for bacteremia: role of protein malnutrition. Ann Surg 1987; 205:681-692.

43. Alverdy JC, Aoys E, Moss GS. Total parenteral nutrition promotes bacterial translocation from the gut. Surgery 1988; 104:186-190.

44. Spaeth G, Berg RD, Specian RD et al. Food without fiber promotes bacterial translocation from the gut. Surgery 1990; 108:240-247.

45. Jones WG, Minei JP, Barber AE et al. Elemental diet promotes spontaneous bacterial translocation and alters mortality from endotoxin challenge. Surg Forum 1989; 40:20-22.

46. Mainous MR, Xu D, Lu Q, Deitch EA. Oral TPN-induced bacterial translocation and impaired immune defenses are reversed by refeeding. Surgery 1991; 110:277-284.

47. Woodruff PWH, O'Carroll DI, Koizumi S, Fine J. Role of the intestinal flora in major trauma. J Infect Dis 1973; 24128(suppl):S290-S294.

48. Winchurch RA, Therpari TN, Munster AM. Endotoxemia in burn patients: levels of circulating endotoxins are related to burn size. Surgery 1987; 102:808-812.

49. Nolan JP. The role of endotoxin in liver injury. Gastroenterology 1975; 69:1346-1356.

50. Rush BF Jr, Sori AJ, Murphy TF et al. Endotoxemia and bacteremia during hemorrhagic shock: the link between trauma and sepsis? Ann Surg 1988; 207:549-554.

51. Howard RT. Microbes and their pathogenicity. In: Simmons RL, Howard RT, eds. Surgical Infectious Disease. New York: Appleton Century-Crofts. 1982:11-28.

52. Morrisson DC, Ryan JL. Bacterial endotoxins and host immune responses. Adv Immunol 1979; 28:293-450.

53. Walker RI, Porvaznik MJ. Disruption of the permeability barrier (zona occludens) between intestinal epithelial cells by lethal doses of endotoxin. Infect Immun 1978; 21:655-658.

54. Walker RI. The contribution of endotoxin to mortality in hosts with compromised resistance: a review. Exp Hematol 1978; 6:172-184.

55. Deitch EA, Berg RD, Specian RD. Endotoxin promotes the translocation of bacteria from the gut. Arch Surg 1987; 122:185- 190.

56. Deitch EA, Berg RD. Endotoxin but not protein malnutrition promotes bacterial translocation of the gut flora in burned mice. J Trauma 1987; 27:161-166.

57. Deitch EA, Li M, Ma JW et al. Inhibition of endotoxin -induced bacterial translocation in mice. J Clin Invest 1989; 84:36-42.

58. Deitch EA, Bridges W, Baker JW et al. Hemorrhagic shockinduced bacterial translocation is reduced by xanthine oxidase inhibition or inactivation. Surgery 1988; 104:191-198.

59. Navaratnam RLN, Morris SE, Traber DL et al. Endotoxin increases mesenteric vascular resistance and bacterial translocation. J Trauma 1990; 30:1104-1115.

60. Wells CL, Maddaus MA, Simmons RL. Role of the macrophage in the translocation of intestinal bacteria. Arch Surg 1987; 122:48-53.

61. Wells CL, Maddaus MA, Erlandsen SL, Simmons RL. Evidence for the phagocytic transport of intestinal particles in dogs and rats. Infect Immun 1988; 56:278-282.

62. Mainous MR, Tso P, Berg RD, Deitch EA. Studies of the route, magnitude and time course of bacterial translocation in a model of systemic inflammation. Arch Surg 1991; 126:33-37.

63. Deitch EA. Simple intestinal obstruction causes bacterial translocation in man. Arch Surg 1989; 124:699-701.

64. Ambrose NS, Johnson M, Burdon DW, Keighley MRB. Incidence of pathogenic bacteria from mesenteric lymph nodes and ileal serosa during Crohn's disease surgery. Br J Surg 1984; 71:623-625.

65. Krause W, Matheis H, Wulf K. Fungemia and funguria after oral administration of Candida albicans. Lancet 1969; 1:598-600.

66. Zeigler TR, Smith RJ, O'Dwyer ST et al. Increased intestinal permeability associated with infection in burn patients. Arch Surg 1988; 123:1313-1319.

67. Deitch EA. Intestinal permeability is increased in burn patients shortly after injury. Surgery 1990; 107:411-416.

68. O'Dwyer ST, Michie HR, Zeigler TR et al. A single dose of endotoxin increases intestinal permeability in healthy humans. Arch Surg 19; 123:1459-1464.

69. Marshall JC, Christou NV, Horn R, Meakins JL. The microbiology of multiple organ failure: the proximal gastrointestinal tract as an occult reservoir of pathogens. Arch Surg 1986; 121:102-107.

70. Hillman KM, ,Riordan T, O'Farrell SM, Tabaqchali S. Colonization of the gastric contents in critically ill patients. Crit Care Med 1982; 10:444-447.

71. Altura BM. Hemorrhagic shock and reticuloendothelial system phagocytic function in pathogen-free animals. Circ Shock 1974; 1:295-300.

72. Nolan JP, Camara DS. Intestinal endotoxins as cofactors in liver injury. Immun Invest 1989; 18:325-337.

73. Formal SB, Noyes HE, Schneider H. Experimental shigella infections III: sensitivity of normal, starved, and carbon tetrachloride-treated guinea pigs to endotoxin. Proc Soc Exp Biol Med 1960; 103:415-418.

74. Driks MR, Craven DE, Celli BR et al. Nosocomial pneumonia in intubated patients given sucralfate as compared with antacids or histamine type 2 blockers: the role of gastric colonization. N Engl J Med 1987; 317:1376-1382.

75. Kudsk KA, Stone JM, Carpenter G, Sheldon GF. Enteral and parenteral feeding influences mortality after hemoglobin-E. coli peritonitis in normal rats. J Trauma 1983; 23:605-609.

76. Peterson SR, Kudsk KA, Carpenter G, Sheldon GF. Malnutrition and immunocompetence: increased mortality following infectious challenge during hyperalimentation. J Trauma 1981; 21:528-533.

77. Wilmore DW, Smith RJ, O'Dwyer ST et al. The gut: a central organ after surgical stress. Surgery 1988; 104:917-923.

78. Mochizuki H, Trocki O, Dominioni L. Mechanism of prevention of post-burn hypermetabolism and catabolism by early enteral feeding. Ann Surg 1984; 200:297-310.

79. Alexander JW, MacMillan BG, Stinnett JD et al. Beneficial effects of aggressive protein feeding in severely burned children. Ann Surg 1980; 192:505-517.

CHAPTER 15

SEPSIS AND GLUCOSE TRANSPORTERS

Cecilia A. Hofmann

INTRODUCTION

In the United States recently, there were more than 400,000 hospital cases of septicemia per year, and the fatality rate for such patients was 25%.[1] The prevalence of sepsis has increased over the past decade, owing particularly to therapeutic advances that are prolonging the lives of growing numbers of immunocompromised or otherwise chronically ill patients. Septic shock thus appears, at least partly, to be a consequence of medical progress and will therefore become an ever-increasing concern in the future.

Profound alterations in glucose homeostasis are foremost among the metabolic derangements that occur in sepsis, and successful therapy for septic shock should be aimed broadly at restoring glucose balance. In sepsis, an early state of hyperglycemia with increased glucose turnover and elevated lactic acid levels progresses later to life-threatening hypoglycemia and lactacidemia.[2] Specific metabolic consequences of sepsis include enhanced peripheral glucose utilization, acceleration of glycogenolysis, decreased glycogen synthesis and depressed hepatic gluconeogenesis. An incomplete understanding of cellular and molecular mechanisms underlying these severe sepsis-induced flaws in glucoregulation has, however, hampered efforts to develop targeted treatments for septic patients.

The recent development of new molecular biology methods and some specific reagents has led to a remarkably-enriched understanding of glucose transport. The aims of this review are therefore to summarize contemporary advances in our grasp of glucose transport regulation and to indicate how this knowledge may help investigators identify specific cellular deficits in sepsis. Improved understanding of altered glucose balance in sepsis should ultimately lead to strategically-developed specific treatment regimens to overcome these harmful changes.

ALTERED GLUCOSE UPTAKE IN SEPSIS

Glucose disposal in peripheral tissues occurs by two complementary processes that appear to be differentially regulated in the septic condition; these are insulin-mediated glucose uptake (IMGU) and noninsulin-mediated uptake (NIMGU).[3,4]

Overall glucose disposal via these processes can be measured, but a change in the whole body glucose disposal rate reflects a net effect of opposing influences, i.e., increased glucose disposal in specific tissues versus decreased glucose disposal in others.

In the fasted condition, NIMGU is the predominant pathway for glucose disposal. Studies by Lang and Dobrescu[4,5] demonstrated that gram-negative infection in rats increased the absolute rate of glucose uptake by insulin-independent mechanisms. The insulinopenic condition, in concert with either euglycemia or hypoglycemia, was associated with sepsis-enhanced uptake and phosphorylation of deoxyglucose by liver, spleen, lung, intestine and skin. Such observations thus demonstrated that sepsis increased NIMGU in macrophage-rich and barrier tissues with a net effect of elevating the rate of total body glucose utilization.

Alternatively, IMGU plays an important role in glucose disposal under the fed condition. Resistance to the normal action of insulin to mediate postprandial glucose disposal has been shown in septic patients[6] and in infected animals.[7] Further results from a study by Lang and Dobrescu[3] indicated that in gram-negative sepsis, the decreased IMGU rate in muscle was primarily responsible for whole body insulin resistance. In this septic situation, the decreased rate of IMGU in muscle was larger than the concomitantly elevated glucose uptake by skin, lung, spleen and intestine. The magnitude of insulin resistance measured in whole animals therefore underestimated the severity of glucose uptake defects in muscle.

Such contrasting effects of the septic condition to decrease glucose uptake in muscle while increasing glucose uptake in other tissues seems paradoxical. However, such differential actions may be readily explained by the exciting realization that multiple forms of glucose transporters exist. This deduction results from cDNA cloning studies demonstrating that glucose transport is mediated by members of a family of structurally related proteins encoded by distinct genes that are expressed in a tissue-specific manner.[8,9]

MOLECULAR AND CELLULAR BIOLOGY OF GLUCOSE TRANSPORT

Glucose represents a major source of metabolic energy, and a transport system for glucose entry is essential in all animal cells. Facilitative glucose transporters are integral membrane proteins present on the cell surface. Such proteins are responsible for transport of glucose down its concentration gradient by facilitated diffusion, an energy-independent process whereby movement of the glucose molecule across the lipid bilayer is accelerated by the transporting protein.[8] Five nonidentical, though structurally similar, facilitative glucose transporter proteins have now been reported with abundance varying in different tissue types.[8,9] Cells of different tissues can apparently adapt glucose uptake to their unique physiologic requirement through this variety of transporters with dif-

Type	Size in Amino Acids	Principal Sites of Expression
GLUT1	492	Many tissues; abundant in placenta, brain, kidney & colon
GLUT2	524	Liver, pancreatic ß-cells, kidney, & small intestine
GLUT3	496	Many tissues including placenta, brain & kidney
GLUT4	509	Skeletal muscle, adipocytes & heart
GLUT5	501	Small intestine

Table 1. Human facilitative glucose transporters.
A numerical system based on the chronological publication of transporter gene sequences is now used to identify different transporter isoforms. Transporter isoforms are similar in structure and size but have differential regulation and tissue expression. The principal sites of expression for each transporter in human tissue are listed.

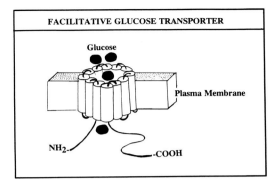

Fig. 1. Model for orientation of facilitative glucose transporters in the plasma membrane. In members of this protein family, 12 transmembrane amino acid sequences have been deduced from hydrophobicity assessments. These highly conserved transmembrane sequences are thought to somehow comprise a channel through which glucose is transported. Less conserved intracellular sequences at the amino- and carboxy-terminal domains are presumably responsible for isoform-specific properties.

fering regulation and expression.

To identify the different transporter isoforms, a numerical system based on the order of cDNA sequence publication is now used. (Table 1) GLUT1 glucose transporter is found in many different cell types and is thought to allow cells to fulfill a basal glucose requirement. GLUT2 plays a key role in glucose homeostasis in liver by mediating bidirectional transport of glucose during opposing physiologic states for glucose uptake or release.[8] GLUT2 also mediates glucose entry into pancreatic ß-cells thus providing for a sensing system that links with insulin secretion. GLUT3, like GLUT1, has a broad tissue distribution although it is relatively abundant in the brain. The GLUT4 protein is expressed only in tissues where glucose uptake is regulated by insulin, i.e., fat, skeletal muscle and heart.[10,11] GLUT5 is observed principally in the small intestine and kidney.[12]

Features of the transporters predict some of their properties. Structurally, there is a 39-65% identity of amino acid sequences between any two human isoforms, and the size of the transporters varies from 492-524 amino acids (Table 1). Based on hydrophobicity assessments, it has been predicted that the fa-

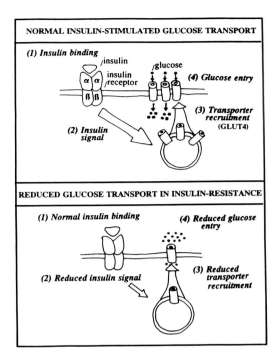

Fig. 2. Insulin action and glucose transport in normal and insulin resistant physiologic states. Insulin's initial action is binding to the extracellular α–subunit of its receptor with resulting signal transduction to intracellular ß-subunits. In response to an as yet undefined cellular signal, glucose transport proteins in intracellular vesicles are translocated and fused with the plasma membrane, thus positioning the transporters to allow glucose entry. Diminished intracellular signalling as well as deficient glucose transporter expression or activity are biochemical lesions that may contribute to lowered IMGU in the insulin-resistant septic condition.

cilitative glucose transporter contains 12 membrane-spanning domains, and that the amino- and carboxy-terminal domains of the protein lie on the cytoplasmic side of the lipid bilayer.[13] By comparison with other transport proteins, it is likely that these transmembrane regions somehow form a channel through which glucose moves, although the precise structure of such a channel remains speculative. (Fig. 1) Highly conserved sequences of the membrane spanning regions presumably support the common function of glucose transport, whereas less well conserved sequences such as those of the amino- and carboxy-termini likely contribute to isoform-specific properties such as transport kinetics and sensitivity to hormone regulation.[8]

The mechanism now considered to be the predominant means for insulin-regulation of glucose uptake in fat and muscle tissue is transporter "recruitment." Extensive studies of such insulin regulation support the hypothesis and model shown in Fig. 2 (upper, whereby the following sequence of events is thought to occur.[14] Insulin binds to the extracellular α-subunit of its plasma membrane receptor, activates the receptor transmembrane ß-subunit and elicits an as yet undefined intracellular signal. In response to the signal, intracellular vesicles containing glucose transporter proteins are translocated to and fuse with the plasma membrane. Fusion of these vesicles with the plasma membrane positions such proteins for transport of glucose across the membrane. Recent studies indicated that GLUT4 was the main transporter isoform thus translocated to the plasma membrane of fat or muscle tissue and is hence primarily responsible for insulin-mediated glucose uptake.[9,15]

While GLUT1 glucose transporters may be similarly recruited to the plasma membrane of adipocytes in response to insulin, the magnitude of such a change is relatively small compared to that of GLUT4 translocation.[9] In adipocytes as in other tissue, GLUT1 seems to be localized normally at the plasma membrane rather than in intracellular vesicles, and therefore appears to play a more important part in basal, i.e., noninsulin-mediated, glucose uptake.

Physiologic states of insulin resistance such as fasting, obesity and diabetes mellitus are characterized by decreased glucose uptake in response to insulin.[9,14] Recent reports on glucose transporter expression in fasted rats and insulin-resistant diabetic mice as well as insulin-deficient diabetic rats have shown that the decreased glucose transport is associated with a specific depletion of GLUT4 mRNA and protein in fat and muscle [16-20] and decreased transporter recruitment after insulin treatment.[19-21] Diminished expression of GLUT4 in fat or muscle of obese and diabetic humans has similarly been reported.[22-24] These findings suggested that decreased expression of GLUT4 glucose transporter might be a biochemical lesion that contributes to insulin resistance (Fig. 2, lower). Since this deficiency can be corrected by refeeding, by treatment with insulin or by treatment with an insulin-sensitizing hypoglycemic drug, a deficient insulin signal may underlie the problem.[16-18]

There have likewise been reports of altered expression of GLUT2 glucose transporter in metabolic states of disrupted glucose homeostasis. In two different animal models for noninsulin-dependent (insulin-resistant) diabetes mellitus, levels of pancreatic ß-cell GLUT2 protein and mRNA expression were reduced.[25-27] Such changes were in concert with insensitivity of ß-cells to glucose for eliciting insulin secretion. Impaired glucose transport into the pancreatic ß-cells may be thus linked to diabetic hyperglycemia.

GLUCOSE TRANSPORTERS IN SEPSIS

To advance our understanding of the pathophysiology of glucose transport in sepsis and endotoxicosis, we recently measured changes in the abundance of mRNA transcripts encoding glucose transporter isoforms in tissues known to be involved in glucose disposal.[28] Six to eight hours following treatment of rats with endotoxin—from *Salmonella enteritidis*—or control saline, tissues including liver, soleus muscle and epididymal fat were rapidly removed from the animals for extraction of RNA. At this selected time, endotoxin-treated animals were in the decompensated phase of shock, i.e., were hypoglycemic and lactacidemic. GLUT1 mRNA abundance was significantly increased in liver (871%), muscle (314%) and fat (660%) from endotoxin-treated animals compared to controls. At the same time, liver GLUT2 mRNA levels were markedly decreased (-58%), thus clearly indicating differential regulation of transporter isoforms. While it is not possible to determine whether such changes in transporter isoform expression reflect or cause changes in glucose transport itself, it is logical to speculate that such changes may be linked with increased peripheral glucose utilization and decreased liver glucose output.

Numerous questions remain unanswered regarding molecular mechanisms underlying endotoxin-mediated alterations of glucose transport. While an increase in GLUT1 mRNA abundance suggests that transporter synthesis may be enhanced, it will be essential to confirm that this change is due to increased transporter transcription rather than increased mRNA stability. Furthermore, it will be necessary to directly determine whether increases in GLUT1 protein levels and glucose transport activity occur concordantly with the RNA changes. Similarly, decreased liver GLUT2 expression must be better understood, and it would be further interesting to assess whether GLUT2 expression is comparably or differentially regulated in the pancreatic ß-cells. To fully understand alterations of peripheral glucose uptake, it will also be necessary to measure expression of GLUT3, another transporter isoform thought to be involved in basal glucose disposal. Finally, full assessment of sepsis-induced changes in GLUT4 mRNA and protein levels in red, white and mixed muscle subtypes will be essential to understanding sepsis-mediated insulin resistance in this tissue.

A key remaining question regarding regulation of glucose transporter expression is "What are the cellular mediators for endotoxin actions?" An early insight was provided by studies of Lee et al[29] showing that monokines from endotoxin-treated macrophages stimulated glucose uptake and glycogen breakdown in myotubes of the L6 skeletal muscle cell line. Such effects required 15 hours, depended on synthesis and insertion of glucose transporters into the cell membrane, and could be emulated by direct treatment of these cells with the monokine tumor necrosis factor. Although not determined, this effect was likely GLUT1-mediated owing to the predominant expression of this transporter isoform in L6 cells. Later studies by others demonstrated increases in GLUT1 mRNA or protein levels in fibroblasts following prolonged exposure (15 hr) to either tumor necrosis factor-α[30] or interleukin-1.[31]

CONCLUSIONS

Fundamental advances in our understanding of glucose transport have been made recently owing largely to the availability of new reagents and study methods. Such changes should facilitate improved understanding of sepsis-induced glucose transport changes. These advances may lead ultimately to development of precisely targeted therapies for improved survival in affected patients.

REFERENCES

1. Increase in national hospital discharge survey rates for septicemia-United States, 1979-1987. Morb Mort Weekly Reports 1990; 39:31-35,.
2. Yelich MR, Witek-Janusek L, Filkins JP. Glucose dyshomeostasis in endotoxicosis: direct versus monokine-mediated mechanisms of endotoxin action. In: Immunobiology and Immunopharmacology of bacterial endotoxins, In: Szentivanyi A, Friedman H, eds. New York: Plenum Publishing Corp., 1986:111-132.
3. Lang CH, Dobrescu C, Meszaros K. Insulin-mediated glucose uptake by individual tissues during sepsis. Metabol 1990; 39:1096-1107.
4. Lang CH, Dobrescu C. Gram-negative infection increases noninsulin-mediated glucose disposal. Endocrinol 1991; 128:645-653.
5. Lang CH, Dobrescu C. Sepsis-induced increases in glucose uptake by macrophage-rich tissues persist during hypoglycemia. Metabol 1991; 40:585-593.
6. Shangraw RE, Jahoor F, Miyoshi H et al. Differentiation between septic and postburn insulin resistance. Metabol 1989; 38:983-989.
7. Lang CH, Dobrescu C. In vivo insulin resistance during nonlethal hypermetabolic sepsis. Circ Shock 1989; 28:165-178.
8. Bell GI, Kayano T, Buse JB et al. Molecular biology of mammalian glucose transporters. Diabetes Care 1990; 13:198-208.
9. Kahn BB, Flier JS. Regulation of glucose-transporter gene expression in vitro and in vivo. Diabetes Care 1990; 13:548-564.
10. Birnbaum MJ. Identification of a novel gene encoding an insulin-responsive glucose transporter protein. Cell 1989; 57:305-315.
11. Fukumoto H, Kayano T, Buse JB et al. Cloning and characterization of the major insulin-responsive glucose transporter expressed in human skeletal muscle and other insulin-responsive tissues. J Biol Chem 1989; 264:7776-7779.
12. Kayano T, Burant CF, Fukumoto H et al. Human facilitative glucose transporters. J Biol Chem 1990; 265:13276-13282.
13. Mueckler M, Caruso C, Baldwin SA et al. Sequence

and structure of a human glucose transporter. Science 1985; 229:941-945.

14. Simpson IA, Cushman SW: Hormonal regulation of mammalian glucose transport. Annu Rev Biochem 1986; 55:1059-1098.

15. Douen AG, Ramlal T, Rastogi S et al. Exercise induces recruitment of the "insulin-responsive glucose transporter." Evidence for distinct insulin- and exercise-recruitable transporter pools in skeletal muscle. J Biol Chem 1990; 265:13427-13430.

16. Hofmann C, Lorenz K, Colca JR: Glucose transport deficiency in diabetic animals is corrected by treatment with the oral anti-hyperglycemic agent pioglitazone. Endocrinol 1991; 129:1915-1925.

17. Berger J, Biswas C, Vicario PP et al. Decreased expression of the insulin-responsive glucose transporter in diabetes and fasting. Nature 1989; 340:70-72.

18. Sivitz WI, DeSautel SL, Kayano T et al. Regulation of glucose transporter messenger RNA in insulin-deficient states. Nature 1991; 340:72-74.

19. Garvey WT, Huecksteadt TP, Birnbaum MJ. Pretranslational suppression of an insulin-responsive glucose transporter in rats with diabetes mellitus. Science 1989; 245:60-63.

20. Klip A, Ramlal T, Bilan PJ et al. Recruitment of GLUT4 glucose transporters by insulin in diabetic rat skeletal muscle. Biochem Biophys Res Commun 1990; 172:728-736.

21. Barnard RJ, Youngren JF, Kartel DS, Martin DA. Effects of streptozotocin-induced diabetes on glucose transport in skeletal muscle. Endocrinol 1990; 126:1921-1926.

22. Sinha MK, Raineri-Maldonado C, Buchanan C et al. Adipose tissue glucose transporters in NIDDM. Decreased levels of muscle/fat isoform. Diabetes 1991; 40:472-477.

23. Garvey WT, Maianu L, Huecksteadt TP et al. Pretranslational suppression of a GLUT4 glucose transporter protein causes insulin resistance in adipocytes from patients with non-insulin-dependent diabetes and obesity. J Clin Invest 1990; 87:1072-1081.

24. Dohm GL, Elton CW, Friedman JE et al. Decreased expression of an insulin-sensitive glucose transporter in muscle from insulin-resistant obese and diabetic patients. Am J Physiol 1991; 260:E459-E463.

25. Thorens B, Flier JS, Lodish HF, Kahn BB. Differential regulation of two glucose transporters in rat liver by fasting and refeeding and by diabetes and insulin treatment. Diabetes 1990; 39:712-719.

26. Thorens B, Weir GC, Leahy JL, Lodish HF. Reduced expression of the liver/beta-cell glucose transporter isoform in glucose-insensitive pancreatic beta cells of diabetic rats. Proc Natl Acad Sci USA 1990; 87:6492-6496.

27. Unger R. Diabetic hyperglycemia: link to impaired glucose transport in pancreatic beta cells. Science 1991; 251:1200-1205.

28. Zeller WP, The SM, Sweet M et al. Altered glucose transporter mRNA abundance in a rat model of endotoxic shock. Biochem Biophys Res Commun 1991; 176:535-540.

29. Lee MD, Zentella A, Pekala PH, Cerami A. Effect of endotoxin-induced monokines on glucose metabolism in the muscle cell line L6. Proc Natl Acad Sci USA 1987; 84:2590-2594.

30. Cornelius P, Marlowe M, Pekala P. Regulation of glucose transport by tumor necrosis factor-alpha in cultured murine 3T3-L1 fibroblasts. Adv Understand Trauma Burn Injury 1991; 30:S15-S20.

31. Bird TA, Davies A, Baldwin SA, Saklatvala J. Interleukin-1 stimulates hexose transport in fibroblasts by increasing the expression of glucose transporters. J Biol Chem 1990; 265:13578-13583.

CHAPTER 16

ACUTE PHASE PROTEINS

Michael E. Gottschalk

Nutritional repletion is an important component of the overall medical care of trauma patients. Delayed wound healing and impaired immune function are just two serious consequences of poor nutrition which can lead to significant morbidity and mortality during the recovery phase posttrauma. The nutritional care of trauma patients is a complex issue since many factors such as the age, nutritional status and health of the individual prior to injury; the type and extent of injury sustained; the ability to provide enteral versus parenteral nutritional support in lieu of the anatomical and physiologic consequences of injury; and the limitations of using traditional nutritional monitors need to be considered. Many of these issues are discussed in other chapters in this monograph. I will focus on the use of acute phase proteins as a monitor of nutritional repletion in trauma patients.

Immediately posttrauma a hypermetabolic, catabolic state exists. Energy requirements depending on the nature of injury can range from 1.5-2 times the basal metabolic rate. Protein needs are also very high, requiring increased amounts of protein to yield a nonprotein calorie to nitrogen ratio in the lower range of 100-150 to 1. Once nutritional therapy is instituted the question is how to best monitor the response to treatment. Overfeeding a patient can be as deleterious as undernutrition. An ideal monitor should respond quickly to changes in nutritional status, be uninfluenced by physiologic changes induced by trauma or sepsis and be easily and reproducibly measurable. Unfortunately such a measurement does not exist so monitoring requires simultaneously following the response of several different parameters. Compared to other disease entities, the physical consequences of trauma can further limit the use of more traditional nutritional measurements.

Posttrauma anthropometric measurements can be difficult to ascertain and may be unreliable as nutritional indices. Body weight may be altered by fluid resuscitation or the application of large dressings, casts, splints and so forth. Daily weights are not always feasible in a critically ill patient. Skinfold thickness is often unattainable, for example in burn patients, and is not a reliable measurement in an edematous patient. Also skin fold thickness responds to changes in nutritional intervention in terms of weeks and not days. Arm muscle circumference or area has similar limitations.

Biochemical indices such as nitrogen balance studies have their own restrictions which can be accentuated by the result of trauma.[1] The multiple trauma or burn patient may have increased extraurinary nitrogen losses from fistulas, wounds, diarrhea or the burn surface area which if unaccounted for will lead to an overestimation of nitrogen balance. Generally nitrogen equilibrium is not attained until 2-12 days after a change in protein intake. Often nutritional support in trauma patients needs to be interrupted to perform diagnostic tests or preoperatively, making it difficult to sustain a consistent day-to-day protein-calorie intake necessary to obtain nitrogen equilibrium for correct interpretation of nitrogen balance studies.

Other biochemical parameters, especially serum proteins have been utilized as monitors of nutritional repletion in trauma patients.[2,3] The goal of nutritional repletion is to provide sufficient calories and protein to compensate for the hypermetabolic, catabolic state thereby improving nitrogen retention. Ideally to be a clinically useful marker of nutritional repletion a change in the concentration of a serum protein should reflect only its synthetic rate which in turn is dependent on the provision of protein and calories. The serum protein should also have a short serum half-life, a small body pool, rapid rate of synthesis and a constant catabolic rate.[4]

Albumin, a frequently utilized nutritional index, has several drawbacks for monitoring nutritional repletion. The half-life of albumin is approximately 21 days, so its response to increased or decreased protein-calorie intake would take weeks and not days. Albumin also has a large body pool with an extravascular to intravascular distribution ratio of 1.5.[4] Redistribution from one space to the other can potentially mask a concurrent change in the synthetic rate of albumin. Even in severe malnutrition states like marasmus the serum albumin concentration may be normal. The serum concentration of albumin can also be affected by nonnutritional entities including liver disease, renal dysfunction and total body water composition. Additionally postinjury many patients often require albumin infusions which will alter its serum concentration unrelated to nutritional support. Serum hepatic secretory proteins with shorter half-lifes are better indicators of short term changes in protein-calorie intake than albumin and correlate more with nitrogen balance.[3,4]

Several studies have evaluated the longitudinal response of short half-life proteins to trauma, however few have evaluated their usefulness in monitoring nutritional support.[1,3] Boosalis et al[3] serially measured protein-calorie intake, nitrogen balance and serum albumin and prealbumin levels in trauma patients from the time of admission until 18 days postinjury. In the short-term prealbumin

was a better indicator of nutritional intervention than albumin. Within one week of increasing protein-calorie intake and improved nitrogen balance the prealbumin concentration increased while the serum albumin level continued to decline over the next two weeks. More studies are needed to document the clinical utility of short half-life proteins during both the immediate posttrauma time period and the convalescent phase.

Prealbumin (transthyretin) is a serum transport protein for thyroid hormone and the vitamin A-retinol binding protein complex.[5,6] It has a short half-life of 18-24 hours. Compared to albumin, prealbumin has a smaller body pool with a greater intravascular to extravascular distribution. Numerous studies in different nontrauma patient groups have demonstrated a consistent correlation between the serum prealbumin concentration and parallel increases or decreases in protein-calorie intake or nitrogen balance.[3,6-8] The response time is usually within the order of several days. Nonnutritional factors including, cirrhosis and hepatitis can lower prealbumin levels. Increased levels of prealbumin occur with chronic renal failure.

Retinol binding protein (RBP) has an even shorter half-life of 12 hours although clinically this does not improve its sensitivity as a nutritional marker over that of prealbumin.[5] RBP transports vitamin A from the liver to peripheral tissues. Serum RBP concentration is dependent on vitamin A stores which regulates hepatic release of RBP. Aside from vitamin A deficiency RBP concentration is decreased in chronic liver diseases, cystic fibrosis, zinc deficiency and hyperthyroidism. Increased RBP levels occur with chronic renal failure. Another commonly used visceral protein as a nutritional index is transferrin. Transferrin's primary function is to transport iron and so its serum concentration is very dependent on the individual's iron status.

Another shortcoming of transferrin is its serum half-life of 7-10 days which like albumin significantly delays its response to changes in nutritional repletion. An increasing concentration of transferrin is a good indicator of positive nitrogen balance, however a decreasing transferrin level is a poor indicator of nitrogen loss.[4] At Loyola University Medical

Center we employ a nutrition panel which measures alpha-1-acid glycoprotein (AAG), prealbumin (PA), transferrin (TF) and albumin. AAG has a serum half-life of 12-18 hours. By serially measuring the serum concentrations of several proteins with different half-lifes together we can better monitor the short and long-term response to nutritional support in conjunction with weekly anthropometric measurements.

For example in a patient with deteriorating weight, skin fold thickness and midarm muscle circumference, the benefit of increasing the daily caloric intake should in several days be reflected by an increase in AAG and PA levels, later followed by an increase TF and finally albumin and improved anthropometric measurements. Conversely with nutritional depletion AAG and PA levels will decrease first without a change in TF, albumin or anthropometric measurements. Measuring several proteins with similar half-lifes eliminates some of the problems in misinterpreting changes in their serum levels due to nonnutritional factors since each protein is affected by different entities. These proteins are measured by nephelometry so results are available in less than 24 hours and only 100 microliters of serum is required for the entire panel. AAG, PA, TF and albumin are part of a larger group of proteins called acute phase proteins whose serum concentrations are affected by trauma.

The acute phase response is an early and unspecific hepatic reaction to systemic tissue injury including inflammation infection, thermal or mechanical trauma, and ischemic necrosis.[9,10] The response pattern is bidirectional with positive acute phase reactants increasing in concentration after injury and negative acute phase reactants decreasing. C-reactive protein (CRP), AAG, alpha-1-antitrypsin, serum amyloid A, fibrinogen, haptoglobulin, ceruloplasmin, complement factor C3 are examples of positive acute phase reactants. The positive acute phase response seems to be a protective response to injury and to serve as a check on the injury induced inflammatory mediated response. These reactants have diverse functions such as antioxidants, proteolytic inhibitors and mediators of coagulation which may in part prevent excessive tissue

damage and hemorrhage as a result of injury. Negative acute phase reactants include the serum transport proteins: albumin, prealbumin, retinol-binding protein and transferrin. Immediately after trauma there is a predictable pattern in the alteration of the acute phase proteins. Initially after injury there is a decrease in the serum concentration of most of the acute phase proteins, both for positive and negative reactants. Redistribution of the protein body pool from the intravascular to extravascular space occurs secondary to an increased microvascular permeability and vascular stasis following trauma and accounts for part of the initial decline in acute phase proteins.[5] The negative acute phase reactant protein concentrations continue to remain depressed for days to weeks after injury due to a decrease in their hepatic synthesis. Albumin reaches a nadir by day 5 posttrauma.

Whether nutritional support in the immediate postinjury phase can alter this response has not be adequately studied. As mentioned before in one study[3] prealbumin concentrations increased within the first week of injury, although lagging behind increased protein-calorie intake and nitrogen balance, while serum albumin levels slowly declined over the same time and were still decreased 18 days after injury. The positive acute phase protein concentrations begin to rise after a lag period of six hours.[5] During this lag phase there is a cascade release of inflammatory mediators such as the cytokines interleukin-1 (IL-1), interleukin-6 (IL-6), tumor necrosis factor (TNF) and cortisol which in turn can stimulate hepatic synthesis of the positive acute phase reactants. The magnitude of the response varies for each individual protein and is different in various animal species. CRP is the earliest acute phase reactant to respond and peaks its serum concentration at 48 hours. The serum protein concentrations of the positive acute phase reactants return to normal by the end of the first week posttrauma.

Only recently have we begun to understand the mechanisms involved in the regulation of the acute phase protein response. Tissue injury initiates a complex array of cellular mediator release including cytokines, prostaglandins, and leukotrienes which may singularly or acting in concert regulate the acute phase response. Using in vitro liver perfusion methods or hepatocyte cell culture systems, studies have started to evaluate the ability of cyotkines to mediate the acute phase response. Much of this work has focused on monitoring mRNA or protein synthesis response to individual or a combination of cytokines. The complete in vivo acute phase response has not been reproduced in vitro. Il-1 stimulates only a subset of the positive acute phase reactants and will inhibit albumin synthesis.[10,11] TNF appears to indirectly mimic the IL-1 response by stimulating IL-1 release.[12] However, TNF in vitro can directly inhibit hepatic albumin synthesis. IL-6 produces a more encompassing response, although not to the magnitude seen in vivo.[10,11]

Following trauma a hypermetabolic, catabolic response occurs which left unabated will lead to depletion of somatic and visceral protein stores, delay wound healing and impair the immune response. Despite increased protein synthesis post-injury the magnitude of protein breakdown is so great that a state of negative nitrogen balance exists. Adequate calorie (based on indirect calorimetry) and protein supplementation during this time period will improve nitrogen retention but not sufficiently to achieve positive nitrogen balance.[13] Nutritional support improves nitrogen retention by enhancing protein synthesis, however there is no effect on whole body protein breakdown.[14] Postinjury there also appears to be less efficient recycling of nitrogen from protein breakdown to new protein synthesis since whole body protein breakdown is greater than the nitrogen needed for new protein synthesis.[13] Protein breakdown is being reprioritized from nitrogen recycling to providing carbon substrates for energy production. The decrease in negative acute phase reactants may be another way the body is reprioritizing metabolism to conserve nitrogen loss by shifting protein synthesis to those proteins necessary for the body to survive the acute injury. Possibly the enhanced protein catabolism post-injury and the negative acute phase response are dually regulated by mediators of the inflammatory response.

In the future nutritional support may involve means of selectively antagonizing the metabolic effects of cytokines and other mediators of the inflammatory response to preserve body protein stores.

References

1. Mattox TW, Brown RO, Boucher BA et al. Use of fibronectin and somatomedin-C as markers of enteral nutrition support in traumatized patients using a modified amino acid formula. JPEN 1988; 12:592-596.
2. Kudlackova M, Andel M, Hajkova H, Novakova J. Acute phase proteins and prognostic inflammatory and nutritional index (PINI) in moderately burned children aged up to three years. Burns 1990; 16:53-56.
3. Boosalis MG, Ott L, Levine AS et al. Relationship of visceral proteins to nutritional status in chronic and acute stress. Crit Care Med 1989; 17:741-774.
4. Church JM, Hill GL. Assessing the efficacy of intravenous nutrition in general surgical patients: dynamic nutrtional assessment with plasma proteins. JPEN 1987; 11:135-139.
5. Fleck A, Colley CM, Myers MA. Liver export proteins and trauma. Brit Med Bull 41:265-273
6. Winkler MF, Gerrior SA, Pomp A, Albina JE. Use of retinol-binding protein and prealbumin as indicators of the response to nutrition therapy. J Amer Diet Assoc 1989; 89:684-687.
7. Brown RO, Buopane EA, Vehe KL et al. Comparison of modified amino acids and standard amino acids in parental nutrtion support of thermally injures patients. Crit Care Med 1990; 18:1096-1101.
8. Tuten MB, Wogt S, Dasse F, Leider Z. Utilization of prealbumin as a nutrtional parameter. JPEN 1985; 9:709-711.
9. Fleck A. Clinical and nutritional aspects of changes in acute-phase proteins during inflammation. Proc Nutr Soc 1989; 48:347-354.
10. Baumann H. Hepatic acute phase reaction in vivo and in vitro. In Vitro Cell Dev Biol 1989; 25:115-126.
11. Steel DM and Whitehead AS. Hetergeneous modulation of acute-phase-reactant mRNA levels by interleukin-1ß and interleukin-6 in the human hepatoma cell line PLC/PRF/5. Biochem J 1991; 277:477-482.
12. Bankey PE, Mazuski JE, Ortiz M, Fulco JM, Cerra FB. Hepatic acute phase protein synthesis is indirectly regulated by tumor necrosis factor. J Trauma 1990; 30:1181-1187.
13. Jeevanadam M, Young DH, Schiller WR. Endogenous protein-synthesis efficiency in trauma victims. Metabolism 1989; 38:967-973.
14. Shaw JHF, Wolfe RR. An integrated analysis of glucose, fat, and protein metabolism in severely traumatized patients. Ann Surg 1989; 209:63-72.

CHAPTER 17

INTRACELLULAR CALCIUM REGULATION:
Derangements During Septic Injury

Mohammed M. Sayeed

INTRODUCTION

"Calcium is to physiologists what DNA is to biochemists." This interesting comment was made by some physiologist a couple of decades or so ago. Today, in 1992, neither physiologists alone can claim a special interest in calcium nor biochemists alone in DNA, but rather all life/health scientists (basic and clinical) share the fascination for the roles of both calcium and DNA in health and disease. Extracellular calcium homeostasis and its hormonal regulation continue to be foci of extensive studies by endocrinologists and metabolic disease experts. Although ultimately linked to extracellular calcium homeostasis, intracellular calcium homeostasis independently plays an important role in the metabolic steady state of cells and in the elicitation of cellular responses specific to a wide variety of hormones. Alternations in intracellular calcium homeostasis can occur in spite of maintained extracellular homeostasis and can lead to alterations in cellular metabolic, secretory, contractile and proliferative functions.

Alterations in cellular calcium regulation have been implicated in a variety of experimental conditions and diseased states, e.g., anoxia, bacterial toxins (leucocidin, streptolysin O), CCl_4 poisoning, vitamin D toxicosis, complement activation, dimethylamino azobenzene carcinogenesis, cystic fibrosis, muscular dystrophy and trauma. These assessments relied mostly on measurements of total tissue or total cellular calcium contents.

Since total calcium measurements include quantities of both intracellular and extracellular calcium, these assessments may or may not be related to changes in the intracellular Ca^{2+} regulation exclusively. More recent studies of cellular Ca^{2+} regulation have included measurements of membrane Ca^{2+} fluxes as well as Ca^{2+} concentrations in the cytosolic compartment of cells. These measurements more specifically implicate changes or disturbances in intracellular Ca^{2+} regulation under experimental conditions or disease states.

Several investigators have, within the last decade or so, assessed intracellular Ca^{2+} regulation and Ca^{2+} dependent cellular functions in various tissues/organs in animals experimentally rendered septic via injections of endotoxin or live gram-negative bacteria. A major objective of this review is to discuss gram-negative septic-injury related changes in cellular Ca^{2+} regulation. A number of such studies were carried out in the author's laboratory and will be discussed in this review. Prior to a discussion of the observed septic related pathophysiologic changes, there will be a discussion of the physiologic phenomenon of intracellular Ca^{2+} regulation. This portion of the review will survey the state of the art knowledge of mechanisms of intracellular Ca^{2+} homeostasis and the involvement of the intracellular Ca^{2+} signal in the elicitation of cellular responses. An understanding of the overall physiology of cellular Ca^{2+} regulation and its participation in hormone specific cell responses is essential for the interpretation and elucidation of alterations observed under pathophysiologic/pathologic conditions.

PHYSIOLOGY OF CELLULAR CA^{2+} REGULATION

INTRACELLULAR CA^{2+} HOMEOSTASIS[1]

Intracellular Ca^{2+} homeostasis refers to maintenance in resting cells of a low cytosolic Ca^{2+} concentration (~100 nM) in spite of approximately 10,000 fold higher concentrations found in the extracellular space (~1 mM) and in the organellar compartment(s) (≥1 mM). Such steep Ca^{2+} concentration gradients across the plasma membrane and the sarcoplasmic/endoplasmic reticular (SR/ER) membrane are evidently maintained through the operation of membrane bound active transport mechanisms balancing passive Ca^{2+} leaks down the concentration gradients. In healthy resting cells such Ca^{2+} leaks through the plasma and SR/ER membranes are much less than that predicted on the basis of Ca^{2+} concentration gradients per se due mainly to a low membrane permeability to Ca^{2+}. Consequently only minimal active Ca^{2+} transport is required across the plasma and organullar membranes in healthy resting cells.

The magnitudes of passive Ca^{2+} movements through the plasma and/or the SR/ER membranes are acutely elevated when the resting cells are stimulated by certain agonists, e.g., catecholamines, vasopressin, acetyl choline or angiotensin II. The elevation of Ca^{2+} concentration occurs transiently. The return of Ca^{2+} concentration to levels found in the resting cells presumably results from the activation of plasma and SR/ER membrane transport mechanisms. The time-dependent profile of elevation of Ca^{2+} concentration and its return to prestimulation level is referred to as intracellular Ca^{2+} transient. The duration of a Ca^{2+} transient with a specific agonist varies from one cell type to the other. The Ca^{2+} transient duration in a given cell type will also vary with one agonist to another.

AGONIST MEDIATED ACTIVATION OF THE INTRACELLULAR CA^{2+} SIGNAL[2]

The mechanisms that generate Ca^{2+} transients are shown in Fig. 1. This figure emphasizes the agonist mediation of both an increased Ca^{2+} influx from the extracellular space and an increased Ca^{2+} efflux from the SR/ER compartment. An intracellular nonmitochondrial compartment other than the SR/ER, referred to as Calciosome, may also participate in the efflux of Ca^{2+}. The increased Ca^{2+} influx through the plasma membrane could result from an agonist mediated "opening" of a receptor-sensitive calcium channel subsequent to sequential interactions between: 1) the agonist and receptor; 2) the agonist-receptor complex and the guanine nucleotide binding protein (G-protein); and 3) the activated G-protein and Ca^{2+} channel. The receptor-sensitive Ca^{2+} channels are often not as highly selective for Ca^{2+} as the voltage sensitive Ca^{2+} channels of excitable cells. Like the voltage-sensitive Ca^{2+} channels, the receptor-sensitive Ca^{2+} channels are blocked by the organic Ca^{2+} channel blockers (dihydropyridines, verapamil, diltiazem) but at considerably higher blocker concentrations. As shown in Fig 1., the activated G-protein interacts also with the membrane enzyme phospholipase C (PLC), which in turn catalyzes the breakdown of membrane phospholipid, phosphotidyl inositol bis-phosphate (PIP_2) to 1,2-diacylglycerol (DAG) and inositol 1,4,5,-triphosphate (IP_3). DAG is retained within the plasma membrane and serves to activate the plasma membrane bound protein kinase C (PKC). IP_3 diffuses to the ER membrane and mediates the release of Ca^{2+} from

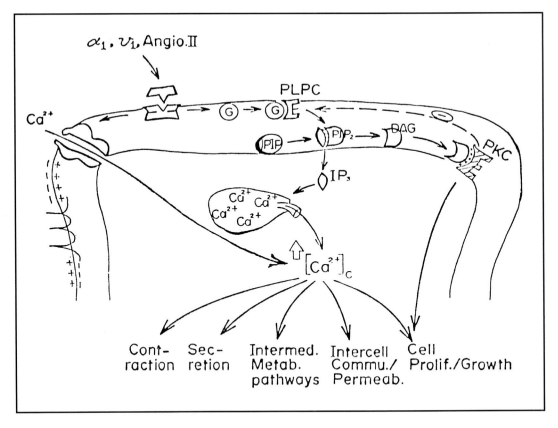

Fig. 1. Mechanisms of intracellular regulation of Ca^{2+}. Figure shows diagrammatic representation of activations of an α_1 adrenergic, v_1, vasopressin, or angiotensin II receptor to lead to an activation of a plasma membrane receptor-sensitive Ca^{2+} channel, and an intramembrane guanine nucleotide binding protein (G). G activation is followed by activation of phospholipase C (PLPC), breakdown of PIP_2 to IP_3 and DAG and activation of protein kinase C (PKC). IP_3 is shown to mediate release of Ca^{2+} from ER vesicles. PIP, phosphotidylinostitol monophosphate, is the precursor of PIP_2. See text for details of mechanisms of intracellular Ca^{2+} regulation.

the ER. While IP_3 plays a relatively clear cut role in agonist-related Ca^{2+} efflux from the ER, the DAG mediated PKC activation is involved in a more complex way in the agonist induced intracellular perturbations. One of the consequences of PKC activation and resulting phosphorylation of certain target proteins is to attenuate the agonist-related PIP_2 breakdown within the membrane. This would result in a negative feedback control of the formation of IP_3 and DAG. Additionally, PKC activation could activate Ca^{2+} extrusion through plasma membrane. This may also be viewed as a mechanism to attenuate the amplitude of the IP_3 mediated Ca^{2+} transient.

Paradoxically, other consequences of PKC activation may be potentiations of cellular responses elicited through the IP_3 mediated Ca^{2+} transients. PKC actions may be temporally separated such that the negative feedback control of IP_3 mediated Ca^{2+} transient may occur more acutely than its potentiation of IP_3 mediated cellular responses.

Role of Intracellular Ca^{2+} Binding Proteins[3]

The increased availability of free Ca^{2+} in the cytosolic milieu subsequent to plasma membrane Ca^{2+} channel activation and/or ER

Ca^{2+} release leads to its binding to a select group of intracellular proteins with high affinity Ca^{2+} binding domains. One such protein which is found ubiquitously throughout the animal kingdom is calmodulin. It may be present both as a free cytosolic protein or in association with other membrane or cytosolic proteins and enzymes. Calmodulin acts as a cellular response switch which is turned on and off by changes in Ca^{2+} concentration over a narrow but specific range (100 nM–1 μM). The Ca^{2+}-calmodulin complex may activate calcium-calmodulin-dependent kinases which in turn phosphorylate certain target proteins. The phosphorylation of target proteins in various cell types serves as the final common pathway for the generation of agonist-specific cellular responses such as activation of a metabolic pathway, contractions, cell-cell communications, cell proliferation and secretion. (Fig. 1)

CONSEQUENCES OF ALTERED INTRACELLULAR Ca^{2+} HOMEOSTASIS:

The foregoing discussion indicates the importance of intracellular Ca^{2+} homeostasis for cells' ability to respond to regulatory agonists. It underscores Ca^{2+} as a physiological mediator serving to turn on and off the switch for various hormone specific cellular responses. The physiological role of Ca^{2+} is dependent entirely on its regulation (within a set range of its cytosolic concentrations, viz. 0.1-1.0 μM) via reversible changes in passive Ca^{2+} movements through ion channels and active movements through pumps in the plasma and SR/ER membranes. Alterations in passive and/or active Ca^{2+} movements before or after agonist interactions with cells can understandably disturb the set range of cytosolic Ca^{2+} concentrations and thereby blunt hormone related responses. An increase in passive Ca^{2+} leak in the resting state cells can result from a pathophysiologic increase in plasma membrane permeability to Ca^{2+} and contribute to an increase in basal cytosolic Ca^{2+} concentration. Alternatively, a failure of active Ca^{2+} extrusion through Ca^{2+} pumping

mechanism within plasma membranes can result in an increase in cytosolic Ca^{2+} concentration. Whether these increases in cytosolic Ca^{2+} concentration in resting cells prior to their hormonal activation can also produce cellular responses is questionable. The elevations of cytosolic Ca^{2+} concentrations after hormonal stimulation of healthy cells occurs in an oscillatory fashion and the frequency of such oscillations is presumed to have a role in the turning on of the "response switch." Since there is no reason to assume oscillatory changes in Ca^{2+} concentration with a non-hormonal increase in Ca^{2+} due to increases in membrane Ca^{2+} permeability, such changes in cytosolic Ca^{2+} are unlikely to result in a specific cellular response. However, experiments using Ca^{2+} ionophore, e.g., A23187, have shown that the ionophore mediated increase in membrane Ca^{2+} flux can lead to cellular responses.

A high concentration of hormone and/or a prolonged exposure of cells to hormones with a sustained activation of receptors and other membrane components of the signal transduction pathway, including the voltage and/or receptor-sensitive plasma membrane calcium channels, may lead to a sustained elevation of cytosolic Ca^{2+} concentration. This would support a high level of cellular response initially but is likely to result in a dampening of the response later on. The failure of return of the cytosolic Ca^{2+} concentrations to a basal level would prevent reactivation of the intracellular Ca^{2+} messenger system.

INTRACELLULAR Ca^{2+} AS A MEDIATOR OF CELL INJURY[4]

A sustained increase in cytosolic Ca^{2+} could have consequences other than an initial enhancement and a later blunting of cellular responses. High intracellular Ca^{2+} concentration can lead to direct activation of certain "lytic" enzymes which are known to remain inactive in healthy cells. Intracellular Ca^{2+} accumulation can activate phospholipases and proteinases. Phospholipases may be implicated in cell membrane injury and proteinases in the possible breakdown of functional proteins. The activation of the hydrolytic enzymes could trigger cell autolysis and contribute to membrane function damage and cell protein depletions. Thus alterations in cellular Ca^{2+} homeostasis could convert the role of Ca^{2+} from that as a physiologic mediator to a mediator of cell injury. Howard Rasmussen, who has made extensive contributions to our understanding of the intracellular role of Ca^{2+}, has likened nature's gift of Ca^{2+} to cells to Prometheus' gift of fire to man. Ca^{2+} can be paradoxically beneficial (physiologic role) and detrimental (pathologic role) as can be fire providing warmth, and causing destruction.

A harmful role of Ca^{2+} in tissue necrosis was recognized by the pathologist Virchow more than 100 years ago. Numerous studies by pathologists have since suggested that tissue calcification is a mark of tissue death. These studies in general do not distinguish whether calcium deposits occur intra- or extracellularly. Relatively recent studies have recognized formation of a calcium containing precipitate inside the cell and organelles after the onset of metabolic and membrane ion and water transport derangements during the course of cell injury. The latter findings evidently support a gross accumulation of Ca^{2+} intracellulary to the level that it can not be buffered by cytosolic ligands, or sequestered in dissolved form inside ER and mitochondria. During the last two decades researchers have demonstrated that intracellular Ca^{2+} accumulation may occur in a graded manner such that Ca^{2+} concentration is progressively elevated along with a progressive loss of cell function until mitochondrial and intracellular calcium salt precipitation occurs. According to this concept, a graded shift in intracellular Ca^{2+} homeostasis may be associated with a graded down regulation of Ca^{2+} depended cellular functions. Thus recent studies have considered potential relationships between cellular Ca^{2+} hemostatic disturbance and cellular functions during initial stages of cell injury prior to onset of irreversible cell damage.

PATHOPHYSIOLOGIC CHANGES IN CA^{2+} REGULATION DURING SEPTIC INJURY

ALTERATION IN TRANSMEMBRANE CA^{2+} TRANSPORT IN THE LIVER IN ENDOTOXIC SHOCK[5,6]

The control of intracellular Ca^{2+} was studied via quantitations of Ca^{2+} efflux, its modulation by norepinephrine and Ca^{2+} uptake by endoplasmic reticulum. Ca^{2+} efflux measurements also allowed for estimations of the size of the intracellular exchangeable Ca^{2+} pool. These studies were carried out in rats which were administered *Salmonella enteritidis* endotoxin at doses which produced in the animals signs and symptoms of shock after four to six hours and a 65% mortality after 24 hours. A group of rats were killed five hours after endotoxin injections, their livers were removed and 0.3 mm thick liver slices prepared. Active plasma membrane ^{45}Ca efflux and intracellular Ca^{2+} pool size were measured using liver slices. Active Ca^{2+} uptake into ER was quantitated using a microsomal fraction. In control rat liver slices, the ^{45}Ca efflux from the intracellular pool was sensitive to iodoacetate demonstrating the metabolic dependency of the efflux process. Ca^{2+} uptake by ER was shown to be ATP dependent. These active movements were unaffected in endotoxin shock. However, the intracellular Ca^{2+} pool size and norepinephrine regulation of Ca^{2+} were adversely affected during shock. An application of 1 μM norepinephrine to control rat liver slices significantly stimulated ^{45}Ca efflux but failed to stimulate efflux in endotoxic rat liver slices. The intracellular Ca^{2+} pool size in endotoxic livers (553±23, SE, μmol/kg) was significantly greater than in controls (413±17). These results suggested that during endotoxic shock there is a depletion of hepatic norepinephrine-mobilized activator Ca^{2+} and an increase in total intracellular Ca^{2+} without any changes in active Ca^{2+} efflux out of cells and into ER.

These changes could be related to endotoxin mediated increases in catecholamines which in turn cause an excessive activation of liver cells in vivo. Consequences of observed Ca^{2+} homeostatic disturbances could cause: 1) an alteration of catecholamine stimulation of the hepatic gluconeogenic response; and 2) an increased susceptibility of liver cells to Ca^{2+} overload.

EFFECT OF CALCIUM BLOCKER DILTIAZEM ON HEPATIC CA^{2+} REGULATION IN ENDOTOXIC SHOCK[7]

Cellular Ca^{2+} regulation was studied not only by measuring Ca^{2+} fluxes but also by quantitating cytosolic free Ca^{2+} concentrations in livers of endotoxic rats (IV *Salmonella enteritidis*). Experiments were carried out also to determine whether endotoxin-mediated alterations in intracellular Ca^{2+} regulation could be abrogated by treatment of rats with the calcium entry blocker, diltiazem. The latter experiments tested the hypothesis that hepatic Ca^{2+} dysregulation in endotoxic shock results from an increased influx of extracellular Ca^{2+} through receptor sensitive calcium channels.

As in previous studies, shock signs and symptoms were observed in rats four to six hours after endotoxin injections. Five hours after injections, rats were killed and hepatocytes isolated for the measurement of cytosolic Ca^{2+} concentrations. Cytosolic Ca^{2+} concentrations were measured before (basal) and after stimulation of cells with epinephrine. To measure cytosolic Ca^{2+}, hepatocytes were loaded with the Ca^{2+} chelator fluorescent dye, quin 2. ^{45}Ca efflux and intracellular Ca^{2+} pool size were measured using liver slices as previously described. The apparent basal cytosolic Ca^{2+} concentrations in endotoxic rat hepatocytes (525±92,SE,nM) was significantly higher than in controls (146±23). A significant increase in basal Ca^{2+} concentration occurred after stimulation with epinephrine (1 and 10 μM) in control rat hepatocytes but not in the hepatocytes from endotoxic rats. In endotoxic rats treated with diltiazem soon after endotoxin injections, basal cytosolic Ca^{2+} concentration was significantly lower than in rats given endotoxin alone. Furthermore, diltiazem treatment of endotoxic rats resulted in a significant epinephrine mediated elevation in cytosolic Ca^{2+} concentration. The total hepatic cellular Ca^{2+} pool in the diltiazem treated rats (427±23, SE, μmol/kg) was significantly lower than in endotoxic shock rats (564±27). Thus diltiazem treatment of rats prevented the endotoxin mediated increases in both the cytosolic Ca^{2+} concentration and total cellular Ca^{2+} pool size. The diltiazem treatment also restored the ability of epinephrine to elevate intracellular free Ca^{2+} concentration which was markedly blunted in rats given endotoxin alone. In summary, these studies clearly demonstrated that a hepatic cellular Ca^{2+} overload with both increased cytosolic Ca^{2+} concentration and total cellular Ca^{2+} pool size occurs during endotoxic shock. Furthermore, the endotoxin-mediated cellular Ca^{2+} overload apparently resulted from an increase in receptor-sensitive Ca^{2+} channel activity as it was prevented when the animals were treated with the Ca^{2+} channel blocker, diltiazem.

EFFECT OF ENDOTOXIC SHOCK ON IP_3 MEDIATED MOBILIZATION OF CA^{2+} FROM ER[8]

As discussed above, an impairment in hormone modulation of intracellular Ca^{2+} regulation occurs in the liver in endotoxic shock. This could be due to alteration in hormone and receptor interactions, and/or G protein and phospholipase C activation resulting in either failure of generation of IP_3 or failure of IP_3 to cause a release of Ca^{2+} from intracellular organelles such as ER. Studies were therefore directed toward a determination of the ability of IP_3 to mediate ER release of Ca^{2+} in hepatocytes from endotoxic shock rats.

The rats injected with *Salmonella enteritidis* endotoxin were killed after the onset of shock signs and symptoms as described above. Hepatocytes from control and endotoxic rats were prepared and treated with saponin which selectively enhances plasma membrane permeability such that exogenous molecules like IP_3 can permeate through it. Saponin permeabilized hepatocytes were then incubated in a medium comparable in its ionic composition to that of the cytosol. Ca^{2+} was added to the medium until a steady state concentration was maintained presumably with an equilibration of Ca^{2+} between medium and ER. Steady state was maintained at comparable Ca^{2+} concentrations in control (130±31, SE, nM) and endotoxic rat (124±18) permeabilized hepatocytes. Addition of IP_3 (1 μM) effected an increase in medium Ca^{2+} (to 257±54) in control but not in endotoxic rat permeabilized hepatocytes. Treatment of endotoxic rats with diltiazem, similarly as described above, resulted in a restoration of an IP_3 mediated increase in medium Ca^{2+} (to 240±41). Thus, IP_3 mobilization of Ca^{2+} from ER may be impaired during endotoxin shock. The previously described increase in cytosolic Ca^{2+} in liver cells of endotoxic rats may play a role in the attenuated IP_3 mediation of ER Ca^{2+} release. It is known that IP_3-mediated ER Ca^{2+} release is dependent on cytosolic Ca^{2+} concentration and that an increase in cytosolic Ca^{2+} to levels above basal can decrease IP_3 and induced ER Ca^{2+} release. It is reasonable to surmise that a buildup of free Ca^{2+} in the cytosolic compartment during endotoxic injury suppresses IP_3 induces ER Ca^{2+} release. The restoration of IP_3 mobilization of ER Ca^{2+} with the diltiazem treatment of endotoxic rats supports the concept of endotoxic cellular Ca^{2+} overload having an adverse effect on intracellular Ca^{2+} mobilization.

INCREASED CA^{2+} INFLUX IN SKELETAL MUSCLE DURING BACTEREMIC SHOCK[9]

Alterations in intracellular Ca^{2+} regulation during septic injury were found not only in the liver but also in the skeletal muscle. Alterations in the skeletal muscle were observed in a septic injury model in which rats were injected with live *Escherichia coli*, IV, to result in the onset of shock signs at 12-16 hours and a mortality of 50% at 24 hours after the injections. ^{45}Ca flux into muscle cells was measured using the isolated soleus muscles. This technique also allowed the assessment of the size of the intracellular exchangeable Ca^{2+} pool. ^{45}Ca loaded muscles were treated with Lanthanum (La^{3+}) in Ca^{2+}-free media to remove extracellular bound and unbound Ca^{2+}. Thus, measurements of ^{45}Ca flux and total exchangeable calcium actually estimated Ca^{2+} flux into the intracellular compartment and the size of the intracellular Ca^{2+} pool. The intracellular Ca^{2+} pool size in the skeletal muscle of bacteremic shock rats (719±58, SE, μmol/kg) was not significantly different from the controls (741±34). This is in contrast to an increase in skeletal muscle cellular exchangeable Ca^{2+} with endotoxic injury. Although endotoxic injury has features in common with gram-negative bacteremic injury, endotoxic animals exhibit more severe cardiovascular and metabolic derangements over a shorter time course than the bacteremic animals. The lack of change in cellular exchangeable Ca^{2+} in the bacteremic rats could be due to the slower progression of the cell injury process. Despite a lack of effect of bacteremic shock on the cellular Ca^{2+} pool size, bacteremic injury caused a significant shift in the Ca^{2+} flux kinetics.

The initial flux in bacteremic rat skeletal muscle was nearly two times the initial rate measured in control rat muscles. The increased initial flux would result in a greater availability of intraorgannular Ca^{2+} and thus in the cytosolic environment. Experiments have also assessed muscle depolarization induced increase in Ca^{2+} flux. On depolarization of isolated muscles with 60 mM K^+, a significantly greater increase was observed in Ca^{2+} flux in bactermic rat skeletal muscles than in muscles of control rats. These latter experiments supported the concept that not only the initial Ca^{2+} flux increased with bacteremic shock but also the voltage-sensitive calcium channel activity. Experiments in which bacteremic rats were treated with the calcium blocker diltiazem ten hours after bacterial injections supported the activation of the skeletal muscle calcium channel during bactermic injury. Diltiazem treatment prevented the increase in initial ^{45}Ca flux.

Concluding Remarks

The above discussion illustrates how sustained increases in cytosolic Ca^{2+} concentration above the basal level found in healthy resting cells could lead to a decline in Ca^{2+} depended cellular responses. Such changes in intracellular Ca^{2+} regulation and Ca^{2+} dependent function are plausibly reversible and represent initial events of the cell injury process under pathologic conditions. These changes are distinguishable from gross cellular accumulation of calcium to lead to tissue calcification typical of irreversible cell damage and death. The state of the art knowledge of regulation of intracellular Ca^{2+} and its participation in the transmission of hormonal signals provides insights into multistep sequential subcellular mechanisms whose disarray under pathologic conditions could lead to a reversible or irreversible cell injury process.

Studies of intracellular Ca^{2+} regulation in the liver and skeletal muscle during a septic injury in animals have supported the concept that this regulatory process is altered reversibly in pathologic states. The observed alterations in Ca^{2+} regulation were prevented when septic animals were treated with the calcium blocker diltiazem. The latter results point to a pathologic hyperfunctioning of a receptor-and/or voltage-sensitive calcium channel to cause cellular Ca^{2+} dysregulation. These results also suggest a potential therapeutic use of calcium blockers to prevent Ca^{2+} dysregulation during septic injury.

References

1. Rasmussen H, Barret P, Smallwood J et al. Calcium ion as intracellular messenger and cellular toxin. Environ Health Persp 1990; 84:17-25.
2. Williamson JR., Monck JR. Signal transduction mechanisms in hormonal Ca^{2+} fluxes. Environ Health Persp 1990; 84:121-136.
3. Nairn AC. Role of Ca^{2+}/calmodulin-dependent protein phosphorylation in signal transduction. In: Nishizuka Y, ed. The Biophysics and medicine of signal transduction. New York: Raven Press, 1990: 202-205.
4. Campbell AK. Intracellular calcium. Chichester: John Wiley and Sons. Chichester. 1983: 393-454.
5. Sayeed MM. Alterations in cellular Ca^{2+} regulation in the liver in endotoxic shock. Am J Physiol 1986; 250: R884-R891.
6. Sayeed MM. Ion transport in circulatory and/or septic shock. Invited Opinion. Am J Physiol 1987; 252: R809-R821.
7. Sayeed MM, Maitra SR. Effect of diltiazem on altered cellular calcium regulation during endotoxic shock. Am J Physiol 1987; 253: R549-R554.
8. Maitra SR, Sayeed MM. Effect of diltiazem on intracellular Ca^{2+} mobilization in hepatocytes during endotoxic shock. Am J Physiol 1987; 253: R545-R548.
9. Westfall MV, Sayeed MM. Skeletal muscle calcium uptake in bacteremic rats. Am J Physiol 1989; 256: R201-R206

CHAPTER 18

WOUND HEALING

Richard L. Gamelli

The cutaneous healing process following wounding immediately calls into play a sequence of epidermal-dermal events that, when successful, redevelops the skin, returning it to its former state. Normal wound healing represents an integrated process in which various cells and cell products work in concert to initiate the reparative mechanisms, which ultimately lead to reestablishment of tissue integrity. Whether the inciting event is a planned surgical incision or a traumatic wound, once begun, normal repair follows a near predictable course.[1] (Fig.1)

The initial phase of wound healing is that which occurs with activation of the coagulation system. Coagulation provides homeostasis and assures survival of the organism to control the ongoing blood loss. Coagulation simultaneously provides cells in the injured area with the stimulus to divide. Additionally, components of the coagulation system serve as attractants for cellular components of the inflammatory response. This supports the notion that repair starts almost instantaneously following injury when a number of factors are released into the injured tissue, most notably, platelet derived growth factor (PDGF) transforming growth factor beta (TGF-ß), platelet factor IV (PF$_4$), and fibroblast growth factor (FGF). These various factors are not only mitogenic stimuli but also potent chemoattractants which recruit leukocytes, monocytes and fibroblasts into the area of injury. The inflammatory cells confer resistance to infection as well as debridement of devitalized tissue and bacteria from the wound. The cell which appears to be most critical to the wound healing process is the macrophage, as suggested by the work of Leibovitch and Ross.[2] The macrophage has become recognized to not only function as a phagocyte but also to be a source for additional cellular factors through its secretion of a number of cytokines which may function as growth factors.[3] Thus not only does the macrophage respond to its environment, it also is capable of significantly modifying it. These factors are responsible for information transfer to fibroblasts and endothelial cells, they can regulate cell movement and cell growth, as well as the basic products of wound cells, to include extracellular matrix production and new blood vessel growth.[1]

A healed wound results when there is a progression from the inflammatory to the remodeling phase. The remodeling phase represents the balance between collagen synthesis and collagen lysis and includes maturation of the overlying epithelium. The factors that are responsible for the cessation of the wound healing process following injury are much less well characterized and remain an area of active investigation.

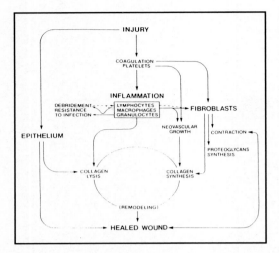

Fig. 1. Schema of the pathways of wound repair.[1]

Wounds, whether they are the result of a surgical incision with primary closure or traumatic defects, are nonuniform. This asymmetry is reflected in both the cellular constituents of the wound and the events of wound healing. Cell types, extracellular matrix and components of the extracellular fluid exist in a gradient across the wound from its center to the edge. The cellular organization of the advancing wound front is typified by macrophages which precede immature fibroblasts. Dividing fibroblasts evolve from the immature fibroblasts and are followed by developing new capillaries. Fibrillar collagen is subsequently deposited by mature fibroblasts and is soon followed by new blood vessel growth.[1]

The macrophage is a cell that is particularly well suited to function within the wound environment. Wounds centrally have no vessels yet present and in essence have a dead space, which is hypoxic, hyperlactated and acidotic. Macrophages release chemotropic substances for capillary endothelial cells in the setting of low pO_2 and/or high lactates. Tumor necrosis factor-alpha, as described by Leibovich, may be the factor released by macrophages in response to wound hypoxia or lactate that is the stimulus for capillary endothelial cells.[4] Tumor necrosis factor in the 5-50 ng range in in vitro studies has been shown to stimulate capillary tube-like activity with cultured endothelial cells. Macrophages also

appear to be responsible, in part, for the high wound lactate levels as they release lactate in large quantities regardless of the degree to which they are oxygenated. The lactate, as well as the low pO_2, have been considered by some important components of the growth environment that exists within the wound. Both oxygen and lactate may well represent controlling mechanisms for new collagen synthesis.[5] Remodelling of the newly synthesized collagen continues over the weeks and months after wound healing has seemingly been completed. Cells which normally exist in other environments without causing fibrosis eventually come to transform the healed wound in to a scar. The degree to which scarring occurs in a wound is a balance between the mechanism responsible for the injury, the genetic makeup of the host, the techniques of wound closure and the anatomic location of the original injury.

Cutaneous Healing

The skin is an apposition of epiderm and mesoderm separated by a thin basement membrane zone (BMZ). This BMZ contains elements from the primary germ cell layers. In the unwounded state, basal keratinocytes are in direct contact with the basement membrane. The BMZ is relatively thin, morphologically separates the epidermis from the dermis and consists of four distinct components. These components include: 1) the plasma membrane of the basal keratinocyte; 2) the lamina lucida which contains laminin; 3) the lamina densa, which is rich in type IV collagen which is a basement membrane specific collagen contributed by epidermal cells; and 4) a sublamina-densa fibrillar zone with anchoring fibrils, single collagen fibers and microfibrillar-like bundles contributed by dermis.[6]

The character of this BMZ tissue has profound effects on the response of keratinocytes during normal homeostases, as well as following injury. Interaction between the cell and the matrix, to which it is exposed, direct and influence the behavior of the basal keratinocytes. Cell matrix interactions have been recognized to include keratinocyte cell attachment, proliferation, and differentiation.

Three of the major matrix molecules, which make up the BMZ are bullous pemphigoid antigen (BPA), laminin and type IV collagen.

BPA is synthesized and deposited extracellularly by human adult keratinocytes without requiring a viable matrix. It has a molecular weight in the range of 220-240 kD. The exact function of BPA is unknown, but of the BMZ components BPA is the one most closely associated with the basal keratinocytes and may be involved with biologic processes such as attachment, proliferation and differentiation.

Laminin is a large (molecular weight 800 kD) noncollagenase cysteine-rich glycoprotein synthesized by epithelial cells. Laminin has an affinity for type IV collagen and heparin sulfate proteoglycans (HS-PG) within the BMZ. For certain cell types, laminin may be an attachment factor to allow cells to anchor to basement membrane collagen.[7]

Type IV collagen is a basement membrane specific collagen that has a native weight of nearly half a million daltons and is important for tissue support. It has been shown that epidermal cells preferentially attach to type IV collagen as opposed to interstitial collagen such as type I collagen.

The interaction of keratinocytes with the underlying matrix in the unperturbed state is characterized by proliferation of basal keratinocytes. Cells above this level which are moving vertically and have lost contact with the matrix are in a state of nonproliferative terminal differentiation. In the unwounded state, the basal cells within the static epidermis are opposed to an intact basal membrane zone that isolates the proliferative pool of keratinocytes (basal cells) from dermal collagen, dermal proteoglycans and increased concentrations of fibronectin. The BMZ also serve as a selective filter that in part controls which soluble factors eventually reach and influence the proliferative keratinocyte. In this manner the BMZ may act as a gate keeper for plasma-derived growth and inhibitory molecules that direct epidermal cell activity.

With cutaneous injury, the BMZ is violated and in its place an early wound matrix forms. This early wound matrix is a mixture of both plasma and dermal components. The temporary matrix bed of a fresh wound has a composition which is distinctly different from that of the intact BMZ. The early wound matrix is characterized by a loss of laminin and type IV collagen. They are replaced by fibronectin, type I collagen, fibrin-fibrinogen and thrombospondin.

Successful closure of a cutaneous injury requires epidermal cells to eventually migrate across the open wound. The epidermis must, therefore, convert from a stationary to migratory epidermis. Examination of keratinocytes at the margin of a wound reveals that there is a time-dependent process for the movement of epidermal cells across the wound. Early changes that have been recognized are thickening of wound margin keratinocytes. By 24 hours, wound orientated cytoplasmic changes have been reported and at 24-48 hours cells are actively migrating across the open wound. Migration of epidermal cells across the open wound is facilitated by the changes that have occurred in the wound bed and its matrix as the result of the wounding process.

Laminin, which is an adhesion factor for keratinocytes and suppresses their migration, is not present following wounding as is in the case of an intact epidermis. Conversely, fibronectin which is found diffusely throughout the dermis and in the intact state and not in contact with keratinocytes, is now readily present in a wound and is a potent stimulus for keratinocyte motility. Studies examining keratinocyte extracellular matrix interactions have shown marked alterations in keratinocyte mobility as a function of the matrix environment. Nickoloff and coworkers have demonstrated that fibronectin significantly promotes keratinocyte mobility in vitro. Additionally, they noted that thrombospondin, a high molecular weight glycoprotein, which is released from the alpha-granules of platelets, had a significant effect on keratinocyte movement. Fibronectin and thrombospondin both significantly augmented keratinocyte mobility as compared to controls. Conversely, laminin depressed keratinocyte mobility as compared to controls, as well as fibronectin or thrombospondin.[8]

The collagen substrate, as shown by Martinet, also further modulates epidermal cellular response to motility factors. In studies examining migration of epithelial cells on different substrates, with or without laminin or fibronectin added to the assay medium, they noted the greatest degree of keratinocyte mobility with the combination of type I collagen and fibronectin.[9] This combination would be most characteristic of the early wound environment. Interestingly, they noted that type IV collagen and type V collagen in combination with fibronectin produced the greatest degree of inhibited epidermal cell migration.

Woodley et al[6] have suggested a conceptual model to represent the wound healing state. In this scheme, epidermal cells respond to violation of the basement membrane zone by changing their primary axis of migration. In contrast to the usual vertical migration during differentiation, following wounding keratinocytes begin to move horizontally over a wound bed matrix composed of the type I collagen, serum fibronectin and elastin. The horizontal migration of epidermal cells continues until wound closure is achieved and reestablishment of a normal BMZ beneath the migrating epidermis.

Keratinocyte migration during the wound healing process may be facilitated by epidermal cell synthesis of type IV collagen. Woodley has proposed that migrating epidermal cells under their leading edge synthesize and deposit type IV collagen. This serves as a point of attachment and mechanical fixation and allows the epidermal cell to pull itself in the direction of the newly formed type IV collagen. At this point the cell reestablishes its configuration by the release of locally active collagenase. This results in the dissolution of the type IV collagen in the immediate subadjacent pericellular zone. The released cell is then capable of type IV collagen resynthesis and repeating the attachment and migration process. In this way, epidermal cells are capable of ratchetting across the open wound.[7]

The net response to wounding of the epidermis and violation of the BMZ are changes in the microenvironment of the basal keratinocytes which promote wound closure. The interaction of keratinocytes with the underlying matrix in the unperturbed state is characterized by epidermal cells that have movement which is primarily vertical, cell division which is arresting and differentiation which is terminal. Upon disruption of the BMZ, epidermal cell movement becomes lateral, cell division is one of proliferation and the cells remains undifferentiated until wound closure is achieved. Upon wound closure and the reestablishment of the BMZ, the migrating epidermis reverts to a stationary epidermis and the wound undergoes maturation with cell movement, again becoming vertical and division arresting, and differentiation occurring.

Growth Factors

The process which occurs following injury results in an orderly progression of cells and events which are thought in part to be regulated by cell-specific attractants. The source of these cell attractants appears to be the migrating cells which produce factors that facilitate recruitment of subsequent cell populations. As an example, platelets which aggregate early during the clotting process release a series of factors which facilitate the movement of macrophages and immature fibroblasts into the early wound matrix. In addition to serving as chemotactic factors, many of these same compounds have considerable mitogenic activity and may function in a dual capacity. Once cells enter the wound environment, proliferation is determined by the type and levels of the growth factors present in the wounds. Numerous studies have shown that various growth factors in high concentrations are often cytolytic. TNF and interferon gamma have been reported by Craig et al as prime examples of this phenomenon.[10] TNF, while it can function as a growth factor and has been found in wounds, has been shown in high concentrations to cause increased inflammation and decreased collagen accumulation. Interferon-gamma is a macrophage activator, but decreases keratinocyte mobility and proliferation.

The source of the growth factors in the wound can occur via a variety of pathways. Some growth factors such as insulin-like growth factor I (IGF$_1$) and insulin-like growth factor II (IGF$_2$) are delivered by the blood in an endocrine-like fashion. Certain other growth factors such as platelet derived growth factors and the transforming growth factors are synthesized by one cell population and used by another in a paracrine-like fashion. Other cell types produce and utilize their secretory products in an autocrine or self-stimulatory manner.[11]

Growth factors have been characterized as either competence or progression factors, dependent upon the stage in the cell cycle in which their primary activity is exerted. Competence factors act early in the cell cycle, moving the cells out of G$_o$ into active proliferation. Progression factors act later in the cell cycle.[12] Platelet derived growth factor and fibroblast growth factor are recognized competence factors, while the insulin-like growth factors, type I and II, are progression factors. Such growth factors have very different individual activities; however, under certain conditions can show strong synergistic activities in promoting cell division. While IGF growth factors alone can not induce cells to proliferate, PDGF at high doses can induce proliferation, perhaps by the induction of IGF$_1$ production.[13] Certain growth factors which act early in the cell cycle may also work through the elevation of cytoplasmic calcium and pH and initiate the transcription of fos and myc genes. These events may represent part of the pathways through which certain growth factors prepare the cells for DNA synthesis and division.

Growth factors exerted their efforts on cells via cell surface receptors. Such receptors show specificity in high affinity binding. A number of these receptors, particularly for EGF, PGF, IGF$_1$, have tyrosine kinase activity as part of their intracellular domain. With growth factor binding, the kinase becomes activated and phosphorylates tyrosine on intracellular cytoplasmic proteins as well as tyrosines on the receptor itself. The phosphorylation of the cytoplasmic proteins leads to their activation and the initiation of the growth factor response. Autophosphorylation of the receptor heightens its affinity for the ligand and, also, may facilitate internalization of the receptor.[14]

GROWTH FACTORS IN WOUND HEALING

The macrophage is central to the normal wound healing process. Macrophages serve as a source of growth factors that have activity for both fibroblastic and epithelial cells in the wound. Additionally, many of the factors released by the macrophage have a marked effect on wound matrix formation. Such peptide factors that have been recognized include transforming growth factor beta, epidermal growth factor somatomedin C and interferon-gamma. These peptide growth factors appear capable of interacting with the extracellular matrix molecules to include fibronectin, thrombospondin and laminin.

Transforming growth factor beta is a 25 kD compound released at the injury site by platelets, macrophages and T-cells. It is capable of significantly enhancing matrix formation. Epidermal growth factor, a 6 kD peptide, initially isolated from mouse submaxillary glands, which is released by macrophages and platelets, increases fibronectin and thrombospondin in the wound environment. Transforming growth factor beta and epidermal growth factor appear to work in a cooperative fashion to increase local fibronectin production in the wound environment. Somatomedin C is capable of increasing keratinocyte mobility and this appears to be associated with an increase in thrombospondin production. Conversely, interferon-gamma is recognized to decrease fibronectin and thrombospondin production and to lead to a reduction in keratinocyte motility and proliferation. Potentially, interferon-gamma may serve as a down-regulator of the wound healing process and be one of the factors responsible for signalling the end to the wound healing process.

In addition to effects on matrix formation, growth factors have been recognized to have profound effects on cellular movement and mitogenesis, as well as production of collagen. Platelet derived growth factor is chemotactic for fibroblast and monocyte/macrophages. PDGF is mitogenic for fibroblast and stimulates fibroblast collagen synthesis as well as collagenase secretion. TGF-ß serves as a chemoattractant for fibroblast and monocyte/macrophages. TGF-ß is mitogenic for fibroblast while inhibitory for epithelial cells. Collagen synthesis as well as collagenase secretion are both stimulated by TGF-ß. Basic fibroblast growth factor serves as a chemoattractant for epithelial cells and fibroblast, as well as being mitogenic for endothelial cells and fibroblast. Epidermal growth factor is a chemoattractant for endothelial cells, as well as being mitogenic for endothelial cells and fibroblasts.[15]

Growth Factor Modification of Wound Healing

Lynch et al examined the effects of isolated, as well as combinations of growth factors to alter cutaneous healing.[16] In a porcine model of partial thickness skin wounds, epidermal thickness, epidermal-dermal interface area, dermal thickness, dermal cellularity and hydroxyproline content were examined in seven-day-old wounds after the application of 500 ng of factor, to include PDGF, IGF, TGF-A, FGF and TGF-B, singularly or in combination. Platelet derived growth factor and insulin-like growth factor was the most potent combination. Wounds treated with the combination evidenced increase in epidermal thickness, dermal thickness and organization and maturation. Additionally, these wounds had a significant increase in their hydroxyproline content. Interestingly, these changes were not associated with any heightening of the inflammatory component within the healing wounds. Schultz et al examined the relative ability of various growth factors to facilitate wound healing in a middermal burn wound performed in a porcine model.[17] Wound reepithelialization was evaluated as percent reepithelialization. In wounds that were allowed to be open and dry and desiccate, significantly reduced degrees of reepithelialization occurrence. When the wound was treated with silver sulfadiazine topical cream, the rate of closure exceeded 50%. The incorporation of transforming growth factor-alpha or vaccinia growth factor into the sulfadiazine cream significantly facilitated wound closure. Vaccinia growth factor is a 24 kD protein that binds to the EGF receptor and stimulates its autophosphoryl–ation. Vaccinia growth factor is created by cells infected with the virus and encodes for a 140-residue polypeptide with approximately 35% sequence homology to both EGF and TGF-α.

Brown and coworkers in a prospective randomized clinical trial used skin graft donor sites to determine whether epidermal growth factor could accelerate the rate of epidermal regeneration in humans.[18] Incorporation of epidermal growth factor into silver sulfadiazine cream when applied to donor sites resulted in a time to 25% or 50% healing that was decreased by one day. The times to 75% or 100% healing were reduced by 1.5 days.

In clinical studies examining the utility of wound derived fluid to facilitate the closure of venous stasis ulcers, Hunt and Knighton showed a significant reduction in the time to wound closure for treated wounds. With this approach, autologous platelet-rich plasma is obtained and the platelets are then stimulated with thrombin to cause release of the alpha-granule contents. The alpha-granules are subsequently isolated and prepared as a topical salve in a microcrystal collagen. A series of nonrandomized clinical and randomized clinical trials have been performed. One reported study in 14 patients with 19 wounds achieved 100% reepithelialization at an average of six weeks. In the placebo group, three of 12 patients healed during the initial eight weeks of trial, however, nine of 12 patients failed to heal within the eight-week trial period. The failed patients were crossed over to the treatment arm and achieved one hundred percent epithelialization of 11 wounds in an average of 6.5 weeks.[19] In a more recently reported study, Herndon et al show that the systemic administration of growth hormone in a dose-dependent fashion markedly decreased the healing time of donor sites in burned children. The same effect, however, was not found in adult burn patients treated with growth hormone. Currently, a multicenter clinical trial is under way examining the utility of growth hormone administration in the pediatric burn patients to facilitate wound healing.[20]

SUMMARY

Wound healing represents an adaptive response of the organism to deal with injury. It is a complex series of cellular and bio-chemical events that lead to reconstitution of the damaged surface. While not the focus of this review, it is markedly different in the adult of the species than in the fetus. Our understanding of the normal wound healing process has provided many insights but still many questions remain resolved. The future hoped-for strategies are to be able to identify patients who are at risk for impaired wound healing due to nutritional deficiency, drug administration such as steroids or chemo-therapy, vascular problems or following radiation therapy. In these clinical situations, impaired wound healing is likely to be present. Our ability to therapeutically intervene to restore healing and prevent wound healing complications would represent a significant therapeutic advance. The potential to improve normal healing so that the time to closure would be shortened for cutaneous wounds or the ultimate strength of a wound improved without the induction of a hyper-trophic scar or keloid, remain additional challenges. Further, the long-term consequences of such treated wounds, with the potential induction of tumors, needs to be carefully monitored and remains of concern as we attempt to manipulate the wound.

REFERENCES

1. Hunt TK. Prospective, a retrospective perspective on the nature of wounds. In: Barbul A, Pines E, Caldwell M, Hunt TK, eds. Growth factor and other aspects of wound healing: Biological and clinical implications. New York: Alan R Liss, 1989.

2. Leibovich SJ, Ross R. The role of the macrophage in wound repair. Am J Pathol 1975; 84:71-100.

3. Whal SM, Wong H, McCartney-Francis N. Role of growth factors in inflammation and repair. J Cell Biochem 1989; 40:193-199.

4. Leibovich SJ, Polverini PJ, Shepard HM et al. Macrophage-induced angiogenesis is mediated by tumor necrosis factor-alpha. Nature 1989; 329:630-632.

5. Knighton DR, Silver IA, Hunt TK. Regulation of wound healing angiogenesis-effect of oxygen gradients and inspired oxygen concentration. Surgery 1981; 90:262-270.

6. Woodley DT, O'Keefe EJ, Prunieras M. Cutaneous wound healing: A model for cell-matrix interactions. J Am Acad Dermatol 1985; 12:420-423.

7. Woodley DT, Bachman PM, O'Keefe ET. The role of matrix components in human keratinocyte reepithelialization. In: Barbul A, Caldwell M, Eaglstein W, eds. Clinical and experimental approaches to dermal and epidermal repair. New York: Wiley-Liss, 1991:129-140.

8. Nickoloff BJ, Mitka RS, Riser BL, Dixit VM, Varani J. Modulation of keratinocyte motility. Am J of Pathology 1988; 132:543-551.

9. Martinet N, Lesile AH, Grotendorst G. Identification and characterization of chemoattractants for epidermal cells. J Invest Dermatol 1988; 90:122-126.

10. Craig RW, Buchan HL. Differentiation-inducing and cytotoxic effects of tumor necrosis factor and interferon-gamma in myeloblastic ML-1 cells. Cell Physiol 1989; 141:466-52.

11. Sporn MB, Todaro GJ. Autocrine secretion and malignant transformation of cells. N Engl J Med 1980; 303:878-880.

12. Pledger WJ, Stiles CD, Antoniades HN, Scher CD. Induction of DNA synthesis in Balb/c 3T3 cells by serum components. Reevaluation of the commitment process. Proc Natl Adac Sci USA 1977; 74:4481-4485.

13. Clemmons DR, Underwood LE, Van Wyk JJ. Hormonal control of immunoreactive somatomedin produced by human fibroblast. J Clin Invest 1981; 67:10-19.

14. Nemeth GG, Bolander ME, Martin GR. Growth Factors and Their Role in Wound and Fracture Healing. In: (eds), Barbul A, Pines E, Caldwell M, Hunt TK, eds. New York: Alan R Liss, 1989: 1-17.

15. Sprugel KH, McPherson TM, Clowes AW, Ross R. Effect of growth factors in vivo. I cell ingrowth into porous subcutaneous chambers. Am J Pathol 1987; 129:601-613.

16. Lynch SE, Colvin RB Antoniades HN. Growth factors in wound healing: Single and synergistic effects on partial thickness porcine skin wounds. J Clin Invest 1989; 84:640-646.

17. Schultz GS, White M, Mitchell R et al. Epithelial wound healing enhanced by transforming growth factor-alpha and vaccina growth factor. Science 1987; 235: 350-351.

18. Brown GL, Nancy LB, Griffin J et al. Enhancement of wound healing by topical treatment with epidermal growth factor. N Engl J Med 1989; 321:76-79.

19. Knighton DR, Ciresi F, Fiegel VD et al. Classification and treatment of chronic nonhealing wounds: Successful treatment with autologous platelet-derived wound healing factors (PDWHF). Ann Surg 1986; 204:322-330.

20. Herndon DN, Barrow RE, Kunkel Broemeling L, Rutan RL. Effects of recombinant human growth hormone on donor-site healing in severely burned children. Ann Surg 1990; 212:424-429.

CHAPTER 19

IMMUNE CONTROL OF WOUND HEALING

Mark C. Regan
Adrian Barbul

Introduction

Following injury the body has three major priorities: limitation of blood loss, prevention of infection and restoration of tissue integrity. Tissue damage induces platelet degranulation and activation of the coagulation cascade, preventing blood loss. This in turn is responsible for initiation of the repair process. The process of wound repair consists of a sequence of inflammation and repair aimed at the restoration of tissue integrity and function. Achieving this goal necessitates both the removal of dead and damaged tissue and the subsequent synthesis and reorganization of replacement tissue.

The wound is well recognized as an area of intense immune activity with elements of both the specific and nonspecific immune system present throughout the healing process. Polymorphoneuclear leukocytes (PMN) are the first blood leukocytes to enter the wound site. They initially appear in the wound shortly after injury and subsequently their numbers increase steadily, peaking at 24 to 48 hours.[1] Their main function appears to be phagocytosis of the bacteria which have been introduced into the wound during injury. The presence of PMNs in the wound following injury does not appear to be essential in order for normal wound healing to take place [2,3] with healing proceeding normally in their absence provided that bacterial contamination has not occurred.

The next cellular immune element to enter the wound are macrophages. These cells are derived from circulating monocytes by a combination of migration and chemotaxis, first appearing within 48 to 96 hours postinjury and reaching a peak around the third day post injury.[1] Their appearance is followed somewhat later by T-lymphocytes which appear in significant numbers around the fifth day postinjury, with peak numbers appearing about the seventh day after injury. In contrast to PMNs, the presence and activation of both macrophages and lymphocytes in the wound is critical to the progress of the normal healing process.[4,5]

The Role of the Macrophage

The macrophage appears to have a dual role at the wound site. Initially they participate in the inflammatory and debridement process superseding the PMN as the major wound phagocyte and later play a regulatory role in the mediation of the fibroblastic phase of healing. It is this latter role which is crucial to the success of the wound healing process. A combination of systemic hydrocortisone to induce systemic monocytopenia and local antimacrophage serum for local elimination of tissue macrophages resulted in a significant impairment of wound debridement and fibroplasia in guinea pigs.[4] Wound fibrin levels were elevated and clearance of fibrin, neutrophils, erythrocytes and other miscellaneous debris from the wound was delayed in treated animals. In addition there was both a delay in the appearance of fibroblasts in the wound and in the subsequent rate of expansion of the wound fibroblast population.[6] In a rat model we have observed a decrease in wound breaking strength and collagen deposition following in vivo macrophage depletion using the mouse anti-rat antimacrophage monoclonal antibody OX-42 which was accompanied by a significant depletion of wound infiltrating macrophages.

Further evidence for macrophage involvement in the regulation of wound healing is provided by the findings that intradermal injection of allogeneic macrophages increases both collagen synthesis and wound breaking strength in 8 day old rat skin wounds,[7] while injection of wound macrophages into rabbit corneas induces angiogenesis and scar formation.[8,9]

Activated macrophages are capable of influencing many aspects of wound healing including the proliferative[6] and synthetic activities of fibroblasts[9] and induction of neovascularization.[10,11]

Macrophages mediate their effects on other wound elements via the release of monokines. These intracellular transmitters are capable of regulating fibroblast and endothelial function. Of the cytokines produced by activated macrophages, TGF-ß[12], TNF-α and IL-1[13] have been detected in significant quantities in the extracellular fluid at the site

of healing. Topical application of TGF-ß[14] and PDGF[15] to healing wounds results in significantly enhanced wound breaking strength. Application of TGF-ß at the time of wounding in rats with steroid induced monocytopenia results in a wound breaking strength not significantly different from non-steroid treated rats; this effect is not seen with topical PDGF application. Neither treatment resulted an increase in the number of macrophages in the wound. TGF-ß appears to act directly on the fibroblasts, inducing type I procollagen gene expression, while the effects of PDGF seem to be mediated indirectly, possibly by attracting further macrophages and inducing the release of other monokines. This hypothesis is supported by observations in models of impaired healing. Following total body irradiation, which induces monocytopenia with selective sparing of skin tissue, there is a significant decrease in wound breaking strength. Topical treatment with TGF-ß[16] but not PDGF[17] results in significantly increased wound strength. By contrast following megavolt electron beam surface irradiation to the skin surface, which impairs skin fibroblasts but spares the bone marrow, TGF-ß[17] has no effect on subsequent healing while PDGF[16] increases wound breaking strength by 50% in parallel with an increase in the number of macrophages and fibroblasts in the healing wound.

IL-1, another macrophage product, has been shown to inhibit collagen synthesis in subcutaneously implanted sponges in rats.[18] While TNF-α has been found to have no effect on wound collagen deposition[19] when administered alone, it acted synergistically with PDGF and inhibited the effects of TGF-ß on collagen deposition. We have found that administration of TGF-α into PVA sponges induces increased collagen deposition, an effect which is abrogated by simultaneous administration of indomethacin. This indicates a possible indirect inflammatory mode of action for TNF-α. On the other hand TNF-α antibody administration, which blocks the effects of TNF-α, also induces an increase in collagen deposition.[20] The data are consistent with a direct inhibitory effect of TNF-α on fibroblast synthetic activity, however this effect is masked by its strong proinflammatory and macrophage activating effects.

THE ROLE OF THE LYMPHOCYTE

Direct evidence for lymphocyte involvement in the control of wound healing is provided by studies examining the effects of in vivo lymphocyte depletion on wound healing parameters. Global T-cell depletion causes marked diminution in wound breaking strength and in the hydroxyproline content of subcutaneously implanted polyvinyl alcohol sponges used as an index of wound reparative collagen deposition.[5,21-22] Selective depletion of the T suppressor/cytotoxic lymphocyte subset causes marked enhancement of wound healing at two and four weeks postwounding. These findings suggest a possible role for the T suppressor/cytotoxic lymphocyte subset in the overall down regulation of wound healing activity. It might be expected that the T helper/effector cells would promote such activity. Selective depletion of this subset, however, has no effect on either wound breaking strength or wound collagen deposition.[5] Simultaneous depletion of T-helper/effector and T suppressor/cytotoxic T-cells lead to significant increases in both wound breaking strength and collagen synthesis.[22] This suggests that an incompletely characterized T-cell population, bearing the T-cell marker but neither the T-helper nor the T-suppressor antigenic determinant, is responsible for the promotion of wound healing since its deletion impairs wound healing.

Further support for these findings is provided by work in the congenitally athymic nude mouse.[23] These animals have a profoundly impaired T-cell dependent immune system and display significantly enhanced wound breaking strength and collagen deposition in response to injury when compared to normal thymus-bearing animals. Administration of the anti-T-cell monoclonal antibody to these athymic animals, in order to deplete the small numbers of extrathymically derived T-cell present, had no effect on either wound healing parameter but confirmed the previously observed significant decreases in wound breaking strength and hydroxypro-

line deposition when administered to normal thymus bearing control mice. T-cell reconstitution of nude mice, by injection of syngeneic T-lymphocytes, resulted in significant decreases in wound breaking strength towards the levels observed in normal controls.

Additional evidence supporting a central role for T-lymphocytes in the control of wound healing is provided by studies which examine the in vivo effects of alternate forms of T-cell manipulation on various parameters of healing. Administration of agents known to enhance T lymphocyte function, such as growth hormone,[24] vitamin A[25] or arginine[26] leads to increases in wound breaking strength and collagen deposition while agents which suppress T-lymphocyte function such as steroids,[27] retinoic acid, citral and cyclosporin A[28] markedly impair wound healing. Modification of T-lymphocyte function by adult thymectomy, which prevents the induction of T-suppressor cells, causes an increase in wound maturation. This effect could be reversed by intraperitoneal placement of autologous thymic grafts in millipore chambers in thymectomized rats.[29] Conversely administration of purified thymic hormones, thymulin (FTS), thymopoietin and thymosin fraction V (TF5), results in impaired wound healing as assessed by wound breaking strength and wound collagen deposition.[30] This data suggests that the thymus exerts an inhibitory effect on normal wound healing, possibly by enhancing T-suppressor cell activation following injury.

Lymphocytes exert many of their effects via cytokines. In vitro studies have shown that lymphokines are capable of modulating many fibroblast functions including migration, replication and collagen synthesis. Some, such as TGF-ß, lymphotoxin or γ-interferon are well characterized, while many other proteins which can modulate in vitro fibroblast activity have not been fully characterized. Both inhibitory and stimulatory lymphokines have been described for many fibroblast functions,[31] however exactly how these various signals interact in vivo is presently unknown.

As mentioned previously, the presence of a number of potential regulators of healing has been confirmed in vivo at the wound site. The presence of biologically active TGF-ß[12] and IL-6 has been shown in early wounds, however neither IL-2, IL-3 nor IL-4 could not be detected.[13] In a similar model we failed to detect either IFN-γ or TGF-ß at ten days post injury.[32] The effects of TGF-ß administration on wound strength have already been mentioned.[33] Similar increases in both fresh and fixed wound breaking strength, with an associated rise in collagen deposition, were seen following administration of human recombinant IL-2 (60,000 U and 140,000 U/day) in rats.[34] In contrast the administration of IFN-γ via subcutaneously implanted osmotic pumps in mice resulted in a decrease in the thickness and collagen content of the capsule which formed around the device.[35]

CONCLUSION

Both in vitro and in vivo studies have demonstrated that the presence of both macrophages and T-lymphocytes at the wound site is essential in order for the normal healing process to occur. Both macrophages and T-lymphocytes possess the capacity to regulate essential steps in the process of wound healing. The presence of macrophages is essential for the initiation and maintenance of wound fibroblast activity. T-cells do not appear to be required for the initiation of the healing process and healing can progress in the absence of T-lymphocytes, however the presence of an intact T-cell immune system is essential for a normal outcome, indicating that the T-cells probably provide a regulatory influence over macrophage induced activities. The exact interaction of these immune cells and their secretory products with other wound elements remains to be fully delineated.

REFERENCES

1. Ross R, Benditt EP. Wound healing and collagen formation. I. Sequential changes in components of guinea pig skin wounds observed in the electron microscope. J Biophysiol Biochem Cytol 1961; 11:677-700.
2. Simpson DM, Ross R. The neutrophilic leucocyte in wound repair. A study with anti-neutrophil serum. J Clin Invest 1972; 51:2009-2023.
3. Simpson DM, Ross R. Effects of heterologous antineutrophil serum in guinea pigs: hematalogical and ultrastructural observations, Am J Pathol 1971; 65:49-102.
4. Leibovich SJ, Ross R. The role of the macrophage in wound repair. A study with hydrocortisone and antimacrophage serum. Am J Pathol 1975; 78:71-100.
5. Barbul A, Breslin JR, Woodyard JP, Wasserkrug HL et al. The effect of in vivo T-helper and T-suppressor lymphocyte depletion on wound healing. Ann Surg 1989; 209:479-483.
6. Leibovich SJ, Ross R. A macrophage-dependent factor that stimulates the proliferation of fibroblasts in vitro. Am J Pathol 1976; 84:501-513.
7. Casey W, Peacock EJ, Chvapil M. Induction of collagen synthesis in rats by transplantation of allogeneic macrophages. Surg Forum 1976; 27:53.
8. Clarke RA, Store RD, Leung DM. Role of macrophages in wound healing. Surg Forum 1976; 27:16.
9. Hunt TK, Knighton DR, Thakral KK, Goodson WH et al. Studies on inflammation and wound healing: Angiogenesis and collagen synthesis stimulated in vivo by resident and activated macrophages. Surgery 1984; 96:48-59.
10. Greenberg GB, Hunt TK. The proliferation response in vitro of vascular endothelial and smooth muscle cells exposed to wound fluid and macrophages. J Cell Physiol 1978; 97:353-360.
11. Polverini PJ, Cotran RS, Gimbrone MA Unanue ER. Activated macrophages induce vascular proliferation. Nature 1977; 269:804-806.
12. Cromack DT, Sporn MB, Roberts AB, Merino MJ et al. Transforming growth factor ß levels in rat wound chambers. J Surg Res 1987; 4-2: 622-628.
13. Ford HR, Hoffman R, Wing EJ, Magee DM et al. Wound cytokines in the sponge matrix model. Arch Surg 1989; 124:1422-1428.
14. Mustoe TA, Pierce GF, Thomason A, Gramates P et al. Accelerated healing of incisional wounds in rats induced by transforming growth factor-ß. Science 1987; 237:1333-1336.
15. Pierce GF, Mustoe TA, Senior RM, Reed J. In vivo incisional wound healing augmented by platelet-derived growth factor and recombinant C-SIS gene homodimeric proteins. J Exp Med 1988; 167:974-987.
16. Mustoe TA, Purdy J, Gamates P, Deuel TF et al. Reversal of impaired wound healing in irradiated rats by platelet-derived growth factor-BB. Am J Surg 1989; 1598:345-350.
17. Cromack DT, Purdy JA, Porras-Reyes B, Mustoe, TA. Acceleration of tissue repair by transforming growth factory: In vivo mechanism of action by selective radiotherapy impaired healing. Surg Forum 1990; 41:630-631.
18. Laato M, Heino J. Interleukin-1 modulates collagen synthesis by rat granulation tissue cells both in vivo and in vitro. Experiential 1988; 44:32-29.
19. Steenfos HH, Hunt TK, Scheuenstuhl H, Goodson WH. Selective effects of tumor necrosis factor-alpha on wound healing in rats. Surgery 1989; 106:171-176.

20. Regan MC, Kirk SJ, Hurson M, Sodeyama M et al. Tumor necrosis factor-α inhibits in vivo collagen synthesis. Surgery 1992; In press.

21. Peterson JM, Barbul A, Breslin RJ, Wasserkrug HL et al. Significance of T lymphocytes in wound healing. Surgery 1987; 102:300-305.

22. Efron JE, Frankel HL, Lazarou SA, Wasserkrug HL et al. Wound healing and T lymphocytes. J Surg Res 1990; 48:460-463.

23. Barbul A, Shaw T, Rotter SM, Efron JE et al. Wound healing in nude mice: A study on the regulatory role of lymphocytes in fibroplasia. Surgery 1989; 105:764-769.

24. Prudden JF, Nishihara G, Ocamp L. Studies on growth hormone III. The effect on wound tensile strength and marked postoperative anabolism induced with growth hormone. Surg Gynecol Obstet 1958; 107:481-482.

25. Ehrlich HP, Hunt TK. Effect of cortison and vitamin A on wound healing. Ann Surg 1968; 167:324-326.

26. Barbul A, Rettura G, Levenson SM, Seifter E. Arginine: A thymotrophic and wound promoting agent. Surg Forum 1977; 28:101.

27. Sandberg N. Time relationship between administration of cortisone and wound healing in rats. Acta Chir Scand 1964; 127:446.

28. Fishel RS, Barbul A, Wasserkrug HL. Cyclosporine A impairs wound healing in rats. J Surg Res 1983; 34:573-575.

29. Barbul A, Sito D, Rettura G, Levinson SM et al. Thymic inhibition of wound healing: Abrogation by adult thymectomy. J Surg Res 1982; 32:338-342.

30. Barbul A, Shaw T, Frankel H, Efron JE et al. Inhibition of wound repair by thymic hormones. Surgery 1989; 106:373-377.

31. Freundlich B, Bamalaski JS, Neilson E, Jimenes SA. Regulation of fibroblast proliferation and collagen synthesis by cytokines. Immunol Today 1986; 7:303-307.

32. Lazarou SA, Barbul A, Wasserkrug HL, Efron G. The wound is a possible source of posttraumatic immunesuppression. Arch Surg 1990; 124:1429-1431.

33. Roberts AB, Sporn MB, Assoian RK. Transforming growth factor type p: Rapid induction of fibrosis and angiogenesis in vivo and stimulation of collagen formation in vivo. Proc Nat Acad Sci 1986; 83:4167-4171.

34. Barbul A, Knud-Hansen J, Wasserkrug HL, Efron G. Interleukin 2 enhances wound healing in rats. J Surg Res 1986; 4-0:315-319.

35. Granstein RD, Murphy GF, Marjolis RJ et al. Gamma-interferon inhibits collagen synthesis in vivo in the mouse. J Clin Invest 1987; 79:1254-1258.

CHAPTER 20

GROWTH FACTORS IN WOUND HEALING

Thomas A. Mustoe

Growth factor research began with the isolation of nerve growth factor 40 years ago. Its place in biology was thought to be unique until epidermal growth factor (EGF) was described 20 years ago by Stanley Cohen. The interest in growth factors has exploded in the last 10 years with an acceleration in the knowledge about the integral role they play in many basic functions including wound healing. Multiple new growth factors have been described within the past five years, which are candidates for promoting wound healing but whose effects have not yet been defined.

Up until 1987, it was widely thought that wound healing could not be stimulated in the noncompromised host by pharmacological methods; manipulations of the wound environment were limited to preventing infection and meticulous surgical technique. For several years prior to that, it had been recognized that platelets contained growth factors, notably platelet derived growth factor (PDGF) and transforming growth factor beta (TGF-ß), that were also found in macrophages and predictably were found in fluid from wounds in measurable quantities. Given their stimulatory effects as growth factors on mesenchymal cells, it was predicted that they might be important in wound healing. With newly available recombinant growth factors in quantities sufficient to test in animals, it became possible to test the hypothesis that growth factors could stimulate healing in the normal animal when given topically. Utilizing initially platelet purified TGF-ß from Michael Sporn's lab, and recombinant PDGF from Amgen as well as platelet purified PDGF from Tom Deuel's lab, we were able to demonstrate accelerated healing of surgical incisions in rats by a single topical application at the time of wounding.[1,2]

Since that time there has been extensive literature documenting improvement of wound healing in a variety of animal models with several growth factors, and in the last two years several human trials have been started although most are still ongoing and FDA approved clinical use on a routine basis is still at least two to three years away. This review will summarize the evidence for efficacy of the best documented growth factors, EGF, PDGF, TGF-ß and basic FGF of the fibroblast growth factor family, as well as a summary of the clinical knowledge to date. It will include some of the newer growth factors with future clinical potential and attempt to prognosticate the role these growth factors may play clinically 10 years from now.

TGF-β: POTENTIAL CLINICAL APPLICATIONS FOR GROWTH FACTORS

TGF-ß designates a group of at least five closely related peptides synthesized in one form or another by virtually all cells. It is found in large quantities in both platelets and macrophages, in wound fluid, and as well as being proliferative for mesenchymal cells under some conditions, it is chemotactic for inflammatory cells including macrophages, activates macrophages and directly stimulates fibroblasts to synthesize collagen, other components of the extracellular matrix and inhibits protein breakdown. In vitro it also inhibits epithelial cell and endothelial cell proliferation. Based on these properties it was a strong candidate for a vulnerary agent, and indeed over the last four years has been repeatedly demonstrated to accelerate healing of surgical incisions (as measured by wound breaking strength) in skin and intestine, in both normal wounds and impaired wounds including steroid treated, adriamycin treated and irradiated wounds. What makes the work potentially clinically applicable was that these results were achieved by a single topical application of TGF-ß at the time of wounding (in either a collagen or methylcellulose vehicle presumably allowing slow release). Topical application or even a suture impregnated with the material could easily be accomplished at the time of surgery even on internal incisions clinically.

In addition to surgical incisions, the other major areas of problem wound healing include chronic wounds (largely leg ulcers and pressure sores) and burns. The latter are treated by grafting and the major wound issues are the healing of the donor sites, and their availability. The availability issue is being addressed by cultured epithelial cells and dermal equivalents and will not be discussed further in this chapter. In ulcers the success of healing is fundamentally related to the ability to form new tissue (granulation tissue), and animal models of dermal ulcers whether they be contractile wound such as on the dorsum of rats or noncontractile ulcers in the rabbit ear,[3]

TGF-ß has been demonstrated to be very active in accelerating healing and stimulating new granulation tissue. An important issue though is that consistent with its in vitro effects, at higher doses, although granulation tissue is stimulated, epithelialization is actually inhibited.

CLINICAL POTENTIAL OF TGF-β

Given TGF-ß's multiple inhibitory effects in vitro and data in animals indicating a biphasic dose response suggesting toxicity at higher doses, its introduction into clinical trials has been delayed in spite of the fact that it remains the most effective growth factor to date in stimulating collagen production and wound breaking strength in the critical first week of incisional healing. Given its promise, it seems likely that it will eventually make it to clinical trials and it remains extremely promising.

An additional issue for consideration in terms of eventual clinical use is the difficulty in demonstrating efficacy in wound healing studies in general in patients given the complexity of the process and the multiple variables such as blood supply, nutrition, age and stress which are all critical in the wound healing process. This problem is magnified when considering surgical incisions whether internal or external in that the only meaningful functional outcome which can be measured readily is the presence or absence of wound dehiscence which in all but the highest risk patients is a rare event. Due to the large number of patients that would be needed for a trial demonstrating differences in wound dehiscence between treatment and control, all current trials are being directed to chronic wounds, and it is likely that surgical indications will not be proven until much later. It can also be anticipated that if a growth factor is approved for a specific clinical indication such as pressure sores, usage will quickly spread to other areas "off label" such as use in clinical incisions.

PDGF: ANIMAL AND CLINICAL STUDIES

PDGF, like TGF-ß is initially delivered to the wound spaces by platelets and may be a critical signal for initiating the presumed growth factor cascade largely governed by inflammatory cells. PDGF is a potent mitogen for mesenchymal cells including fibroblasts and smooth muscle cells and is a chemoattractant for inflammatory cells and fibroblasts. In animal models it has been demonstrated to increase breaking strength moderately (30-50%) at seven days postwounding, with its greatest effects seen consistently at two to three weeks postwounding and remarkably extending up to 90 days postwounding after a single topical application. Unlike TGF-ß its effects on surgical incisions are macrophage dependent as demonstrated in macrophage depleted steroid and total body irradiated models. PDGF is also a potent inducer of granulation tissue in a "dead space" model such as a Hunt-Schilling chamber model of healing, as well as in a noncontracting dermal ulcer model.[3] Although epithelial cells contain no receptors for PDGF, epithelialization is also promoted in this model as well as granulation tissue indicating the importance of granulation tissue ("neodermis") for epithelialization perhaps in part by secondary release of growth factors from the granulation tissue such as KGF (keratinocyte growth factor) produced by fibroblasts and highly stimulatory for epithelialization.

PDGF: CLINICAL TRIALS AND APPLICATIONS

Based on the potential shown by PDGF in the animal trials, clinical trials have been initiated by more than one company starting out in pressure ulcers.[4] Although only 5 patients of the 23 in the trial (primarily a phase 1 safety trial) received a therapeutic dose of PDGF, the preliminary results did show an acceleration in wound healing in the treatment group,[4] with an estimated 10-day acceleration in healing (36-26 days) at a dose of 1 $\mu g/cm^2$ surface area of wound. In terms of animal studies predicting clinical efficacy this is the same dose efficacious in the rabbit ear dermal ulcer model suggesting that indeed animal models are useful to predict clinical efficacy and that some of the multiple other growth factors showing activity in animal studies may find clinical uses. The study is of course highly preliminary, and phase II and

phase III studies which take at least a couple of years to complete will have to be equally optimistic for the drug to reach the market. Studies in the other big group of chronic wounds, venous leg ulcers are sure to follow.

FGF IN WOUND HEALING

Basic FGF, the best studied member of the seven-member FGF family of structurally closely related peptides, has been most widely studied in vitro for its marked angiogenic properties of stimulation proliferation of endothelial cells. It also stimulates fibroblasts and indeed is unique among candidate growth factors in its ability to stimulate all cell types involved in soft tissue repair including keratinocytes.

In animal models, bFGF has consistently augmented wound healing processes as measured in dead space models. Although we have not seen effects in a normal rat skin incision, when given to diabetic rats increases in breaking strength have been seen. In ulcer models in diabetic mice as well as rabbit ear dermal ulcers, bFGF has been demonstrated to accelerate healing as well as be a potent angiogenic agent.

An important clinical wound healing problem is the deleterious effect of hypoxia caused by local tissue scarring such as in venous ulcers or diabetic ulcers, or due to inadequate inflow due to peripheral vascular disease. Angiogenic agents such as bFGF have been proposed as particularly attractive to stimulate healing under these conditions, but a recent study underwritten by Synergen for bFGF in leg ulcers was dropped for lack of clinical effects. An explanation for this result may lie in recent work (unpublished observations) from our laboratory in the rabbit ear dermal ulcer model demonstrating a complete lack of efficacy under ischemic conditions, while under nonischemic conditions it was quite effective. To further bolster the validity of this observation, efficacy was restored when the ischemic ulcer animals were treated with hyperbaric oxygen. Based on these observations, pressure sores, which are not normally hypoxic unless there is extensive local scarring might be predicted to respond to bFGF, but the results of clinical trials still have not been made public. bFGF is actually collagenolytic in some animal models including the rabbit ear dermal ulcer model, which makes it unlikely that it will find utility in the treatment of surgical incisions.

EGF IN WOUND HEALING

EGF, perhaps the best studied growth factor on the molecular and cell receptor level, is most notable for its potent effects on epithelial cell proliferation. In vitro it has also been demonstrated to have some stimulatory effects on mesenchymal cells and has shown some ability to increase granulation tissue in dead space animal models. There have even been some scattered reports of some efficacy in a surgical incisional model when continuously delivered. Nevertheless, in our rabbit ear dermal ulcer model, the effects on epithelial cells predominated and no effects were seen on granulation tissue.

EGF was the first growth factor to get into clinical trials, and the first clinical report of efficacy was encouraging. In 1989, Brown et al[5] reported a two day acceleration of skin graft donor sites treated topically with EGF compared to paired control sites on the same patients, which reached statistical significance and was hailed as the beginning of a new era of clinical growth factor therapy. Since that time, a similar study utilizing healthy male volunteers failed to demonstrate an effect. It is possible that EGF will find eventual use in the treatment of burn donor sites, an impaired host situation where a relatively deficiency of growth factor is more likely to exist. However demonstration of clinical efficacy of healing of widely meshed grafts may be very difficult, and unless there is a demonstrated benefit such as shortened hospital stay in terms of donor site healing the clinical usefulness is still uncertain.

Another area in which EGF has shown promise is the healing of corneal ulcers in animals. Yet human trials have been in progress for at least three years without reporting of positive effects as of yet, which probably means that the results up until now have not been all that encouraging.

TGF-α, which has the same cell surface receptor as EGF or other growth factors that act primarily on epithelial cells, may have advan-

tages not yet demonstrated, but there is much less animal data, and no ongoing clinical trials.

OTHER GROWTH FACTORS

Several other growth factors have shown some efficacy in animal trials and are active in vitro in stimulating some of the cells involved in wound healing, but have been less extensively studied and no clinical trials have yet been reported. These include insulin growth factor I (IGF-1) which has been demonstrated to be normally present in wounds. By itself, it has not been effective in incisional healing but when combined with insulin growth factor binding protein type I, it has shown efficacy in a rat linear incisional model (Jyung, Mustoe, Clemmons, unpublished observations). Growth hormone (GH) given systemically induces IGF-1 production, and systemic administration of GH shows considerable promise as a wound healing agent, perhaps through local IGF-1 effects but also likely through its metabolic effects in minimizing tissue catabolism in stress or malnourished states. Herndon et al[6] has demonstrated healing of skin graft donor sites subjected to multiple skin graft harvests by two to three days resulting in a significant reduction in the length of hospitalization. There is considerable potential for widespread use of GH in the aged, malnourished and any patient subject to a major stress resulting in a catabolic nutritional state to minimize wound healing complications in major surgical or trauma patients.

Other factors deserving mention as potential clinical wound healing agents include KGF, (keratinocyte growth factor), a member of the FGF family with potent effects on epithelial cells, VPF, (vascular permeability factor), an angiogenic factor recently described, PD-ECGF (platelet-derived endothelial cell growth factor), another specific endothelial cell mitogen purified from human platelets which has accelerated healing in the rabbit ear dermal ulcer model, GMCSF (granulocyte-macrophage colony stimulating factor) which has been approved for clinical use given systemically to raise white cell counts but which also stimulates surgical incisional healing in normal and impaired states when given topically (Jyung, Wu, Mustoe, unpublished observations), and the interleukins IL-1 and IL-2 which act on lymphocytes but also activate macrophages, and for which clinical trials will likely be proposed.

The field is evolving very quickly. The wound healing complex if dressings, hospitalization, nursing care and medical services are included is a multibillion dollar industry. The market for a growth factor that will promote healing of chronic wounds is potentially huge which of course is the reason there has been such intense interest by the biotechnology industry in putting growth factors into clinical trials. Surgical incisions heal by collagen deposition across a coapted wound, while pressure sores heal via contraction, granulation tissue production and smaller amounts of epithelialization in well vascularized wounds. Leg ulcers are usually ischemic by local or large vessel factors, and contraction plays a minimal role so that epithelialization as well as granulation tissue formation is potentially a rate limiting step. It is quite likely that different growth factors will find utility in different clinical situations, but it will be very difficult to sort these factors out clinically given the tremendous variability of wound healing even under ideal laboratory conditions.

The importance of oxygen in wound healing is covered in Chapter 18, but the interaction of hypoxia with growth factors has already been alluded to earlier in reference to our work with bFGF. Another area ripe for investigation and potential clinical utility is the interaction of growth factors with hyperbaric oxygen. We have found that either PDGF or TGF-ß when combined with hyperbaric oxygen are able to totally reverse the ischemic deficit in a rabbit ear dermal ulcer model (Zhao, Mustoe, unpublished observations) while either by itself is only partially effective. It is quite likely that other treatment combinations in the future will extend the utility of growth factors and make the area an exciting field with tremendous evolution within the next decade.

One area of clinical use that deserves mention is the use in multiple "Wound Healing Centers" of PDWHF, the company name for material derived from autologous platelets harvested from blood samples and treated to release the growth factors, PDGF, TGF-ß and several other proteins which may contribute to wound healing. The centers have been commercially successful, combining multiple principles of good wound care including aggressive debridement and revascularization of ischemic limbs combined with PDWHF. Their success in treating chronic wounds has been excellent, but the role of PDWHF apart from the other therapeutic measures still has not been determined in published, prospective, randomized trials. However, the approach that a cocktail of growth factors may be superior to single growth factor therapy is quite attractive, and utilizing the bodies own combination is a rational approach.

A final caveat in the clinical use of growth factors lies in the appropriate increasing attention to cost-benefit analyses in medicine. A treatment that accelerates the healing of a leg ulcer by one week will find widespread use if its cost is less than the nursing care or dressings would have been for the week. On the other hand, if recombinant growth factor technology adds thousands to the cost of healing a chronic wound, their use will be limited.

REFERENCES

1. Mustoe TA, Pierce GF, Thomason A, Gramates P et al. Accelerated healing of incisional wounds in rats induced by transforming growth factor-ß. Science 1987; 237:1333-1335.
2. Pierce GF, Mustoe TA, Senior RM, Reed J et al. In vivo incisional wound healing augment by platelet-derived growth factor and recombinant c-sis gene homodimeric proteins. J Exp Med 1988;167:974-987.
3. Mustoe TA, Pierce GF, Morishima C, Deuel TF. Growth factor induced acceleration of tissue repair through direct and inductive activities in a rabbit dermal ulcer model. J Clin Invest 1991; 87:694-703.
4. Robson MC, Phillips LG, Thomason A, Altrock BW et al. Recombinant human platelet-derived growth factor-BB for the treatment of chronic pressure ulcers. Lancet 1992.
5. Brown GL, Nanney LB, Griffen J, Cramer AB et al. Enhancement of wound healing by topical treatment with epidermal growth factor. N Engl J Med 1989; 321:76-79.
6. Herndon DN, Barrow RE, Kunkel KR, Broemeling L et al. Effects of recombinant human growth hormone on donor site healing in severely burned children. Ann Surg 1991; 214:424-431.

CHAPTER 21

THE CURRENT STATUS OF SKIN SUBSTITUTES

John C. Fitzpatrick
William G. Cioffi, Jr.

INTRODUCTION

Early excision and placement of autograft is generally accepted as the standard of care for patients with deep burns. However, due to lack of available donor sites, this may be a technically difficult proposition in patients with extensive burns. Inability to provide adequate early coverage of the burn wound places the patient at risk for the development of infection. An open wound also perpetuates the hypermetabolic state resulting from the initial insult and places the patient at risk for additional complications. This has been the impetus behind an extensive search for a satisfactory skin substitute over the last 50 years.

SKIN SUBSTITUTE REQUIREMENTS

The ideal skin substitute will need to satisfy many criteria for performance and function. It will need to be exceptionally durable, with the same elasticity, tensile strength and resistance to shear of normal skin. Physically, it must allow normal rates of evaporative water and heat loss. Functionally, it should prevent hypertrophic scarring and joint contracture and minimize cosmetic scarring. It should decrease wound pain to allow effective physical therapy and joint motion to occur. The material should be nonantigenic and compatible with healing tissues to allow ingrowth of a blood supply. It should adhere to the wound to decrease bacterial density and prevent further bacterial contamination. Adequate wound adherence will also help prevent further physical injury to the wound bed. The material should also encourage orderly wound repair in partial thickness injuries (which may heal on their own). The material should either undergo normal remodeling with minimal tissue reaction or be totally inert and not inhibit tissue remodeling in the normal tissues surrounding the burn. Finally, it should have a long shelf life with minimal storage requirements, be inexpensive and not transmit disease.

Unilaminate Skin Substitutes

Historically, many attempts have been made to develop a unilaminate skin substitute (using films or sheets of cellulose, polyvinyl alcohol polymers, ethylene oxide polymers, nylon and polytetrafluoroethylene) with a notable lack of success to date. Practically, this type of skin substitute is very appealing because most of the products developed have a long shelf life with minimal storage requirements, are easily applied, relatively inexpensive and do not transmit disease. Unfortunately, wound adherence is variable and usually minimal with the dressing being sealed at the wound edge by the formation of a serous crust. Submembrane suppuration is the usual outcome, especially in full thickness wounds when residual nonviable tissue is present. Fragmentation of the material at the time of removal is also a common occurrence with the residual fragments forming a nidus for infection and inflammation in the wound. In short, unilaminate membranes have been a disappointment as skin substitutes, and much work remains to be done to improve their durability and wound adherence before they become clinically useful alternatives for temporary wound coverage.

Bilaminate Skin Substitutes

Bilaminate skin substitutes come in many different forms, and may be broadly classified as synthetic, natural biologic or processed biologic. Synthetic substitutes consist of materials such as the polytetrafluoroethylene/nylon mesh developed by Levine. Natural biologic substitutes consist of such materials as porcine xenograft, fresh or frozen human allograft or human amnion. Processed biologic substitutes consist of such materials as the numerous Silastic/collagen membranes and all of the combinations of epidermal and dermal substitutes listed in Table 1.

Synthetic Skin Substitutes

Synthetic bilaminate skin replacements, such as that developed by Levine et al, generally consist of some type of inner layer (nylon or polytetrafluoroethylene) bonded to a Silastic or polytetrafluoroethylene outer layer. The inner layer must form a framework for the ingrowth of fibroblasts and formation of a neodermis suitable for eventual placement of an epidermal layer, yet be removable in its entirety without fragmentation of the material or destruction of the neodermis which has formed in its pore structure. The outer layer emulates the epidermal functions of water vapor conservation, protection from trauma and impermeability to bacteria and liquid water. To date, synthetics have not demonstrated performance equivalent to allograft or autograft except on wounds which were incompletely debrided of necrotic tissue; the use of the synthetic skin substitutes resulted in more rapid debridement of necrotic tissue than was achieved with allograft or xenograft.

Natural Biologic Skin Substitutes

Natural biologic materials such as xenograft and allograft possess many of the desired performance characteristics for ideal skin substitutes. Their best qualities include resistance to evaporative water and heat loss, good wound adherence with resistance to bacterial wound colonization and the ability to encourage orderly wound repair. Their in-

Epidermis	Dermis
Thin autograft	Collagen/glycosaminoglycan
Suction blisters (epidermis only)	Collagen gels with fibroblasts added
Cultured keratinocytes	Cultured fibroblasts on synthetic carriers
Silastic (prior to grafting)	Allograft (epidermis free)

Table 1. Processed biologic skin replacement combinations.

adequacies include antigenicity resulting in rejection, limited shelf life with significant requirements for proper storage, expense, limited availability and the possibility for disease transmission.

Attempts have been made in the past to utilize immunosuppression to induce immunologic tolerance of allograft. Studies in animals demonstrated that tolerance and long term graft survival could be successfully induced by the use of immunosuppressive drugs and donor bone marrow prior to grafting with donor skin. Several attempts have been made to form a permissive environment in humans utilizing azathioprine, antithymocyte globulin, and cyclosporine A, with some success. The side effects of these drugs, particularly the first two, including acute problems such as pancytopenia and infection, as well as potential long-term problems reported in the conventional transplantation literature (including malignancy) have dampened enthusiasm for this method of skin substitution.

Xenograft products (and amnion) are useful for encouraging reepithelialization of partial-thickness wounds but do not encourage dermal repair of full-thickness wounds; rather, they cause the development of granulation tissue. Allograft, either fresh, frozen or lyophilized, can be used for coverage of both partial-thickness and full-thickness wounds. Vascular and fibroblastic ingrowth into allograft results in excellent adherence and optimal decrease in the wound bacterial density. "Take" of allograft has been used as a predictor of autograft survival in patients with extensive burns and limited donor sites to minimize the chance of graft loss. The ability of allograft dermis to "take" and form a framework for dermal healing has been exploited in full-thickness wounds to provide a bed for the application of very thin autograft, epidermal blisters and cultured keratinocytes with variable success (vide infra). The possibility of disease transmission—hepatitis, human immunodeficiency virus, malignant skin neoplasms, hematologic malignancies and bacterial infections—as well as the limited shelf life and storage requirements for fresh allograft limit its usefulness. These problems are overcome to a certain extent by the use of frozen or lyophilized allograft but at the cost of decreased efficiency of "take" and antibacterial action.

PROCESSED BIOLOGIC SKIN SUBSTITUTES

Processed biologic materials include both epidermal replacements and combinations of epidermal and dermal replacements to provide complete skin substitutes. These materials are particularly important in the extensively burned patient with limited donor sites. The ability to produce graftable tissue from the limited donor sites is essential to the survival of those patients with catastrophic burns who survive the initial resuscitation period.

EPIDERMAL SUBSTITUTES

Autograft skin (0.008-0.010 inch) is widely used at this time for grafting patients with extensive thermal injury and is the standard to which all epidermal substitutes must be compared. Advantages include complete tissue compatibility, definitive wound closure to limit the risk of infection, better durability than any other skin substitute (although not ideal), lower cost and lack of disease transmission. Due to limited donor sites, though, the graft is of necessity often widely meshed, and the interstices heal by confluence of scar epithelium. No dermal regeneration has been demonstrated in the interstices of meshed skin grafts, and wound contraction secondary to scar formation is a major difficulty. Suction blisters of epidermis have been placed on excised burn wound in a patchwork fashion to achieve coverage of the wound surface and result in a similar confluence of scar epithelium between the epidermal islands. The use of cultured autologous keratinocytes is an exciting innovation which permits rapid and enormous expansion of the number of donor keratinocytes to help achieve coverage in patients with extensive burn injury. Theoretically, such epidermal sheets may be placed in a confluent fashion to provide complete seamless coverage of the burn wound, no matter how extensive the injury. However, their use is somewhat marred by inconsistent "take" on the burn wound—especially nonplanar nonanterior surfaces or surfaces which are completely free of dermis, the time (up to four weeks) required to raise cells for application to the wound and the limited viability of the cells after they have been removed from their culture medium for maturation, transport and application. They also suffer from lack of durability in comparison to normal skin. The presence of dermis seems to increase both the take and the durability of the cultured keratinocytes and this correlates well with observations that the best take and cosmetic results are found when cultured cells are applied to partial thickness rather than full thickness burn wounds. As a result of the lack of take and the lack of durability of the keratinocytes that do take, there may be impairment of other crucial parts of burn rehabilitation, such as physical and occupational therapy, for an extended period of time.

Dermal Replacements

Dermal replacements may prove to be the vital link in the search for the ideal skin substitute. The failure of cultured keratinocytes applied to the wound bed following a full thickness excision may be secondary to the absence of a dermal analogue. The importance of the dermis, from the standpoints of providing a nutrient supply (including paracrine factors) to the epidermis, maximizing durability of the healed skin and minimizing the degree of scarring has been realized and is the impetus for research in this area.

Fetal Wound Healing

Intense interest has been focused on the process of fetal skin wound healing, which has been noted to occur without scarring. Initial observations documented a lack of wound contraction in some fetal models of wound healing. Subsequent studies have confirmed rapid dermal regeneration and normal dermal-epidermal histology without evidence of scar formation in either the epidermal or dermal layers. Hypotheses concerning this novel wound healing have centered on the role of: 1) the increased content of extracellu-

lar matrix glycosaminoglycans (such as hyaluronic acid) and glycoproteins (such as fibronectin) in amniotic fluid which fosters a permissive environment for both cellular proliferation/migration and the orderly deposition of collagen fibrils; and 2) the increased content of peptide growth factors such as transforming growth factor TGF-α, TGF-ß, hyaluronic acid stimulating activity factor and epidermal growth factor in amniotic fluid which may assist in the rapid and orderly wound healing which occurs in fetal skin.

Collagen and Glycosaminoglycans

Collagen, low in antigenicity and readily available from commercial sources, has been used alone and in collagen/glycosaminoglycan matrices (bonded to various materials such as polyurethane and Silastic films for ease of handling) to serve as an extracellular mold for the ingrowth of fibroblasts in the process of formation of a neodermis. Various glycosaminoglycans have been used to alter the final neodermal viscoelastic and pore size properties; these include chondroitin-6-sulphate, dermatan sulphate and hyaluronic acid. Fibronectin (a glycoprotein) increases the incorporation of hyaluronic acid in collagen sponge which is important to maintain proper pore size and three-dimensional orientation between collagen fibrils thus allowing fibroblast migration to take place. Both chondroitin-6-sulphate and dermatan sulphate have been noted to increase the mechanical strength of the collagen layer, and to influence the rate of cell replication. Recently, the addition of synthetic adhesion peptides containing the sequence arginine-glycine-aspartic acid (the cell attachment site for many extracellular matrix molecules) to collagen/glycosaminoglycan membranes has been shown to increase the attachment of keratinocytes to the membranes and increase the number of fibroblasts present in the membrane pores. The interactions between the cellular and extracellular matrix components comprising the dermis remain incompletely defined. When those interactions of greatest importance to the function of the dermis have been identified and can be applied to the production of a neodermis the development of a clinically useful dermis may be possible.

Collagen Gels and Fibroblasts

Collagen gels with cultured autologous fibroblasts (or allogeneic fibroblasts, as reported by Hull, Finley, and Miller) have been used to form a neodermis. Recently cultured keratinocytes have been added to form a complete skin replacement. This is a logical sequel to the formation of a neodermis alone, which requires the addition of some form of epidermal component (either thin autograft or cultured keratinocytes) to effect closure of a wound. Although appealing, this approach has been hampered by the extended period of time required for in vitro expansion of the cells and construction of the graft, as well as disappointing "take" of the finished product. The disappointing "take" may be inherently related to the time required for production of the graft, as this allows a marked inflammatory response to occur in the excised wound bed (or in the unexcised burn wound) which impairs the rapid vascularization and biologic union of the graft with the wound bed which is required for viability of the graft. Modifications of the present techniques to improve both the rapidity of cellular expansion and the "take" of the finished product will be necessary before this technology is practical.

Cultured Fibroblasts and Synthetic Carriers

Cultured fibroblasts seeded into various carriers (such as Dexon or Vicryl mesh) have been used to provide a dermal replacement which results in the generation of a neodermis more rapidly and with less inflammation than has been possible up to this time with the various collagen/glycosaminoglycan dermal substitutes. These materials are just now entering clinical trials, and no randomized prospective studies comparing these dermal substitutes with other substitutes have been performed. Forthcoming work will determine the ability of these products to establish a neodermis and will also shed light on the relative importance of the extracellular matrix in the formation of the neodermis.

Allograft

Allograft skin, which once was viewed as only a biologic dressing, may prove to be an ideal dermal analogue. As the immunobiology of skin has been further investigated (and as was suspected by Medawar and Gibson) it has become clear that only the Langerhans cell of the epidermis expresses class II major histocompatibility complex products which are essential for rejection to occur. It appears that these cells are depleted in stored allograft skin, especially in frozen products. Cuono and colleagues in 1986 reported the successful closure of wounds by placement of autologous cultured keratinocytes (or autograft) on the exposed dermis of previously placed adherent allograft skin from which the epidermis had been removed. This method of dermal substitution is particularly attractive for several reasons. Allograft may be easily stored for relatively long periods of time and is available without extensive preparation at the time of surgery. It presents an unaltered extracellular matrix to encourage orderly wound healing. Its durability and physical properties are acceptable for temporary wound coverage. It adheres well to the wound bed and lowers bacterial density in the wound while preventing further contamination. Finally, it is slowly replaced by the patients' own tissue as fibroblasts invade the donor dermis and normal turnover of the extracellular matrix occurs. The principal concern about the use of allograft at this time centers about the possibility of disease transmission, in spite of careful testing; a secondary drawback is cost. Finally, it is not a definitive closure, since keratinocytes must be placed at a later time to complete the healing process.

Investigators in China have addressed this issue in two related fashions; a slurry of autologous epithelium and allograft dermis is produced and poured on the excised wound bed in order to achieve closure, or autologous keratinocytes are placed in grooves cut in allogeneic dermis which is then placed on the excised wound in the same fashion as allograft.

After the allogeneic epidermis separates, the autologous epithelium effects coverage of the allogeneic dermal surface. Approximately 70 to 80 days are required for complete healing. No allograft rejection has been noted, consistent with the observations of Hull utilizing collagen gel/allogeneic fibroblast dermal replacements and those of Cuono utilizing whole allogeneic grafts covered with autologous keratinocytes after removal of the allogeneic keratinocytes. These reports await confirmation by others, and the precise origin of the epithelial cover is undetermined at this time.

CONCLUSION

The ideal skin substitute remains undeveloped. The presently available materials, including dermal analogues, imperfectly mimic the functional and cosmetic properties of the natural skin they are replacing. The combination of a dermal analogue with cultured keratinocytes appears to be the most promising of the current approaches to the problem. The current technology falls short of the concept of "a suit of skin off the rack," which may never be realized due to the limiting factors of the rate of cell division and cell maturation. As the processes underlying fetal skin formation, fetal wound healing and the immunobiology of the skin become better understood, it may be possible to manufacture a nonantigenic skin replacement. At that time, a clinically useful skin substitute will be a reality.

SELECTED READING

1. Alsbjörn B. In search of an ideal skin substitute. Scand J Plas Reconstr Surg 1984; 18:127-133.
2. Boyce ST, Glafkides MC, Foreman TJ, Hansbrough JF. Reduced wound contraction after grafting of full-thickness burns with a collagen and chondroitin-6-sulfate (GAG) dermal skin substitute and coverage with Biobrane. J Burn Care Rehab 1988; 9(4):364-370.
3. Burke JF. Observations on the development and clinical use of artificial skin—an attempt to employ regeneration rather than scar formation in wound healing. Jap J Surg 1987; 17(6):431-438.
4. Cooper ML, Hansbrough JF, Spielvogel RL et al. In vivo optimization of a living dermal substitute employing cultured human fibroblasts on a biodegradable polyglycolic acid or polyglactin mesh. Biomaterials 1991; 12(3): 243-248.
5. Cooper ML, Hansbrough JF, Foreman TJ. In vitro effects of matrix peptides on a cultured dermal-epidermal skin substitute. J Surg Res 1990; 48(6):528-533.
6. Cuono CB, Langdon R, Birchall N et al. Composite autologous-allogeneic skin replacement: Development and clinical application. Plastic Reconstr Surg 1987; 80(4):626-635.
7. Doillon CJ, Wasserman AJ, Berg RA, Silver FH. Behaviour of fibroblasts and epidermal cells cultivated on analogues of extracellular matrix. Biomaterials 1988; 9(1):91-96.
8. Gallico III GG. Biologic skin substitutes. Clin Plastic Surg 1990; 17(3):519-526.
9. Heimbach D, Luterman A, Burke J et. al. Artificial dermis for major burns. Ann Surg 1988; 208(3):313-320.
10. Hull BE, Finley RK, Miller SF. Coverage of full-thickness burns with bilayer skin equivalents: A preliminary clinical trial. Surgery 1990; 107(5):496-502.
11. Longaker MT, Adzick NS. The biology of fetal wound healing: A review. Plastic Reconstr Surg 1991; 87(4):788-798.
12. Pricolo VE, Caldwell MD, Mastrofrancesco B, Mills CD. Modulatory activities of wound fluid on fibroblast proliferation and collagen synthesis. J Surg Res 1990; 48(6):534-538.
13. Pruitt BA, Levine NS. Characteristics and uses of biologic dressings and skin substitutes. Arch Surg 1984; 119(3): 312-322.
14. Tompkins RG, Burke JF. Progress in burn treatment and the use of artificial skin. World J Surg 1990; 14(6):819-824.
15. Yannas IV, Burke JF, Warpehoski M et. al. Prompt, long-term functional replacement of skin. TASAIO 1981; 27:19-23.
16. Yannas IV. What criteria should be used for designing artificial skin replacements and how well do the current grafting material meet these criteria? J Trauma 1984; 24(9 Supp): S29-S39.

CHAPTER 22

TREATMENT OF ENDOTOXIC SHOCK IN THE YOUNG TRAUMA VICTIM:
Immunotherapy and Prophylaxis

Masakatsu Goto
Toyokazu Yoshioka
W. Patrick Zeller

INCIDENCE OF TRAUMA

Trauma continues to be a major medical and social problem. Trauma is the leading cause of mortality in children aged 1 to 19 years.[1] In 1986, 22,411 children died due to injury in the United States. Death rate due to trauma in the United States is similar to other developed countries. Trauma caused about 40% of all deaths in one- to four-year-old children, and 70% of all deaths in five- to 19-year-old children. Motor vehicle accident (MVA) trauma is the most common cause of fatal injury in children. Death due to MVA was 45% of all trauma death. The incidence of fatal trauma has not decreased in the last 20 years although death due to other diseases in childhood has declined.

Major causes of immediate death following trauma are hemorrhage and head injury. When compared to the body weight, head weight is disproportionally greater in children than the adult. Supportive systems such as ligaments and the skeleton are underdeveloped in pediatric patients. Thus, the head is easily traumatized in childhood.

Common causes of delayed death following trauma are multiple organ failure (MOF) and septic shock. Increased incidence of gram-negative infection in patients with severe trauma and injury is related to suppressed immunity. Therefore, treatment of gram-negative sepsis/septic shock has been a major task for management of patients with severe trauma and injury.

HOST DEFENSE

The host defense system is immature in children. Monocyte/phagocyte cells (macrophages) and polymorphonuclear leukocytes (PMN) play an important role in phagocytosis and detoxification of invading organisms and toxins. Macrophage and PMN populations are decreased in the young. Macrophage and PMN function is also decreased in the young.[2,3] Since the macrophage is the primary cell responsible for the detoxification of endotoxin,[4] decreased macrophage cell number and function in the young contributes to the susceptibility to endotoxin.

Lymphocyte function is also immature in the young. It has been shown that immunoglobulin release from B-cells is reduced in the young. Immunoglobulin may neutralize bacterial toxicity including endotoxin and help chemotaxis of phagocytic cells. Thus, decreased immunoglobulin concentration is responsible in part for the decreased host defense in the young. Decreased immunoglobulin release from B-cells in the young is due to immature B-cell function and T-cell function. It is thought that decreased T-cell function is due to less exposure to antigens in the young when compared to the adult. Hayward and Lydyard[5] demonstrated immature B-cell function in the young by showing a lack of immunoglobulin release in B-cell incubated with adult T-cells.

Complement also plays a role in chemotaxis and phagocytosis of the PMN. Complment levels are reduced in the newborn. Hepatic dysfunction occurs during severe trauma. Thus, acute phase protein production is suppressed and complement is decreased.

Gram-Negative Sepsis/Septic Shock

Gram-negative sepsis/septic shock is the most common cause of death in the late phase of trauma. When the young trauma victim gets sepsis/septic shock, the mortality rate increases to 50%-80%.[6]

Endotoxin (Lipopolysaccharide: LPS), which constitutes outer membrane of gram-negative bacteria, is responsible for shock associated with gram-negative infection. Mediators such as tumor necrosis factor (TNF), interleukin-1 (IL-1) and interleukin-6 (IL-6) are involved in the pathophysiology of endotoxic shock.[7-9] TNF is released by endotoxin stimulation and then induces IL-1 release. Endotoxin has been detected in plasma of gram-negative septic shock in the adult and

also in the young. Sequential release of monokines/cytokines during gram-negative sepsis/septic shock has been shown in pediatric patients with gram-negative sepsis/septic shock.[10]

Since cardiovascular and glucoregulatory changes are life-threatening during endotoxic shock, hemodynamics and glucose metabolism have been extensively studied. The pathophysiology of endotoxic shock has been shown to be different in the young than in the adult. The hyperdynamic state followed by the hypodynamic state is commonly seen in adult sepsis/septic shock. However, the hyperdynamic state is not often seen in newborn septic shock. In experimental models of newborn septic shock, mean arterial pressure is maintained and systemic vascular resistance is elevated in the initial period even though cardiac output is markedly decreased. Heart rate is not always increased during newborn septic shock.[11]

The hypermetabolic state is found in the initial period of sepsis/septic shock and then is followed by the hypometabolic state.[12] Hyperglycemia is induced during the hypermetabolic states. Plasma catecholamine, glucocorticoid and glucagon levels are increased in the hypermetabolic state. Thus these stress hormones appear to contribute to the hyperglycemia. Increased glucose utilization and decreased gluconeogenesis cause the hypoglycemia. Since plasma insulin level increases during adult septic shock, hyperinsulinemia has been thought to be responsible for the hypoglycemia. However, in young animal models of endotoxic shock, hyperinsulinemia has not been detected although hyper- and hypoglycemia are present. (Table 1) Thus, glucoregulatory responses are different in the young than in the adult.

In animal models, suckling rats were 350 times more sensitive to endotoxin than adult rats.[12] Major sites of gram-negative bacterial invasion are wounds. At times wounds in the trauma victim are not infected by gram-negative bacteria but sepsis/septic shock may ensue. A potential mechanism for sepsis/septic shock is the translocation of bacteria and/or endotoxin from the gastrointestinal tract to the circulation. Since the young victim has an

		hour		
		0	**2**	**4**
10 day old	Glucose (mg/dl)	94±2	112±4	52±3
	Insulin (µm/ml)	27±2	16±1	15±2
28 day old	Glucose (mg/dl)	163±3	152±10	72±18
	Insulin (µm/ml)	9±1	52±17*	13±3

S. enteritidis LPS at the dose of LD90 was intraperitoneally administered. While plasma insulin concentration was increased in 28-day-old rats, plasma insulin concentration was not increased in 10-day-old rats. * p<0.01 vs Time 0.

Table 1. Plasma glucose and insulin concentration.

	Plasma LPS (ng/ml) at 30 min	Plasma Glucose (mg/kg) at 4 hours
Low Dose (LD20*)	84±15	64±3
High Dose (LD90*)	113±14@	57±4@

Plasma endotoxin (LPS) and glucose concentrations in 10-day-old rats were measured after an intraperitoneal injection of LPS at low dose or high dose. Intravenous endotoxin administration has been shown to induce dose-related pathophysiology. This result demonstrates that plasma LPS and glucose concentrations correlates the dose of LPS ip administration.
*20% and 90% mortality at 24 hours;
@ p<0.05 vs Low Dose .

Table 2. Plasma LPS and glucose concentration.

immature host system, even a small amount of bacterial and/or endotoxin translocation could cause sepsis/septic shock.

The event of endotoxic shock is endotoxin-dose related.[11,12] In experimental newborn animals, a highly lethal dose of endotoxin induces hyperglycemia and then hypoglycemia. A low lethal dose of endotoxin induces hyperglycemia but not hypoglycemia. These responses are related to plasma endotoxin levels in the early phase following an intraperitoneal injection of endotoxin in 10-day-old rats. (Table 2)

IMMUNOTHERAPY, PROPHYLAXIS, TOLERANCE IN ENDOTOXIC SHOCK

Endotoxin triggers TNF release resulting in sequential release of cytokines and shock. Neutralization of endotoxin may be the most important strategy for the treatment of endotoxic shock. Increased plasma TNF is an early physiologic response during endotoxic shock. Neutralization of TNF may blunt sequential pathophysiologic events of endotoxic shock. Beneficial effects of anti-TNF antibody treatment have been reported in experimental sepsis/septic shock. However, since TNF effects have not been well characterized, anti-TNF antibody treatment in human patients has not been used extensively.

In the treatment of endotoxic shock, immunotherapy with antiendotoxin antibodies was reported as early as 1949. Antibody treatment prevented local Shwartzman reaction, intravascular coagulation and death which were induced by endotoxin. Specific antibodies such as anti-O antigen antibodies were also useful for the treatment of endotoxic shock. However, anti-O antigen antibodies may not crossreact with other endotoxins. Thus, anti-O antibodies have been used for classification of bacteria. However, anti-O antibody has been developed for endotoxin of *H. influenzae* type b and has been used for the prophylaxis of *H. influenzae* type b infection.

Endotoxin (lipopolysaccharide) is made up of three components consisting of repeated polysaccharide (O-antigen), inner polysaccharide and lipid A. Core-glycolipid (inner polysaccharide and lipid A) is known to be conserved in gram-negative bacteria. Thus, anti-core-glycolipid antibodies have been successfully developed to neutralize multiple endotoxins. Anti-core-glycolipid antibodies are called anti-LPS antibodies.

Adhikari et al[13] successfully treated septicemia of low birth weight neonates with immunotherapy. These results indicated that anti-core-glycolipid polyclonal antibodies were effective in the treatment of endotoxic shock and gram-negative infection in the young. However, since availability of polyclonal antibodies is a limiting factor in clinical practice, monoclonal antibodies have been extensively studied.

Ziegler et al[14] also developed anti-core-glycolipid antibodies, using mutant *E. coli* LPS J5. Mutant J5 has less unwanted effects than smooth *E. coli* LPS. Therefore, J5 was used for the antigen in animals and humans. Anti-J5 monoclonal antibody (HA-1A) was also shown to be effective for the treatment of human sepsis/septic shock.[15] However, the mortality and morbidity following HA-1A treatment remained high. The high mortality has been explained to be due to delayed treatment.

The structure of lipid A is highly conserved within the cell membrane of gram-negative organisms. Since lipid A is responsible for the toxic effects of lipopolysaccharide, anti-lipid A antibodies may be beneficial for the treatment and prophylaxis of gram-negative sepsis/septic shock. It is generally accepted that anti-lipid A monoclonal antibodies cross-react with lipid A derived from other organisms. However, the effects of anti-lipid A monoclonal antibodies on lipopolysaccharide or gram-negative organisms are conflicting. Anti-lipid A monoclonal antibodies have been reported to react differently to glycolipid, lipopolysaccharide and gram-negative organisms, abolishing the action of lipopolysaccharide. Other laboratories have reported that anti-lipid A monoclonal antibodies do not decrease the action of lipopolysaccharides. Potential explanation for these conflicting results are: lipid A contains

various antigenic epitopes, hydrophilic components of lipopolysaccharide could conceal the attachment of some monoclonal antibodies to lipid A and intrinsic differences in the monoclonal antibody.

We[16] demonstrated that anti-lipid A monoclonal antibodies (IgG and IgM) were effective for the treatment of suckling rat endotoxic shock. (Table 3) Therefore, the action of anti-lipid A antibodies on lipopolysaccharide or gram-negative organisms may be antibody dependent. We[16] also demonstrated that prophylaxis with anti-lipid A monoclonal antibodies was effective in suckling rat endotoxic shock. (Table 4) Since severe trauma such as multiple injury has a high risk for sepsis/septic shock, prophylactic immunotherapy could be considered as a potential for the high-risk trauma patient. Since lipid A has only minor heterogeneity, anti-lipid A antibodies may be more useful than anti-O antigen antibodies or anti-core glycolipid antibodies for endotoxic shock prophylaxis.

Effects of this passive immunity may be effective for the prophylaxis of endotoxic shock

LPS	90%
LPS+A78S1	33%*
LPS+A523	22%*

A78S1: anti-lipid A monoclonal IgG
A523: anti-lipid A monoclonal IgM
*p<0.01 vs LPS

Table 3. 24-hour mortality in 10-day-old rats.

LPS	60%
LPS+A78S1*	13%@

*A78S1: anti-lipid A monoclonal IgG; @ p<0.01. A78S1 was intraperitoneally injected to pregnant rats on the 17th gestational day for prophylaxis of newborn rat endotoxic shock. Newborn rats received an intraperitoneal injection of endotoxin. Twenty-four hour mortality was observed.

Table 4. 24-hour mortality in 0-day-old rats.

only for a short period. Antibodies may induce second antibody formation. Therefore,
passive immunity may have disadvantages
when compared to active immunity although
passive immunity has an advantage in immediate therapy. Active immunization may be
more appropriate for prevention from gram-
negative sepsis/septic shock, especially in the
young.

Hyporesponsiveness to LPS, endotoxin
tolerance, has been noted for decades. Two
phases of LPS tolerance are classified: the early
phase and the late phase. The late phase of
LPS tolerance is due to antibody production.
In early endotoxin tolerance the reticuloendothelial cells mediate the protection. However, the mechanism of early endotoxin
tolerance still has not been fully understood.

We have demonstrated that early endotoxin tolerance is induced in suckling rats.
We also have reported that when endotoxin is
administered repeatedly, tolerance to endotoxin is increased.[17] These results suggest that
endotoxin administration may induce early
endotoxin tolerance in the young. In experimental animals, anti-LPS antibody is present
two to three weeks after LPS injection. Our
previous study showed that serial endotoxin
injection induced early endotoxin tolerance
and also anti-LPS antibody formation in adult
rats.[17] Therefore, early endotoxin tolerance
and antibody formation could theoretically
be induced in the young by endotoxin injection. *E. coli* J5 has been successfully used in
human volunteers for antibody production.
Therefore, J5 may be useful for prophylaxis in
the young with severe trauma and without
gram-negative infection, inducing early endotoxin tolerance and anti-LPS antibody formation. We feel that immunomodulation is a
potentially important treatment modality for
child trauma care.

REFERENCES

1. Division of injury control, center for environmental health and injury control: Childhood injuries in the United States. Am J Dis Child 1990; 144:627-646.
2. Orlowski JP, Sieger L, Anthony BF. Bactericidal capacity of monocytes of newborn infants. J Pediatr 1976; 89:797-801.
3. Kugo M, Sano K, Uetani Y, Nakamura H. Superoxide dismutase in polymorphonuclear leukocytes of term newborn infants and very low birth weight infants. Pediatr Res 1989; 26:227-231.
4. Filkins JP. Comparison of endotoxin detoxification by leukocytes and macrophages. Proc Soc Exp Biol Med 1971; 137:1396-1400.
5. Hayward AR, Lydyard PM. B-cell function in the newborn. Pediatr 1979; 64(Supple):758-764.
6. Jarvis WR. Epidemiology of nosocomial infections in pediatric patients. Pediatr Infect Dis J 1987; 6:344-351.
7. Beutler B, Cerami A. The endogenous mediator of endotoxic shock. Clin Res 1987; 36:192-197.
8. Dinarello CA. Interleukin-1. Rev Inf Dis 1984; 6:51.
9. LeMay DR, LeMay LG, Kluger MJ, D'Alecy LG. Plasma profiles of IL-6 and TNF with fever-inducing doses of lipopolysaccharide in dogs. Am J Physiol 1990; 259:R126-R132.
10. Waage A, Brandtzaeg P, Halstensen A et al. The complex pattern of cytokines in meningococcal septic shock. Association between interleukin-6, interleukin-1 and fetal outcome. J Exp Med 1989; 169:333-338.
11. Goto M, Griffin AJ, Chiemmongkoltip P et al. Endotoxin shock in newborn dogs: Serial hemodynamic studies. J Lab Clin Med 1988; 112:109-117.
12. Zeller WP, Goto M, Witek-Janusek L, Hurley RM. Mortality, temporal substrate, and insulin responses to endotoxic shock in zero, ten, and twenty-eight day old rats. Surg Obstet Gynecol 1991; 173:375-383.
13. Adhikari M, Coovadia HM, Gaffin SL, Broch-Utene JG et al. Septicaemic low birth weight neonates treated with human antibodies to endotoxin. Arch Dis Child 1985; 60:382-384.
14. Ziegler EJ, McCutchan A, Fierer J et al. Treatment of gram-negative bacteria and shock with human antiserum to a mutant Escherichia coli. N Eng J Med 1982; 307:1226-1230.
15. Ziegler EJ, Fisher CJ, Sprung CL et al. Treatment of gram-negative bacteria and septic shock with HA-1A human monoclonal antibody against endotoxin. N Eng J Med 1991; 324:429-436.
16. Goto M, Zeller WP, Mathews H, Hurley RM. Prophylactic immunotherapy in newborn rat endotoxicosis. Circ Shock 1989; 28:357-367.
17. Goto M, Zeller WP, Hurley RM, Jong JS, Lee CH. Prophylaxis and treatment of newborn endotoxic shock with anti-lipid A monoclonal antibodies. Circ Shock 1991; 35: 60-64.

CHAPTER 23

HEMOSTASIS IN THE TRAUMA PATIENT

Jeanine M. Walenga
Areta Kowal-Vern
Jawed Fareed
Richard L. Gamelli

Trauma patients often experience coagulopathies due to their injuries alone, but which may also be complicated by underlying disorders, previous medications, alcohol, etc. In particular, thermally injured patients are at risk of hemorrhage and thrombosis secondary to tissue injury, sepsis and infection. Disseminated intravascular coagulation (DIC) and vasculitis is not uncommon in these patients; thrombotic disorders can lead to poor wound healing (microthrombi), amputation or demise.

In the diagnosis of these disorders, the clinical coagulation laboratory has traditionally focused on bleeding disorders rather than hypercoagulability. Diagnostic testing typically consists of the PT, APTT, fibrinogen, platelet count, bleeding time and FSP assays. These tests have proven useful in screening for low levels of coagulation factors or platelet dysfunction in identifying obvious bleeding abnormalities and relatively significant fibrinolysis. However, they are not specific enough to identify the locale and nature of these abnormalities nor do they detect a hypercoagulable (thrombotic) state. Cellular interactions, in particular that of the vascular endothelium, are not taken into account by these assays.

Recent developments allow for a molecular approach to investigate hemostatic activation with more specific and sensitive biochemical analyses.[1,2] Previously unknown parameters of the coagulation and fibrinolytic systems, endothelium, platelet function and cellular activation can now be quantitated. (Table 1) In addition, low molecular weight peptides generated by specific enzymatic reactions within either the coagulation, fibrinolysis or platelet systems have been identified. (Table 1) The measurement of these hemostatic markers provides a reliable tool for detecting specific early events which lead to hemorrhagic or hypercoagulable disorders.[3-6]

If a coagulopathy can be identified early and its origin specified (before clinical conditions become established), targeted treatment can be provided. Quantitation of the hemostatic markers can aid in these diagnoses. Furthermore, some of these markers are thought to play a role in cell growth and wound healing. Better understanding of these mechanisms opens new avenues of diagnosis and treatment in the trauma patient population.

α_2-Antiplasmin	α_2-AP
α_2-Macroglobulin	α_2-Mac
Activated partial thromboplastin time	APTT
Angiotensin converting enzyme	ACE
Antiphospholipid antibody	APA
Antithrombin III	AT III
ß-Thromboglobulin	ßTG
C_1-esterase inhibitor	C_1Inh
Cyclic AMP	CAMP
D-dimer	D-di
Endothelin	ET
Endothelium derived relaxing factor	EDRF
Extrinsic pathway inhibitor	EPI
Factor VII	FVII
Fibrin(ogen) split products	FSP
Fibrinopeptide A	FPA
Fragment 1.2 (prothrombin derived)	F1.2
Heparin cofactor II	HC II
Kallikrein	Kal
Kinin	Kinin
Modified antithrombin	ATM
Plasmin-antiplasmin complex	PAP
Plasminogen	Plg
Plasminogen activator inhibitor	PAI
Platelet factor 4	PF4
Platelet derived growth factor	PDGF
Platelet activating factor	PAF
Pre-kallikrein	PK
Prostacyclin	PGI_2
Protein C	PrC
Protein S	PrS
Prothrombin time	PT
Thrombin-antithrombin complex	TAT
Thromboxane B_2	TxB_2
Tissue plasminogen activator-plasminogen activator inhibitor complex	tPA-PAI
Tissue plasminogen activator	tPA
Tissue factor	TF
Urokinase-like plasminogen activator	uPA
Von Willebrand's factor	VWF

Table 1. Hemostatic parameters.

STATE OF THE ART

The Coagulation System

Hemostasis, the maintenance of blood in a fluid state, is based on an intimate interrelationship between several physiologic systems. (Fig. 1) A balance of cellular blood elements, coagulation and fibrinolytic enzymes, inhibitors and cofactors, vascular integrity and the rheologic properties of blood not only keeps blood in a fluid state but allows for localized coagulation when blood vessel damage has occurred.[7]

The coagulation cascade is composed of a series of linked proteolytic reactions beginning at the site of factor VII-tissue factor (extrinsic system) or through the kallikrein-kinin system associated with the immune and other physiologic responses (intrinsic pathway). (Fig. 2) The PT and APTT assays screen for normal levels of these enzymes. Additional plasma factors which act as important inhibitors to the coagulation cascade have been identified; however, PT/APTT assays are not sensitive to these proteins. Four important inhibitors are described below.

AT III plays a central role in the regulation of the coagulation system, strongly inhibiting thrombin and factor Xa. It also inhibits factors XIIa, XIa, and Va, kallikrein, C_1-Inh and plasmin. Qualitative abnormalities and quantitative deficiencies of AT III are associated with an increased risk of

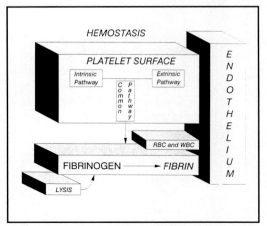

Fig. 1. Diagrammatic representation of the interrelationships of the coagulation, fibrinolytic, platelet and vascular endothelial systems.

thrombosis.[8] The therapeutic efficacy of heparin depends on the presence of AT III such that persons lacking this inhibitor fail to respond to heparin therapy appropriately.

Protein C is a plasma factor which inhibits factors Va and VIIIa and stimulates fibrinolysis. It is activated by thrombin bound to vascular endothelium. Individuals with protein C deficiency have an increased incidence of thrombosis.[9] Protein S is a cofactor of Protein C activation.

HC II is another inhibitor of thrombin distinguishable from AT III. Heparin also interacts with HC II to inhibit thrombin. Recent studies have associated a low circulating level of HC II with clinical thrombosis.[10]

EPI, also called lipoprotein associated coagulation inhibitor (LACI), is the only known inhibitor of factor VIIa-tissue factor. EPI prevents thrombotic complications in many inflammatory and infectious disease states.[11] The full role of EPI in thrombosis is currently under investigation.

When the coagulation system is activated, certain products of the enzymatic reactions are generated.[2] A profile of the molecular markers generated during coagulation activation may be helpful in identifying patients with a prethrombotic state and may provide useful data on the bleeding or thrombotic risk status of a patient. The following markers described below are produced with thrombin generation.

When prothrombin is converted to thrombin, a small protein (F1.2) is cleaved from the prothrombin molecule. Elevated levels have been identified in patients with ongoing thrombosis.[12,13]

Thrombin, once formed, readily binds to natural inhibitors such as AT III. Low levels of complexes of TAT normally circulate in blood. During a thrombotic episode, higher than normal levels of TAT are formed.[12] In addition, when thrombin has been generated,

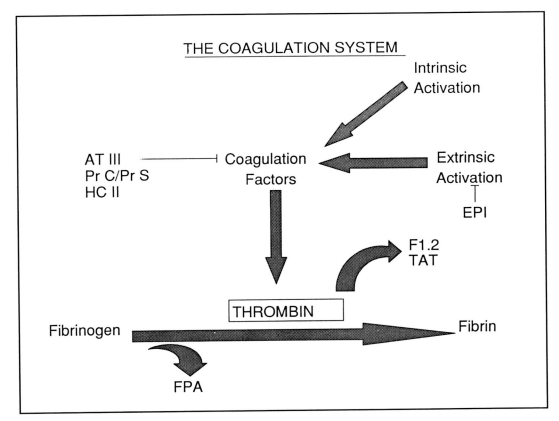

Fig. 2. Flow diagram of the components of the coagulation system.

another marker is formed. The reaction of AT III and thrombin produces a modified AT III molecule (ATM) which can be measured.

Thrombin cleavage of fibrinogen yields two small soluble peptides: FPA and FPB. Thus FPAs are cleaved from fibrinogen before FSPs are formed. Moreover, FPAs are specific indicators of thrombin activity on fibrinogen, whereas FSPs can be derived from fibrinogen or fibrin. Thus assay of FPA provides an early, specific indication of thrombin activation and a hypercoagulable state,[2,14] not an indication of fibrinolytic activation.

FIBRINOLYTIC SYSTEM

The fibrinolytic system is equally as important to normal hemostasis as the coagulation system. The activators, inhibitors and hemostatic markers generated during fibrinolytic activation are described below in Fig. 3.

Plasminogen is the precursor of plasmin, the active enzyme of the fibrinolytic path-

way. Abnormal plasminogen or plasminogen deficiencies have been described in individuals with thromboembolic diseases or a consumptive coagulopathy.[15] It is essential to have adequate plasminogen levels for effective thrombolytic therapy.

Plasminogen activators are a heterogeneous group of serine proteases that convert plasminogen to plasmin. tPA is the major component of the fibrinolytic system. It is synthesized in the endothelium and can be found in plasma. uPA is another important activator. Plasminogen activator levels are increased in certain pathologic bleeding states. Decreased levels are correlated with thromboembolic diseases and myocardial infarction.[16]

The inhibitor of tPA, PAI, is as important as tPA for adequate fibrinolytic activity. Elevated levels can be associated with a thrombotic tendency.[17] α_2-Antiplasmin is an important inhibitor of plasmin which binds to plasma or fibrin-bound plasmin thereby inactivating it. Decreased levels can lead to

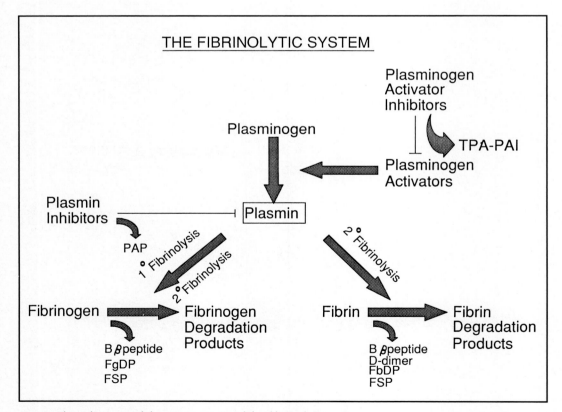

Fig. 3. Flow diagram of the components of the fibrinolytic system.

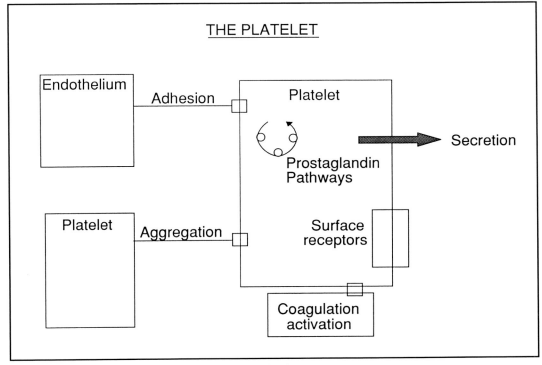

Fig. 4. Flow diagram of the components of the platelet system.

excessive fibrinolysis and bleeding.[18] α_2-Macroglobulin is also an inhibitor of plasmin. It has a wide spectrum of protease inhibiting activity forming complexes with thrombin, plasmin and kallikrein. α_2-Macroglobulin may also have a regulatory role at cell surfaces or on endothelium.

When the fibrinolytic system has been activated generating plasmin, PAP complex levels are elevated in the blood.[19] Increased levels have been reported in sepsis and DIC,[20] (and personal communication Drs. M. Levi and J.W. ten Cate, University of Amsterdam). tPA-PAI complexes are also elevated in blood during fibrinolytic activation.

Plasmin progressively degrades fibrin or fibrinogen, releasing a series of peptides from the B chain in a first step. The generated fragments are Bß-related peptides that include Bß 1-118, Bß 1-42 and Bß 15-42. Subsequent cleavage yields larger fragments X, Y, D and E from the D and E domains. Bß-related peptides are elevated in DIC and primary fibrinolysis.[21]

As stated previously, FPA and FPB are released upon thrombin's action on fibrino-

gen. This exposes polymerization sites on the central "D" and "E" domains of the remaining fibrinogen molecule. The fibrinogen molecule is further cleaved by thrombin (or plasmin) generating the X, Y, D and E fragments. These fragments are the FSPs, commonly measured to indicate the level of fibrinolytic activation. The cleaved fibrinogen molecules assemble side-to-side and end-to-end, joining at the exposed sites resulting in crosslinked fibrin.

D-dimer is derived from crosslinked fibrin following the enzymatic action of plasmin. This differs from the FSP fragments which are derived from either fibrinogen or fibrin by either thrombin or plasmin activity. Thus elevated levels of D-dimer are specifically indicative of ongoing coagulation activation (fibrin formation) with subsequent fibrinolytic activation (generation of plasmin) and breakdown of the formed clot. The D-dimer assay is also more sensitive than the FSP assay. Elevated levels are found with DIC, fibrinolytic activation, thrombolytic therapy and myocardial infarction.[5,12,21]

Platelets

The platelet is the first line of defense against bleeding. One of the main functions of platelets is the formation of a platelet plug to arrest bleeding and maintain vascular integrity. On the other hand, platelets can become hyperactivated and present a risk factor for the development of a thrombotic event. Various markers related to the activation of platelets are described in Fig. 4.

The membrane surface of the platelet is composed of different glycoproteins (GPIb, GPIIb, GPIIIa, GPIIIb) and an inner phospholipid layer. The glycoproteins, which serve as receptors to mediate the surface contact reactions of the platelet (stickiness, shape change, adhesion, internal contraction and aggregation), are exposed upon activation of the platelet.[7] In particular, platelet factor 3 (PF3), a phospholipid, is exposed which is necessary for the binding of coagulation factors to facilitate thrombin generation. The presence of these receptors can be quantitated. Certain platelet disorders lead to thrombocytopenia induced by antibodies directed towards the platelet, e.g., heparin induced. There are several laboratory techniques which can be used to identify this problem.

Platelet function can be assessed in the laboratory using different agents to induce aggregation of platelet-rich plasma. Von Willebrand's factor, essential for initial adhesion of the platelet to the vessel wall via a specific glycoprotein (GPIb), can also be quantitated by this technique.

The internal granules of the platelet contain numerous proteins which play a role in hemostasis. Alpha granules contain PF4, ßTG, PDGF, fibronectin, albumin, fibrinogen and factors V and VIII. The beta or dense granules contain ADP, serotonin, Ca^{+2} and phosphates. Measurement of these release products in the plasma can be used to identify platelet activation.

PF4 functions as an anti-heparin substance and a cell growth regulator. Elevated levels have been observed during inflammatory states, venous thrombosis, myocardial infarction, myeloproliferative syndrome and diabetes.[2,14] Heparin treatment also mobilizes PF4. This can have an adverse effect on the anticoagulant, reducing its efficacy. ßTG is similar in action to PF4.[2,14]

Prostaglandins are directly associated with the function of platelets. PGI_2 (prostacyclin) is a potent platelet anti-aggregating agent and vasodilator derived from the endothelium. TxA_2 is a potent platelet aggregating agent and vasoconstrictor stored in platelet granules. The stable metabolite of TxA_2, TxB_2, is measurable. Prostaglandins are also associated with the functioning of the cardiovascular, pulmonary, immunologic, gastrointestinal and other systems.

Leukotrienes are substances of a similar nature as prostaglandins derived from white blood cells. These are being studied for their role in thrombotic diseases. PAF (1-0-alkyl-2-acetyl derivative of phosphorylcholine) is a lipid probably derived from the platelet itself which induces platelet aggregation and secretion. The function of PAF is not completely understood, but it may have a significant clinical role.

Endothelium

The endothelium contributes a major role in hemostasis. Besides providing a non-thrombogenic surface, it serves in a poly–functional capacity. The endothelium can induce or suppress clot formation. Normal fibrinolytic activity is dependent on functioning vascular endothelium. tPA, PAI, von Willebrand's factor and PGI_2 are derived from the endothelium. These cells also generate glycosaminoglycans, and they also take part in the activation of protein C. By measuring these substances, an indirect measure of the functional integrity of the endothelium can be obtained.

A newly identified endothelium derived protein is endothelin, a vasoactive peptide with potent vasoconstrictor action.[22] Endothelin release may be stimulated by fractured thrombi rather than evolving thrombi.[23] The mechanism of generation of endothelin, its function and the clinical relevance of elevated levels is currently under investigation. Endothelium also produces various vasodilating factors which are collectively known as endothelial-derived relaxing factors (EDRFs).

ACE is the enzyme found in the lung vasculature which converts angiotensin I to angiotensin II and inactivates bradykinin. Angiotensin II is a very potent vasoconstrictor.

OTHER MECHANISMS

The role of leukocytes in hemostasis is currently being investigated. It is known that neutrophils are a major source of proteolytic enzymes and oxygen free radicals. Activation of neutrophils, lymphocytes and/or macrophages may stimulate hemostatic activation.[24,25] Blood viscosity plays a role in normal hemostasis.[3] In some individuals, immunoglobulins are produced against phospholipids creating a thrombotic tendency known as antiphospholipid antibody (APA) syndrome.[26]

An important and rapidly expanding area is that of cytokines. Cytokines are a unique cascade system of peptides. They act as mediators in infection, host defense, response to injury and tissue destruction by mobilizing acute phase proteins of the immunologic and hemostatic systems. The cytokines are modified by interferons, prostaglandins, corticosteroids and environmental stimuli such as hypoxia.[27]

It is hypothesized that tumor necrosis factor (TNF) is one of the earliest responders to cellular activation such that upon physical injury (burn, crush) or the presence of a foreign antigen (bacteria) the cell (lymphocyte or macrophage-monocyte) is stimulated and TNF is released, as a signal transducer, to activate the same or another cell to release one or several interleukins (IL's). The IL acts as a messenger to specific cells to produce an inflammatory or other activation response. For example, systemic IL-6 production is induced locally by TNF and IL-1ß release.

To the extent that current knowledge exists it is suggested that TNF, IL-6 and IL-1ß play a role in modulating the hemostatic system, whereas, IL-2 has no known role as yet. Specifically IL-6 is known to stimulate a peripheral neutrophilia, a lymphopenia and a reticulocytosis,[28] TNF may increase fibrinolytic activity by increasing tPA antigen,[29] and activated leukocytes induce fibrin depo-

Parameter	Day 1	Day 5
COAGULATION SYSTEM:		
PrC	↓	↓
PrS	↓	↓
AT III	↓	N
TAT	↓	N
FVII:antigen	↓	N
FVII:coagulant	↓	N
CONTACT SYSTEM:		
Kinin	↓	N
Kal	↓	↓
C_1Inh	↓	N
FIBRINOLYTIC SYSTEM:		
D-Di	↑	↑
Plg	↓	N
α_2-AP	N	N
tPA	↑	↑
PAI	↑	↑

n=60; For abbreviations see Table 1.

Table 2. Coagulation parameters of thermally injured patients compared to normals.

sition and platelet activation. The platelet release reaction promotes leukocyte adherence which leads to a positive feedback mechanism. Activated monocytes release thromboplastin (a procoagulant material) which induces the coagulation response. Studies, of course, are necessary to prove these concepts.

STUDIES IN THERMAL INJURY PATIENTS

Although some investigators have studied a limited number of coagulation parameters, the hemostatic abnormalities of trauma and burn patients have not been comprehensively defined and correlated with clinical outcome. We have conducted a large scale study at the Shock-Trauma Institute of Loyola to characterize the hemostatic changes that occur in the thermally injured patient and how they correlate with the degree of injury, the healing process, and associated disorders such as DIC, thrombosis and bleeding.[30-33] Our preliminary results are given below.

A. Coagulation and Contact System Parameters

Burn Groups:	PrC	PrS	ATIII	TAT	FVII:c	FVII:ag	Kal	Kinin	C$_1$-Inh
<20% vs. 20-40%									
<20% vs. >40%		*	*		*	*	*		*
<20% vs. 0%	*	*				*			*
20-40% vs. >40%			*		*	*	*	*	*
20-40% vs. 0%	*	*	*	*		*			*
>40% vs. 0%	*	*	*		*	*	*		*

B. Fibrinolytic Parameters

Burn Groups:	Plg	PAI	tPA	D-di
<20% vs. 20-40%				
<20% vs. >40%	*	*	*	
<20% vs. 0%				*
20-40% vs. >40%	*	*	*	
20-40% vs. 0%				*
>40% vs. 0%	*	*	*	*

* Significant at 97% (ANOVA-Scheffe-F-test); n=60. For abbreviations see Table 1.

Tables 3A & B. Statistical significance of hemostatic markers.

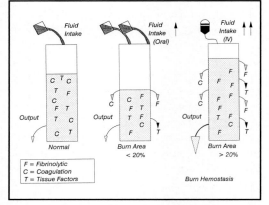

Fig. 5. Interactions between the coagulation and fibrinolytic systems in the thermal injured patient.

Sixty patients admitted to the Loyola University Burn Center within 24 hours of injury were studied (June 1990-June 1991). Blood samples from 47 males/13 females (average age 37) were collected in the first 48 hours and 5-7 days later. The data was categorized by % burn (2° + 3°): <20%, n=22; 20%-40%, n=18; >40%, n=20. Routine clot based assays, synthetic substrate (functional) assays and ELISA (immunoassays) were used to determine the levels of hemostatic markers of coagulation and fibrinolysis. Cytokines, platelet factors, prostaglandins and endothelin were measured by radioimmunoassays.

Following thermal injury, a general upregulation of the production and utilization of the coagulation and fibrinolytic parameters, increased fibrinolytic debris and a decrease in the natural anticoagulants such as AT III, PrC, and PrS was observed. The combined effect of the changes in the coagulation and fibrinolytic systems resulted in a hypercoagulable state and increased thrombotic risk.[30] (Tables 2, 3 and Fig. 5) The FVII:c/FVII:ag ratio was significantly elevated in all groups compared to normal volunteers, during the entire first week following the burn, further indicating a hypercoagulable state.

Most strikingly, this activation process resulted in a consumption of the regulatory mediators. AT III values were significantly decreased with the severity of the burn; however, they increased dramatically over the five days postburn. The subjects' age and percent burn accounted for 48% of the variance in AT III values.

In certain populations, F1.2 and ATM have been shown to be predictive of increased thrombotic risk when they are elevated.[12,13] However, by one-factor ANOVA statistical analysis of burn patients with DIC compared to the other burn patients, F1.2 and ATM were not of predictive value for DIC. In a second statistical analysis, these patients were evaluated on the basis of percent burn area: <20%, 20-40%, >40%. By this analysis,

ATM showed slight significance (p <0.05) as a marker of DIC but only in patients with ≥40% burn area. Thus, compared to ATM, TAT, D-dimer, AT III, Protein C and Protein S, F1.2 was the least sensitive marker of DIC in thermal injury patients.

Plasmin-antiplasmin complex (PAP) is known to be elevated in inflammation and infection.[20] It was evaluated in the burn patients to determine if it is a predictor of infection. Within the span of two weeks, there were 16 episodes of infection in 14 patients requiring antibiotics and a 13% (8/60) mortality. In the <20% burn group, there were three infections with an average PAP level of 10nM/L, 4 infections in the 20-40% group (mean PAP = 11.7 nM/L); and 9 infections in the >40% group (mean PAP level = 12 nM/L). Of the 16 episodes of infection or sepsis, PAP was elevated in 10 patients (63%). Normal PAP levels range 2.5-8.0 nM/L.

PAP was elevated on day 5 during the clinically stabilized phase regardless of percent burn and did not appear to correlate with the type of burn, inhalation or fibrinolytic state. Since PAP was also elevated in thermal injury patients who did not have sepsis or serious infection, this data suggests that PAP is not a specific predictor of infection in burn (p <0.1).

Platelet activation studies indicated an increase in TxB_2 levels as the burn wound size increased; however, the obtained values did not indicate major platelet activation. The levels of PGI_2 were well below normal. This may be attributed to either decreased production or altered functionality of the endothelium. A trend of increasing PGI_2 and extent of body surface area of burn has been observed.

Since PGI_2 levels were below normal and TxB_2 levels were relatively normal, it can be inferred that there was no suppression of a mechanism to activate the platelets. Other studies revealed that these platelets were stimulated but without granular release. Although our other studies have shown a hypercoagulable state in thermal injury patients, the data of this study indicates that this is not due to platelet activation.

Our studies of cytokines in this patient population have revealed several interesting correlations to the clinical presentation. There appears to be an effect of IL-1ß, IL-6 and TNF but not IL-2 on the hemostatic mechanisms associated with thermal injury. These newly available data add pieces to the complex puzzle which need to be synthesized into a working cascade. Our work is presently being expanded.

The thrombotic risk of thermal injury patients increases the chance that the burn wound zone of coagulation will propagate during the first 48 hours and at the time of sepsis, resulting potentially in an increase in the depth of injury. The hypercoagulable state appears to increase in severity as the extent of burn wound size increases and returns to more stable levels in the majority of patients by 5-7 days postinjury, barring any complications. The incorporation of molecular markers of hemostatic activation and cytokines has greatly aided in understanding the mechanisms involved in the recovery from thermal injury. This knowledge can help in the diagnosis and treatment of these patients.

SUGGESTED DIRECTION

Based on the information obtained from the quantitation of hemostatic markers and cytokines, several treatment regimens can be suggested to reduce clinical complications, to treat ongoing pathologies and to promote healing.

Heparin alone has not been effective in preserving tissue viability in animal experimentation or averting the ongoing intravascular clotting in massive burns. Fibronectin given in a fresh-frozen plasma infusion was also considered beneficial in burn patients without the realization at the time that coagulation factors were also replenished during the infusion. Uncontrolled pilot studies of patients in septic shock have shown that AT III and heparin infusions have increased survival.[34,35]

In order to decrease the thrombotic risk in these patients, future trials replacing AT III, particularly in ≥40% burn group, may show a decrease in mortality and morbidity. AT III has been beneficial in patients with

Antithrombotic

Antithrombin III concentrate

Dermatan sulfate

Heparan sulfate

Heparin

Heparinoids

Hirudin

Hirulog

Low molecular weight heparins

Protein C concentrate

Peptides

Synthetic oligosaccharides

Thrombomodulin

Antiplatelet

Fish oil products

GP IIb/IIIa inhibitors

Prostanoid modulators

Recombinant peptides

Endothelium Modulators

Defibrotide

DDAVP

Growth factor peptides

Other

Viscosity modulators

C_1-Inhibitor concentrate

Table 4. New antithrombotic agents.

septic shock and DIC. Similarly, protein C concentrates may also be effective. Recombinant and synthetic inhibitors of thrombin such as hirudin, hirulog and oligopeptides may also be useful in the control of these processes.

Congenital C_1Inh deficiency is known to precipitate the occurrence of angioneurotic edema. Since C_1Inh was significantly depressed in our patients, it is interesting to speculate what role this may play in the initial edema formation. Concentrates of C_1I are available in Europe. It may be of interest to test the clinical usefulness of this treatment in burn injuries.

Many new antithrombotic agents are under development. These agents will either replace heparin in those patients resistant to treatment or will be used to more effectively target the cause of the thrombotic disorder.[36-38] These agents have less bleeding complications and do not induce thrombocytopenia as a side effect.

Although heparin has not been a successful treatment of clotting disorders in thermally injured patients, it possesses certain cell regulatory properties. The new low molecular weight heparins which have an antithrombotic effect equal to that of heparin, but a reduced anticoagulant effect, may prove more clinically useful than heparin in trauma patients.[36] In addition, heparan sulfates, dermatan sulfates and heparinoid mixtures (mostly chondroitin sulfate) may be beneficial as well.[37,39] This entire area will be greatly advanced in the near future with the ability to identify and quantitate cytokines.

Another drug, currently available in Italy for treatment of peripheral vascular disease is defibrotide (Crinos, Milan, Italy). This drug is a polydeoxyribonucleotide derivative obtained from mammalian lung mucosa. The apparent mechanism of action of defibrotide is to regulate cell function enhancing PGI_2 production and fibrinolytic activity. Other ongoing studies suggest that defibrotide may be an effective treatment in microangiopathy and hemolytic uremic syndrome. Studies in cancer therapy (cell growth regulation) are also in progress. Recently this drug has been approved for oral usage in patients with various thrombotic disorders. Since this agent does not produce any anticoagulant effect, yet it does produce an antithrombotic effect, it may be of major value in the treatment of sepsis and trauma.

A list of some of the newer antithrombotic drugs is given in Table 4. Many of these drugs have a significant effect on the vascular system. Thus vascular insufficiency, fibrinolytic deficit and platelet activation can be target-controlled by the proper use of these agents. Many of these drugs are often given in conjunction with other drugs such as vasodilators, antibiotics and hemodynamic stabilizers. Recently, it has been discovered that these latter drugs also have an effect on hemostatic parameters. Thus the observed pathologic events in a patient with thermal injury or trauma may be due to secondary factors as well. The use of various markers of hemostatic activation may help in the differential diagnosis of the pathogenic trigger.

The current recommendation is that thermally injured patients and trauma patients in general be evaluated for hemostatic abnormalities using the newly identified markers. The present global PT, APTT and fibrinogen are useful screening assays but have proven to be too low in sensitivity to detect a hypercoagulable state and are very nonspecific. One should delineate the activation state of the hemostatic system by studying the platelet-, fibrinolytic- and coagulation-associated markers and tissue injury-associated factors. The interrelationships among these markers and factors and their relevance to the prethrombotic state is an important consideration in the overall management of the trauma patient and for targeted pharmacologic treatment. Knowledge of the cytokine changes that occur in these patients at the various stages of their recovery will also bring much useful information to define their clinical course and identify beneficial treatments.

The degree of subclinical activation of hemostasis should vary depending on the severity and extent of the burn/trauma and other underlying complications. If a subclinical prethrombotic state can be diagnosed in these patients, it may be possible to reduce or eliminate microthrombi formation which can impair the healing process, DIC complications or overt thrombotic complications leading to loss of limb or demise. By identifying the specific cause of the disorder, targeted treatment, particularly with the newly developed agents, can be utilized.

References

1. Fareed J, Bick RL, Squillaci G et al. Molecular markers of hemostatic disorders: Implications in the diagnosis and therapeutic management of thrombotic and bleeding disorders. Clin Chem 1983; 29:1641-1658.
2. Fareed J (ed): Molecular markers of hemostatic disorders. Semin Thromb Hemost 1984; 10:215-340.
3. Lowe GDO, Wood DA, Douglas JT et al. Relationships of plasma viscosity, coagulation and fibrinolysis to coronary risk factors and angina. Thromb Haemost 1991; 65(4):339-343.
4. Meade TW, Brozovic M, Chakrabarti RR et al. Haemostatic function and ischaemic heart disease: Principal results of the Northwick Park heart study. Lancet 1986; 2:533-537.
5. Thompson SG, van de Loo J, Haverkate F, on behalf of the ECAT Angina Pectoris Study Group. Principal results of the ECAT angina pectoris study. Thromb Haemost 1991; 65:Abst 468.
6. Heinrich J, Schulte H, Balleisen L et al. Predictive value of haemostatic variables in the PROCAM-study. Thromb Haemost 1991; 65:Abst 466.
7. Corriveau DM, Fritsma GA. Plasma proteins: Factors of the hemostatic mechanism. In: Hemostasis and Thrombosis in the Clinical Laboratory. Ed. Corriveau DM, Fritsma GA. JB Lippincott, 1988:34-66.
8. Marciniak E, Farley CH, DeSimone PA: Familial thrombosis due to antithrombin III deficiency. Blood 1974; 43:219-231.
9. Seligsohn U, Berger A, Abend M et al. Homozygous protein C deficiency manifested by massive venous thrombosis in the newborn. N Engl J Med 1984; 310:559-562.
10. Duckert F, Tran TH, Marbet GA. Association of hereditary heparin cofactor II deficiency with thrombosis. Lancet 1985; 2:413-414.
11. Sandset PM, Sirnes PA, Abildgaard U. Factor VII and extrinsic pathway inhibitor in acute coronary disease. Br J Haematol 1989; 72:391-396.
12. Boneu B, Bes G, Pelzer H et al. D-dimers, thrombin-antithrombin III complexes and prothrombin fragments 1+2: Diagnostic value in clinically suspected deep vein thrombosis. Thromb Haemost 1991; 65:28-32.
13. Bauer KA, Rosenberg RD. The pathophysiology of the prethrombotic state in humans: Insights gained from studies using markers of hemostatic system activation. Blood 1987; 70:343-350.
14. Nichols AB, Owen J, Kaplan KL et al. Fibrinopeptide A, platelet factor 4, and beta-thromboglobulin levels in coronary heart disease. Blood 1982; 60:650-654.
15. Scharrer I, Robbins K, Wohl R et al. Investigations on two congenital abnormal plasminogens (Frankfort I and Frankfort II): Their relationship to thrombosis. Thromb Haemost 1983; 50(1) Abst 806.
16. Gram J, Jespersen J. A selective depression of tissue plasminogen activator (t-PA) activity in euglobulins characterizes a risk group among survivors of acute myocardial infarction. Thromb Haemost 1987; 57(2):137-139.
17. Hamsten A, Walldius G, Szamosi A et al. Plasminogen activator inhibitor in plasma: Risk factor for recurrent myocardial infarction. Lancet 1987; 2:3-9.
18. Aoki N, Saito H, Kamiya T et al. Congenital deficiency of α_2-plasmin inhibitor associated with severe hemorrhagic tendency. J Clin Invest 1979; 63(5): 877-884.

19. Collen D, Wiman B. Fast-acting plasmin inhibitor in human plasma. Blood 1978; 51(4),563-569.

20. Velasco F, Torres A, Andres P, Duran MI. Functional activities and concentrations of plasmin inhibitors in normal subjects and D.I.C. patients. Thromb Haemost 1982; 47(3):275-277.

21. Lawler CM, Bovill EG, Stump DC et al. Fibrin fragment D-dimer and fibrinogen Bß peptides in plasma as markers of clot lysis during thrombolytic therapy in acute myocardial infarction. Blood 1990; 76(7):1341-1348.

22. Patrignani P, Maschio AD, Bazzoni G et al. Inactivation of endothelin by polymorphonuclear leukocyte-derived lytic enzymes. Blood 1991; 78(10):2715-2720.

23. Stewart DJ, Kubac G, Costello KB, Cernacek P. Increased plasma endothelin-1 in the early hours of acute myocardial infarction. JACC 1991; 18(1):38-43.

24. Mehta J., Nichols WW, Mehta P: Neutrophils as potential participants in acute myocardial ischemia. J Am Coll Cardiol 1988; 11:1309-1316.

25. Dinerman JL, Mehta JL, Saldeen TGP et al. Increased neutrophil elastase release in unstable angina pectoris and acute myocardial infarction. JACC 1990; 15(7):1559-1563.

26. Gavaghan TP, Krilis SA, Daggard GE et al. Anticardiolipin antibodies and occlusion of coronary artery bypass grafts. Lancet 1987; 2:977-978.

27. Ghezzi P, Dinarello CA, Bianchi M et al. Hypoxia increases production of interleukin-1 and tumor necrosis factor by human mononuclear cells. Cytokine 1991; 3:189-194.

28. Ulich TR, del Castillo J, Gus K. In vivo hematologic effects of IL-6 on hematopoiesis and circulating numbers of RBCs and WBCs. Blood 1989; 73:108.

29. Silverman P, Goldsmith GH, Spitzer TR et al. Effect of tumor necrosis factor on the human fibrinolytic system. J Clin Oncol 1990; 8:468-475.

30. Kowal-Vern A, Gamelli RL, Walenga JM et al. The effect of burn wound size on hemostasis: A correlation of the hemostatic changes to the clinical state. J Trauma, in press 1992.

31. Kowal-Vern A, Warpeha R, Gamelli R et al. Hemostatic abnormalities in thermal injury patients. Blood 1990: 76(10):Abst 1691.

32. Kowal-Vern A, Walenga JM, Gamelli R et al. Platelet activation in thermally injured patients assessed by thromboxane B_2 and 6-Keto-PGF$_{1\alpha}$. Thromb Haemost 1991; 65(6):Abst 2286.

33. Kowal-Vern A, Warpeha R, Gamelli R et al. Interleukin-1ß and tumor necrosis factor-α in thermal injury patients. Blood 1990; 76(10):Abst 2037.

34. Ono, I. Alteration of coagulation and fibrinolysis after burn injury and significance of anticoagulation therapy using heparin and antithrombin III concentrate. Hokkaido Igaku Zasshi 1987; 62:108-121.

35. Seitz R, Wolf M, Egbring R, Havemann K. The disturbance of hemostasis in septic shock: Role of neutrophil elastase and thrombin, effects of antithrombin III and plasma substitution. Eur J Haematol 1989: 43:22-28.

36. Fareed J (ed): Heparin and its derivatives. Parts I and II. Semin Thromb Hemost 1988: 11(1 and 2):1-236.

37. Fareed, J, Walenga JM, Breddin HK et al (eds): Newer strategies in the management of thrombotic disorders. Parts I-III. Semin Thromb Hemost 1989: 5(2-3):99-479.

38. Walenga JM, Fareed J (eds): Development of non-heparin glycosaminoglycans as therapeutic agents. Parts I and II. Semin Thromb Hemost 1991:17(suppl 1 and 2):1-239.

CHAPTER 24

HEMATOPOIETIC RESPONSE

Thomas P. Paxton
Richard L. Gamelli

Immunosuppression following trauma is a major factor in the increased risk for postinjury septic complications. Defects in both humoral and cell-mediated immunity concomitant with an alteration in the production and function of hematopoietic cells is largely responsible for the increased incidence of posttraumatic septic events. It has also become recognized that there are significant alterations in cell secretory products. These so called cytokines represent vital links of communication between cellular components within the host defense system. Modulating these cytokine pathways could yield new treatment options for patient care and management. Knowledge of posttraumatic changes in the immune system and the process of hematopoiesis suggest the possibility of the hematopoietic growth factors as future adjunctive therapeutic agents both singly and in combination with conventional antimicrobial therapy. The goal of such an approach is to alter the course of posttraumatic infectious episodes by controlling in tandem the production and function of specific myeloid and lymphoid elements to improve overall host resistance.

POSTINJURY IMMUNOSUPPRESSION

Nonspecific and specific immune defects following major trauma include demonstrable qualitative and quantitative dysfunction in neutrophils, macrophages and lymphocytes along with decreased complement levels and antibody production. Alterations in the proliferative response of cellular components, in addition to the qualitative changes, further compromise host defense mechanisms.[1-5,7,13,47]

Nowhere is this marked depression in immune response more evident than in the thermally injured patient. The skin, being the primary barrier to invading microorganisms, is eliminated. Concomitant inhalation injury may damage the mucociliary apparatus, contributing to a higher incidence of life-threatening pneumonia. Other potential sources of sepsis include the genitourinary and gastrointestinal tract with translocation of bacteria or bacterial products. Cellular defects include a decrease in neutrophil chemotactic and phagocytic abilities as well as depression of bactericidal activity. Macrophage dysfunction includes a decrease in phagocytosis and IL-1 production, and an increase in monocyte PGE_2 synthesis.[10,12,15,16,17,21] Alteration of lymphocytic function includes an increased T_8-suppressor cell/T_4-helper cell ratio, a decrease in gamma interferon production and suppressed natural killer cell activity.[10,21]

The prostaglandin PGE_2 plays a key role in augmentation of T_8-suppressor cell activity, by depression of monocyte IL-1 and T_4-helper cell IL-2 production.[14,16,18] γ-Interferon has been noted to be decreased for up to several weeks following major trauma which has been postulated to result in reduced antigen presentation and inadequate IL-1 production by the macrophage.[12]

Humoral immune response is hindered by inadequate complement levels and insufficient immunoglobulin production leading to an important reduction in opsinization of invading organisms. Myelopoietic defects include a decrease in circulating colony-stimulating factor levels along with a decline in the production of marrow progenitor cells. Evidence exists that posttraumatic sepsis exacerbates this defect in granulopoiesis.[10]

Local and systemic infection following severe burns, traumatic injuries and operative procedures continues as a major source of patient morbidity and mortality. Sepsis remains the commonest cause of death following severe thermal injury.[10,20] Polk reported that 75% of all deaths following thermal injury were secondary to sepsis.[6] Also, Baker at al reported that 78% of posttraumatic non-neurological deaths were the result of septic complications.[5] The exact cause of global immunosuppression following major traumatic injury is not known at present, however, the demonstrable dysfunction in granulocyte chemotactic, phagocytic and antibody-dependent, cell-mediated cytotoxicity (ADCC) mechanisms in combination with an inadequate bone marrow response is no doubt a major contributor. Recombinant DNA technology has made available for clinical trials the various colony-stimulating factors which would allow modulation of the hematopoietic process in an effort to alter the immune response to injury.[22]

HEMATOPOIESIS

Pluripotent stem cells present in the bone marrow are the earliest recognizable cells in the hematopoietic process. Undifferentiated stem cells are capable of indefinite self-renewal and randomly differentiate into early multipotential progenitor cells committed to either the myeloid or lymphoid subpopulations of hematopoietic precursors. The myeloid and lymphoid stem cells by way of multilateral proliferation and unilateral differentiation produce lineage-specific progenitors of erythroid, megakaryocytic, lymphoid and phagocytic cells.[8] Lineage-specific progenitors lose their capacity for self-renewal, and further differentiation is influenced by the hematopoietic growth factors.[8,22] It is not known precisely what initiates the early proliferation and random differentiation of pluripotent stem cells. Functionally mature cells, also present in the bone marrow, such as endothelial cells, fibroblasts, macrophages, T-lymphocytes and B-lymphocytes may have a role in regulation and support of stem cells.[2]

These functionally mature cells produce an array of cytokines and hematopoietic growth factors. Activated macrophages in response to injury or inflammation produce IL-1 and tumor necrosis factor (TNF) which further stimulate the production of IL-6 and the growth factors now known as granulocyte-macrophage colony-stimulating factor (GM-CSF) and granulocyte colony-stimulating factor (G-CSF).[22,23,24] These specific growth factors appear to support the proliferation and survival of lineage-specific progeny and do not induce stem cell differentiation.[22]

HEMATOPOIETIC GROWTH FACTORS

The colony-stimulating factors (CSFs) are a group of glycoproteins produced by T-lymphocytes, fibroblasts, endothelial cells and macrophages. Their primary action is the stimulation and growth of hematopoietic progenitor cells, promotion of cell viability and biological activity, and regulation of the terminal differentiation of precursor cells. Cell membrane receptors for one or multiple CSFs permit control of the cell-mediated response to infection and interaction of growth factors in directing the development of early and late precursors.[25] The colony-stimulating factors primarily responsible for phagocytic production are IL-3 (also known as multi-CSF), GM-CSF, G-CSF and macrophage colony-stimulating factor (M-CSF). Other cytokines such as IL-4, IL-5, IL-6, and erythropoietin acting synergistically with the above glycoproteins to stimulate increased production of functionally mature phagocytes and erythrocytes and to promote the proliferation of progenitor cells in normal hematopoiesis.[25,26] Not all CSFs act at the same stage of hematopoiesis. IL-3 and GM-CSF along with IL-4 and IL-6 are more important for the proliferation and differentiation of multipotential hematopoietic progenitors. Both G-CSF and M-CSF are late-acting lineage-specific growth factors responsible for stimulation of neutrophil and macrophage formation.[22,25] Interleukin-5, IL-3, and GM-CSF are responsible for the maturation of eosinophilic precursors and activation of mature eosinophils.[27]

ERYTHROPOIETIN

Erythropoietin (Epo) is a glycoprotein produced by the kidney in response to hypoxia and anemia. Epo is primarily responsible for the terminal differentiation and maturation of erythroid progenitors. These progenitors are in the later stages of maturation and respond to minute changes in Epo levels.[22] Recombinant technology has produced a readily available supply of Epo which has been used with impressive results in patients with chronic renal failure and intractable anemia.[93] Chronic dialysis patients treated with recombinant Epo demonstrated increased hemoglobin and hematocrit levels and lessened the need for regular transfusions.[94] Epo continues to be a valuable therapeutic tool in the treatment of anemia and renal failure.

INTERLEUKINS

Interleukin-1 (also known as hemopoietin-1) is a monokine produced by activated monocytes usually in combination with TNF in response to bacterial endotoxin (LPS). Acting alone, IL-1 has no proliferative action on hematopoietic precursors. However, in combination with other cytokines it becomes an important mediator of the hematopoietic response to injury or infection. Interkeukin-1 acting synergistically with IL-3 increases the proliferation and differentiation of pluripotential stem cells. In addition, IL-1 increases the production of hematopoietic growth factors such as GM-CSF and G-CSF from activated monocytes, macrophages, endothelial cells and fibroblasts.[28-32] (Table 1) Sieff et al showed an increase in GM-CSF and G-CSF mRNA from fibroblasts and human umbilical vein endothelial cells (HUVE) in response to IL-1 and TNF stimulation.[30,32] Silver et al demonstrated fewer positive blood cultures and significantly improved survival in a murine model of thermal injury sepsis when using recombinant human IL-1.[28] Fibroblasts stimulated with IL-1 produce IL-6 and G-CSF, and in combination with these, may play an important role in stimulating dormant stem cells to leave the G_0 resting phase and begin proliferation.[22]

Interleukin-3 supports multipotential progenitor cells in the earliest stages of hematopoietic development which are not yet responsive to GM-CSF or G-CSF.[33] Interleukin-3 is a single chain glycoprotein produced solely by activated T_4-helper lymphocytes.[25] Leary et al showed that IL-3 supported multilineage stem cells, granulocyte-macrophage, granulocyte, macrophage, erythroid, basophilic, eosinophilic and megakaryocyte colony formation.[35] Evidence exists that as cells become more differentiated they become less responsive to IL-3 stimulation. Lopez et al showed that G-CSF was much more effective in supporting granulocyte colony formation than was IL-3.[36] However, evidence also exists that when IL-3 is combined synergistically with growth factors GM-CSF, G-CSF and IL-6, there is a marked stimulation of hematopoiesis and greater increase of all myeloid lineages than when each growth factor is used alone. Using a murine model, Ogawa demonstrated a significantly shorter lag time for multipotential blast cell colony formation using IL-3 in combination with IL-6 and G-CSF compared to IL-3 alone.[22] Seiff et al using IL-3 with G-CSF yielded a higher frequency of granulocyte colony production than when using either growth factor individually.[37] In addition, significantly lower doses of both IL-3 and GM-CSF are needed when used synergistically

Inter-leukin (IL-1)	Alternative Name	Approx. Molecular Weight	Source	Target	Action
IL-1	—	15,000	antigen presenting cells	helper T-cells	helps activate
IL-2	T-cell growth factor	15,000	some helper T-cells	all activated T-cells	stimulates proliferation
IL-3	multi-CSF	25,000	some helper T-cells	various hemopoietic cells	stimulates proliferation
IL-4	B-cell stimulating factor (BSF-1)	20,000	some helper T-cells	B-cells, T-cells, masT-cells	helps activate and promotes proliferation; increases class II MHC molecules on B-cells
IL-5	B-cell growth factor-2 (BCGF-2)	50,000 (dimer)	some helper T-cellss that make IL-4	B-cells, eosinophils	promotes proliferation and maturation
IL-6	B-cell stimulating factor (BSF-2)	25,000	some helper T-cells and macrophages	activated B cells, T-cells	promotes B-cell maturation to Ig-secreting cells; helps activate T-cells
γ-interferon	—	25,000 (dimer)	some helper T-cells that make IL-2	B-cells, macrophages endothelial cells	induces class II MHC molecules and activates macrophages

(Used with permission: Alberts B, Bray D, Lewis J et al. Molecular Biology of The Cell. New York; Garland Publishing Inc., 1989.)

Table 1. Properties of some interleukins.

possibly demonstrating the ability of IL-3 to increase the population of early progenitors responsive to the later-acting more specific CSFs.[33] Similar results have been achieved using erythropoietin and M-CSF for erythroid and macrophage lineages.[38,39]

Gillio et al demonstrated the potential clinical benefit of IL-3 when used singly or in combination therapy with GM-CSF by accelerating recovery of absolute neutrophil and total white blood cell counts in cyclophosphamide-treated primates.[40] The before-mentioned theory of IL-3 increasing the number of early progenitors responsive to later-acting growth factors is substantiated by data from Yang and Clark.[41] Using IL-3 pretreatment in nonhuman primates (macaques) for seven days, they demonstrated a marked increase in white blood cell counts (50,000-60,000) for two weeks using subsequently administered low dose GM-CSF. Absolute numbers of multiple lineage groups were elevated including basophils, a cell not normally found to be elevated with GM-CSF treatment alone. Also noted was an increase in circulating reticulocytes and platelets.[41] These above-mentioned studies and many others not included here indicate the need for further research and clinical trials in human subjects.

Similar to IL-1, in vitro studies have shown IL-4 alone does not stimulate proliferation of hematopoietic precursors. However, no doubt exists as to the ability of IL-4 to augment the proliferative effects of other growth factors in certain progenitor cells.[25,42,43]

IL-4 used in combination with IL-6 and Epo stimulated a marked increase in erythroid colonies with numbers comparable to or greater than those produced with IL-3 and Epo.[42] Also, IL-4 has been shown to double IL-6 dependent granulocyte-macrophage (GM) colony formation as well as increasing colony size.[42] Peschel and others reported that IL-4 in combination with G-CSF also augmented the proliferation of GM progenitors in addition to multipotential and erythroid precursors when combined with Epo.[44]

Interleukin-5 is a late-acting growth factor produced by activated T-lymphocytes. The hematopoietic role of IL-5 is in the terminal differentiation of eosinophils. Ogawa showed proliferative effects of IL-3, GM-CSF and IL-5 on eosinophilic precursors. IL-3 and GM-CSF supported larger more immature eosinophil colonies compared to IL-5 supported cultures.[22] This data and the original work done by Sanderson et al confirmed IL-5 as a lineage-specific growth factor necessary for the proliferation of eosinophilic precursors and biological activity of mature cells.[22,45]

Interleukin-6 previously known as B-cell stimulatory factor enhances immunoglobulin secretion from B-lymphocytes.[33] Like many other cytokines, IL-6 is produced by T-cells, fibroblasts and macrophages and synergistically interacts with other growth factors in regulating progenitor cell growth and differentiation.[42] Rennick et al demonstrated that IL-6 increased GM colony formation when combined with G-CSF, IL-3 or IL-4. Their results also showed that progenitor cells responsive to IL-6 and G-CSF or IL-6 and IL-4 were more mature than progenitors sensitive to IL-6 and IL-3. IL-6 in combination with GM-CSF or M-CSF did not increase the proliferation of early progenitor cells.[42] Both Rennick[42] and Ikebuchi et al[46] increased megakaryocyte and erythroid cell colonies using IL-6 together with IL-3 or IL-4. In addition, IL-6 along with IL-4 and Epo can effectively control erythrocyte development without the influence of IL-3 or GM-CSF.[42] IL-6, therefore, acts with multiple other growth factors at different stages of hematopoiesis to augment the proliferation of primitive stem cells as well as lineage-specific precursors.

GRANULOCYTE-MACROPHAGE COLONY-STIMULATING FACTOR

Granulocyte-macrophage colony-stimulating factor (GM-CSF) is a glycoprotein produced by activated T-lymphocytes, endothelial cells, macrophages and fibroblasts in response to antigen stimulation and/or the synthesis of TNF and IL-1.[25,65,80,81] (Table 2)

GM-CSF stimulates the proliferation of all myeloid progenitors especially the granulocyte, monocyte/macrophage and eosinophil lineages.[81-83] High-affinity GM-CSF receptors have been identified in small numbers on myeloid cell membranes and have also been demonstrated on small cell carcinoma, myeloid leukemia cells and on neural crest cells.[84,91] In addition, GM-CSF may act with other cytokines in the production of megakaryocytes and erythroid progenitors. Donahue et al using GM-CSF with delayed addition of erythropoietin enhanced production of erythroid precursors.[85]

GM-CSF enhancement of biological activity in mature neutrophils, monocytes/macrophages and eosinophils includes improved chemotaxis and phagocytosis, neutrophil oxidative metabolism, antibody-dependent, cell-mediated cytotoxicity (ADCC), arachidonic acid production and increased macrophage tumoricidal capabilities.[86-90] Monocyte production of IL-1 and TNF are also increased in response to GM-CSF stimulation.[86] This global augmentation of biological activity undoubtedly plays a pivotal role in host response to inflammation and infection.

GRANULOCYTE COLONY-STIMULATING FACTOR

Granulocyte colony-stimulating factor is a lineage-specific late-acting mediator of hematopoietic response. In vivo and in vitro studies show that human G-CSF stimulates the production of mature neutrophilic granulocytes from committed hematopoietic precursors in both humans and mice. G-CSF is responsible for the proliferation, differentiation and activity of mature neutrophils.[59] Human recombinant G-CSF (rhG-CSF) is now produced in large quantities and available for use in clinical trials in the immunosuppressed or traumatized patient.

Producers of G-CSF include monocytes, fibroblasts, endothelial cells, and neutrophils.[65-67] High affinity receptors for G-CSF have also been found on myeloid leukemia cell and small cell carcinoma cell lines.[59] Stimulators for production of G-CSF in vitro include IL-1,[67] endotoxin (LPS),[68] TNF-alpha,[69] γ-interferon[70] and GM-CSF.[61]

Enhancement of mature neutrophilic function is the major role of G-CSF. G-CSF has been shown to augment function by promoting chemotaxis,[60] by greatly increasing antibody-dependent cell-mediated cytotoxicity (ADCC)[62,63] and by stimulating superoxide production in response to the chemoattractant *f*-Met-Leu-Phe (f-MLP).[59,64] Also, Avalos et al reported rhG-CSF increased arachidonic acid production from neutrophils.[59]

Clinical trials with G-CSF and rhG-CSF have included patients with transitional cell carcinoma,[73] idiopathic neutropenia,[71] cyclic neutropenia[72] and the neutropenia associated with hairy cell leukemia.[75] Patients treated

with rhG-CSF following chemotherapy for transitional cell carcinoma demonstrated significantly shorter periods of neutropenia and required fewer days of antibiotic coverage.[73] Small cell lung cancer patients receiving chemotherapy had fewer infectious episodes when treated with rhG-CSF.[76] G-CSF improved survival in neutropenic mice infected with *Escherichia coli*, *Serratia marcescens*, *Staphylococcus aureus*, *Pseudomonas aeruginosa* and *Candida albicans*.[74,77,78]

MONOCYTE COLONY-STIMULATING FACTOR

Monocyte colony-stimulating factor (M-CSF or CSF-1) is a cytokine produced by macrophages, fibroblasts and endothelial cells and is responsible for the proliferation and differentiation of macrophage precursors as well as the viability of mature mononuclear phagocytes.[25,48,49,50] Bone marrow stromal cells as well as mature macrophages and monocytes produce M-CSF when stimulated by other cytokines such as IL-1, IL-3 and GM-CSF.[52,65] γ-Interferon and TNF-α also stimulate M-CSF production during an inflammatory response.[50,51] These growth factors may in-

Factor	Size (in mouse)	Target Cells	Producing Cells
Erythropoietin	51,000 daltons	CFC-E	kidney cells
Interleukin-3 (IL-3)	25,000 daltons	pluripotent stem cell most progenitor cells, many terminally differentiated cells	T lymphocytes, epidermal cells
Granulocyte/ macrophage CSF (GM-CSF)	23,000 daltons	GM progenitor cells	T lymphocytes, endothelial cells, fibroblasts
Granulocyte CSF (G-CSF)	25,000 daltons	GM progenitor cells and neutrophils	macrophages, fibroblasts
Macrophage CSF (M-CSF)	70,000 daltons (dimer)	GM progenitor cells and macrophages	fibroblasts, fibroblasts endothelial cells

(Used with permission: Alberts B, Bray D, Lewis J et al. Molecular Biology of The Cell. New York: Garland Publishing Inc. 1989.)

Table 2. Some colony-stimulating factors (CSFs) that influence blood cell formation.

crease the number of M-CSF receptors on early progenitor cells thereby increasing the number of cells destined for the mononuclear lineage.[50] The control of genetic and receptor expression is beyond the scope of this text. However, evidence exists in a murine model that the mononuclear cells themselves may regulate the amount of growth factor present in serum at any one time. Hence, they control their numbers via a feedback mechanism to the bone marrow progenitor cells.[50,53]

Functional control of mature monocytes by M-CSF includes promoting chemotaxis,[54] enhancement of phagocytic activity, increased cell size and cytoplasmic vacuolization, tumor cell cytolysis and increased production of peroxide and superoxide anions.[50,55,56] In addition, Lee et al demonstrated increased resistance to viral infection in murine macrophages with M-CSF.[57] In contrast, M-CSF along with GM-CSF may augment viral replication of the human immunodeficiency virus (HIV) in mononuclear cells and in a clinical setting could be detrimental to AIDS patients as a hematopoietic modifier.[58] Whether acting directly or indirectly with other cytokines, M-CSF is an important mediator of white blood cell and macrophage response to inflammation and infection and warrants further exploration of its therapeutic potential.

THERAPEUTIC POTENTIAL OF CSFs

Clinical trials have demonstrated the therapeutic potential of the colony-stimulating factors. GM-CSF, G-CSF and other CSFs used in vitro and in vivo have shown that it is possible to augment the host response to disease, inflammation, infection or trauma. Thermal injury or mechanical trauma can lead to an immunosuppressed state and an increased risk of septic complication and mortality. Myeloid growth factors may provide a way to up-regulate the host defense system by expanding the number of host response cells while also improving their biological activity.

The immunomodulating effects of the hematopoietic growth factors are the subject of intense research. Antin et al, using rhGM-CSF, treated patients with aplastic anemia and myelodysplastic syndrome and demonstrated temporary augmentation of granulocyte, monocyte and reticulocyte counts.[92] In this trial, rhGM-CSF proved more effective in treating patients with myelodysplastic syndrome, perhaps due to a greater number of stem cells and progenitors in the myelodysplastic marrow.[92] The colony-stimulating factors have proven useful in treating chemotherapy-induced neutropenia by allowing higher doses and more frequent cycling of antineoplastic agents. O'Reilly and Gamelli reported improved hematopoietic recovery following 5-FU administration in a murine model.[100] Mice treated with recombinant murine GM-CSF (rmGM-CSF) 24 and 36 hours after receiving 5-FU have increased total white blood cell, granulocyte and monocyte counts at seven days when compared to controls (5-FU only). Gabrilove et al treated 27 patients with transitional cell carcinoma using rhG-CSF before or after chemotherapy.[95] The authors showed a dose-dependent increase in absolute neutrophil counts with a shorter period of chemotherapy-induced neutropenia. In addition, rhG-CSF significantly reduced the need for antibiotic coverage and allowed a greater number of patients to receive planned chemotherapy on schedule. The incidence and severity of mucositis was also reduced.[95]

Additional forms of neutropenia may benefit from CSF administration. Furukawa and others using rhG-CSF successfully treated a patient with chronic idiopathic neutropenia previously unresponsive to prednisolone and oxymethalone.[96] Similarly, Vadhan-Raj increased absolute eosinophil and monocyte counts in a patient with congenital neutropenia treated with rhGM-CSF. An increase in neutrophils was not seen and was attributed to an intrinsic defect in neutrophil maturation, as rhGM-CSF in other studies has produced a marked increase in all myeloid lineages.[97]

There is evidence to support the use of CSFs in treating the immunosuppression associated with bone marrow transplantation. Brandt et al reported using rhGM-CSF to treat 19 patients with breast cancer or melanoma undergoing autologous bone marrow transplantation following high-dose chemotherapy.[98] Patients receiving a 14-day continuous infusion of rhGM-CSF demonstrated a significantly shorter period of neutropenia compared to controls. No major toxic effects were noted.[98] Furthermore, CSFs may provide a desperately needed adjunct in the treatment of acquired immunodeficiency syndrome (AIDS) by increasing the number and biological activity of host defense cells. rhGM-CSF administration to neutropenic patients with AIDS revealed dose-dependent increases in circulating neutrophil, monocyte and eosinophil counts.[99]

Another application for which the CSFs may prove to be of benefit is in the augmentation of immune response following major thermal injury or severe mechanical trauma. Our laboratory has published multiple studies using GM-CSF and G-CSF in an effort to up-regulate the host response to infection and trauma.

The clinical use of the CSFs in humans has resulted in only mild side effects. The most frequent side effects encompass a viral-type syndrome producing low grade fevers, myalgias, headaches and chills. Bone pain involving the hips, sternum and lower back is a frequent occurrence.[81] Devereux et al described a reproducible transient leukopenia within 30 minutes following GM-CSF administration with spontaneous recovery within one hour.[101] Higher doses have resulted in pleural and pericardial effusions and generalized edema.[102] Jaiyesimi et al recently reported a single case of acute anaphylaxis with G-CSF.[103] These side effects have been reversible with the discontinuation of the drug.

As mentioned previously, sepsis remains the major cause of mortality in the severe thermally injured patient. Sartorelli et al in a murine model of *Pseudomonas* burn wound sepsis demonstrated a significant increase in neutrophil counts and improved chemotaxis in burn/infected animals treated with G-CSF.[60] Similarly, Mooney and others using the same model of burn wound sepsis and G-CSF reported increased mean survival times and a significantly enhanced myelopoietic response when compared to nontreated animals. An increase in the total white blood cell and

neutrophil counts, and preservation of granulocyte-macrophage progenitor cells were felt to be the events responsible for the improved outcome in treated animals.[19]

Combining the effect of G-CSF with routine antimicrobial therapy may be the next advancement in treating the immunosuppressed trauma patient. Silver et al combined the G-CSF-induced improvement in neutrophil biological activity with gentamicin in treating burn/infected mice. They found that either treatment modality when used alone increased survival over nontreated groups but when used in combination (G-CSF + gentamicin) demonstrated an additive effect and significantly improved survival as compared to all groups.[73] In splenectomized mice rendered more susceptible to encapsulated organisms, rhG-CSF was given prior to a challenge with a *Streptococcal pneumonia* aerosol. rhG-CSF treated mice clearly demonstrated an improved survival likely due to enhanced alveolar neutrophil and macrophage clearance of *pneumococci*.[83] It is hoped that this finding will be substantiated in clinical trials examining rhG-CSF's ability to decrease the incidence of nosocomial pneumonia.

Summary

The hematopoietic growth factors are a group of glycoproteins responsible for stem cell renewal, proliferation and differentiation of bone marrow progenitor cells, and the terminal differentiation and biological activity of mature granulocytes and lymphocytes. Numerous clinical studies have already confirmed their beneficial role in the treatment of various forms of neutropenia, aplastic anemia, myelodysplastic syndrome, chronic renal failure and the immunosuppression surrounding chemotherapy, radiotherapy and bone marrow transplantation. Potentially, the colony-stimulating factors may have utility in the treatment of immunosuppression following thermal injury or severe mechanical trauma by enhancing the biological activity of mature phagocytic cells and stimulating the proliferation and differentiation of lineage-nonspecific and lineage-specific precursors.

REFERENCES

1. Polk HC, George CD, Wellhausen SR et al. A systematic study of host defense processes in badly injured patients. Ann Surg 1986; 204: 282, 1986.
2. Meakins JL, McLean APH, Kelly R et al. Delayed hypersensitivity and neutrophil chemotaxis: Effect of trauma. J Trauma 1978; 18: 240.
3. O'Mahony JB, Palder SB, Wood J et al. Depression of cellular immunity after multiple trauma in the absence of sepsis. J Trauma 1984; 24: 869
4. Wang BS, Heacock EH, Wu WV et al. Generation of suppressor cells in mice after surgical trauma. J Clin Invest 1980; 66: 200.
5. Baker CC, Oppenheimer L, Stephens B et al. Epidemiology of trauma deaths. Am J Surg 1980; 140: 144.
6. Polk HC. Concensus summary on infection. J Trauma 1979; 19: 894.
7. Grogan JB, Miller RC. Impaired function of polymorphonuclear leukocytes in patients with burns and other trauma. Surg Gynecol Obstet 1973; 137: 784.
8. Nathan DG. Regulation of hematopoiesis. Pediatr Res 1990; 27: 423.
9. Gabrilove J, Jahnbowski A, Fain K et al. A phase I/II study of rhG-CSF in cancer patients at risk for chemotherapy-induced neutropenia. Blood 1987; 70(suppl 1): 135a.
10. Mooney DP, Gamelli RL. Sepsis following thermal injury. Compr Therap 1989; 15: 22.
11. Davis JM, Dineen P, Gallin JI. Neutrophil degranulation and abnormal chemotaxis after thermal injury. J Immunol 1980; 124: 1467.
12. Miller CL, Fink M, Wu JY, Szabo G et al. Mechanisms of altered monocyte prostaglandin E_2 production in severely injured patients. Arch Surg 1988; 123: 293.
13. Peterson V, Hansbrough J, Buerk C et al. Regulation of granulopoiesis following severe thermal injury. J Trauma 1983; 23: 19.
14. Luger A, Graf H, Schwarz H et al. Decreased serum interleukin-1 activity and monocyte interleukin-1 production in patients with fatal sepsis. Crit Care Med 1986; 14: 458.
15. Ninnemann JL, Stockland AE. Participation of Prostaglandin E in immunosuppression following thermal injury. J Trauma 1984; 24: 201.
16. Faist E, Mewes A, Baker CC et al. Prostaglandin E_2 (PGE$_2$)-dependent suppression of interleukin (IL-2) production in patients with major trauma. J Trauma 1987; 27: 837.
17. Faist E, Mewes A, Strasser T et al. Alteration of monocyte function following major injury. Arch Surg 1988; 123: 287.
18. Unanue ER, Beller DI, CY L et al. Antigen presentation:Comments on its regulation and mechanism. J Immunol 1984; 132: 1.
19. Mooney DP, Gamelli RL, O'Reilly M, Hebert J. Recombinant human granulocyte colony-stimulating factor and pseudomonas burn wound sepsis. Arch Surg 1988; 123: 1353
20. Howard RJ. Effect of burn injury, mechanical trauma, and operation on immune defenses. Surg Clin N Am 1979; 59: 199.
21. Miller SE, Miller CL, Trunkey DD. The immune consequences of trauma. Surg Clin N Am 1982; 62: 167.
22. Ogawa M. Effects of hematopoietic growth factors on stem cells in vitro. Hematol Onc Clin North Am 1989; 3: 453.
23. Clark SC, Kamen R. The human hematopoietic colony-stimulating factors. Science 1987; 236: 1229.
24. Broudy VC, Kaushansky K, Harlan JM et al. Interleukin-1 stimulates human endothelial cells to produce granulocyte-macrophage colony-stimulating factor and granulocyte colony-stimulating factor. J Immunol 1987; 139: 464.
25. Gregory SH, Magee DM, Wing EJ. The role of colony-stimulating factors in host defenses. Proc Soc Exp Biol Med 1991; 197:349.
26. Wing EJ, Shadduck RK. Colony-stimulating factor. In: Torrence PF, ed. Biological Response Modifiers: New approaches to disease intervention. New York: Academic Press, 1985: 219-243.
27. Nakayama N, Hatake K, Miyajima A et al. Colony-stimulating factors, cytokines, and hemopoiesis. Curr Opin Immunol 1989; 2: 68.
28. Silver GM, Gamelli RL, O'Reilly M, Hebert J. The effect of interleukin 1α on survival in a murine model of burn wound sepsis. Arch Surg 1990; 125: 922.
29. Zsebo KM, Yuschenkoff VN, Schiffer S et al. Vascular endothelial cells and granulopoiesis: interleukin-1 stimulates release of G-CSF and GM-CSF. Blood 1988; 71: 99.
30. Sieff CA, Tsai S, Faller DV. Interleukin 1 induces cultured human endothelial cell production of granulocyte-macrophage colony-stimulating factor. J Clin Invest 1987; 79: 45.
31. Zucali JR, Dinarello CA, Oblon DJ, Gross M et al. Interleukin 1 stimulates fibroblasts to produce granulocyte-macrophage colony-stimulating activity and prostaglandin E_2. J Clin Invest 1987; 77: 1857.
32. Sieff CA, Niemeyer CM, Mentzer SJ, Faller DV. Interleukin-1, tumor necrosis factor, and the production of colony-stimulating factors by cultured mesenchymal cells. Blood 1988; 72: 1316, 1988.
33. Garnick MB, O'Rielly RJ. Clinical promise of new hematopoietic growth factors: M-CSF, IL-3, IL-6. Hem Onc Clin North Am 1989; 3: 495.
34. Koike K, Ihle JN, Ogawa M. Declining sensitivity to interleukin-3 of murine multipotential hemopoietic progenitors during their development: application to a culture system that favors blast cell colony formation. J Clin Invest 1986; 77: 894.
35. Leary AG, Yang YC, Clark SC et al. Recombinant gibbon interleukin-3 supports formation of human multilineage colonies and blast cell colonies in the culture: comparison with human granulocyte-

macrophage colony-stimulating factor. Blood 1987; 70: 1343.

36. Lopez AF, Dyson PG, To MJ et al. Recombinant human interleukin 3 stimulation of hematopoiesis in humans: loss of responsiveness with differentiation in the neutrophilic myeloid series. Blood 1988; 72: 1797.

37. Sieff CA, Niemeyer CM, Nathan DG et al. Stimulation of human hematopoietic colony formation by recombinant gibbon multi-colony stimulating factor or interleukin-3. J Clin Invest 1987; 80:818.

38. Sonoda Y, Yang YC, Wong GG et al. Erythroid burst-promoting activity of purified recombinant human GM-CSF and interleukin-3: studies with anti-GM-CSF and anti-IL-3 sera and studies in serum-free culture. Blood 1988; 72: 1381.

39. Zhou BYQ, Stanley ER, Clark SC et al. Interleukin-3 and interleukin-1α allow earlier bone marrow progenitors to respond to human colony-stimulating factor 1. Blood 1988; 72: 1870.

40. Gillio AP, Laver J, Abbout M et al. IL-3 prevents neutropenia following 5-fluorouracil and cyclophosphamide induced myelosuppression in cynomolgus primates. Blood 1988; 72: 117a.

41. Yang YC, Clark SC. Interleukin-3: molecular biology and biologic activities. Hematol Onc Clin North Am 1989; 3: 441.

42. Rennick D, Jackson J, Yang G, Wideman J et al. Interleukin-6 interacts with interleukin-4 and other hematopoietic growth factors to selectively enhance the growth of megakaryocytic, erythroid, myeloid, and multipotential progenitor cells. Blood 1989; 73: 1828.

43. Rennick D, Yang G, Muller-Sieburg C, Smith C et al. Interleukin 4 (B-cell stimulatory factor 1) can enhance or antagonize the factor-dependent growth of hemopoietic progenitor cells. Proc Natl Acad Sci USA 1987; 84: 6889.

44. Peschel C, Paul WE, Ohara J, Grren I. Effects of B cell stimulatory factor-1/interleukin 4 on hematopoietic progenitor cells. Blood 1987; 70: 254.

45. Sanderson CJ, Warren DJ, Strath M. Identification of a lymphokine that stimulates eosinophil differentiation in vitro. Its relationship to interleukin-3 and functional properties or eosinophils produced in culture. J Exp Med 1985; 162: 60.

46. Ikebuchi K, Wong GG, Clark SC et al. Interleukin-6 enhancement of interleukin-3 dependent proliferation of multipotential hemopoietic progenitors. Proc Natl Acad Sci USA 1987; 84: 9035.

47. Gamelli RL, Hebert JC, Foster RS. Effect of burn injury on granulocyte and macrophage production. J Trauma 1985; 25: 615.

48. Stanley ER, Guilbert LJ, Tushinski RJ et al. CSF-1—A mononuclear phagocyte lineage-specific hemopoietic growth factor. J Cell Biochem 1983; 21: 151.

49. Sieff CA. Hemopoietic growth facotrs. J Clin Invest 1987; 79: 1549.

50. Rettenmier CW, Sherr CJ. The mononuclear phagocyte colony-stimulating factor (CSF-1, M-CSF). Hematol Onc Clin North Am 1989; 3: 479.

51. Seelentag WK, Mermod JJ, Montesano R et al. Additive effects of interleukin 1 and tumor necrosis factor-alpha on the accumulation of the three granulocyte and macrophage colony-stimulating factor mRNAs in human endothelial cells. EMBO J 1987; 6: 2261.

52. Fibbe WE, van Damme J, Billiau A et al. Interleukin 1 induces human marrow stromal cells in long-term culture to produce granulocyte colony-stimulating factor and macrophage colony-stimulating factor. Blood 1988; 71: 430.

53. Bartocci A, Mastrogiannis DS, Migliorati G et al. Macrophages specifically regulate the concentration of their own growth factor in the circulation. Proc Natl Acad Sci USA 1987; 84: 6179.

54. Wang JM, Griffin JD, Rambaldi A et al. Induction of monocyte migration by recombinant macrophage colony-stimulating factor. J Immunol 1988; 141: 575.

55. Ampel NM, Wing EJ, Wahhed A, Shadduck RS. Stimulatory effects of purified macrophage colony-stimulating factor on murine resident peritoneal macrophages. Cell Immunol 1986; 97: 344.

56. Wing EJ, Ampel NM, Waheed A, Shadduck RS. Macrophage colony-stimulating factor (M-CSF) enhances the capacity of murine macrophages to secrete oxygen reduction products. J Immunol 1985; 135: 2052.

57. Lee MT, Warren MK. CSF-1-induced resistance to viral infection in murine macrophages. J Immunol 1987; 138: 3019.

58. Gendelman H, Orenstein JM, Martin MA et al. Efficient isolation and propagation of human immunodeficiency virus on recombinant colony-stimulating factor 1-treated monocytes. J Exp Med 1988; 167: 1428.

59. Avalos BR, Gasson JC, Hedvat C, Quan S et al. Human granulocyte colony-stimulating factor: biologic activities and receptor characterization on hematopoietic cells and small cell lung cancer cell lines. Blood 1990; 75: 851.

60. Sartorelli KH, Silver GM, Gamelli RL. The effect of granulocyte colony-stimulating (G-CSF) upon burn-induced defective neutrophil chemotaxis. J Trauma 1991; 31: 523.

61. Gabrilove JL, Jakubowski AJ. Granulocyte colony-stimulating factor: preclinical and clinical studies. Hematol Onc Clin North Am 1989; 3: 427.

62. Vadas MA, Nicola NA, Metcalf D. Activation of antibody-dependent cell-mediated cytotoxicity of human neutrophils and eosinophils by separate colony-stimulating factors. J Immunol 1983; 130: 795.

63. Lopez AF, Nicola NA, Burgess AW, Metcalf D et al. Activation of granulocyte cytotoxic function by purified mouse colony-stimulating factors. J Immunol 1983; 131: 2983.

64. Yuo A, Kitagawa S, Okabe T, Urabe A et al. Recombinant human granulocyte colony-stimulating

factor repairs the abnormalities of neutrophils in patients with myelodysplastic syndrome and chronic myelogenous leukemia. Blood 1987; 70: 404.

65. Ernst TJ, Griffin JD. Regulation of colony-stimulating factor production by normal and leukemic human cells. Immunol Res 1989; 8: 202.

66. Seelentag WK, Mermod JJ, Vassalli P. Interleukin-1 and tumor necrosis factor-alpha additively increase the levels of granulocyte-macrophage and granulocyte colony-stimulating factor (CSF) mRNA in human fibroblasts. Eur J Immunol 1989; 19: 209.

67. Lindemann A, Oster W, Riedel D et al. GM-CSF induces secretion of 'monokines' by human polymorphonuclear neutrophils. Blood 1987; 70(Suppl): 223.

68. Moore MAS, Gabrilove JL, Sheridan AP. Therapeutic implications of serum factors inhibiting proliferation and inducing differentiation of myeloid leukemic cells. Blood Cells 1983; 9: 125.

69. Munker R, Gasson J, Ogawa M et al. Recombinant human tumor necrosis factor induces production of granulocyte-macrophage colony stimulating factor. Nature 1986; 323:79.

70. Herrmann F, Cannistra SA, Griffin JD. T cell monocyte interactions in the production of humoral factors regulating human granulopoiesis in vitro. J Immunol 1986; 136: 2856.

71. Jakubowski AA, Souza L, Kelly F, Fain K et al. Effects of human granulocyte colony-stimulating factor in a patient with idiopathic neutropenia. N Engl J Med 1989; 320: 37.

72. Hammond WP IV, Price TH, Souza LM, Dale DC. Treatment of cyclic neutropenia with granulocyte colony-stimulating factor. N Engl J Med 1989; 320: 1306..

73. Silver GM, Gamelli RL, O'Reilly M. The beneficial effect of granulocyte colony-stimulating factor (G-CSF) in combination with gentamicin on survival after pseudomonas burn wound infection. Surgery 1989; 106: 452.

74. Matsumoto M, Matsubara S, Matsuno T et al. Protective effect of human granulocyte colony-stimulating factor on microbial infection in neutropenic mice. Infec Immun 1987; 55: 2715.

75. Glaspy JA, Baldwin GC, Robertson PA, Souza I et al. Therapy for neutropenia in hairy cell leukemia with recombinant human granulocyte colony-stimulating factor. Ann Int Med 1988; 109: 789.

76. Brochund MH, Scarffe JH, Thatcher N et al. Phase I/II study of recombinant human granulocyte colony-stimulating factor in patients receiving intensive chemotherapy for small cell lung cancer. Br J Cancer 1987; 56: 809.

77. Cohen AM, Hines DK, Korach ES, Ratzkin BJ. In vivo activation of neutrophil function in hamsters by recombinant human granulocyte colony-stimulating factor. Infect Immun 1988; 56: 2861.

78. Kobayashi Y, Okabe T, Uzumaki H et al. Differentiation therapy of myelodysplastic syndrome by granulocyte colony-stimulating factor. Clin Res 1988; 36: 412A.

79. Wang JM, Chen ZG, Colella S, Bonilla MA et al. Chemotactic activity of recombinant human granulocyte colony-stimulating factor. Blood 1988; 72: 1456.

80. Keslo A, Metcalf D, Gough NM. Independent regulation of granulocyte-macrophage colony-stimulating factor and multi-lineage colony-stimulating factor production in T-lymphocyte clones. J Immunol 1986; 136: 1718.

81. Mitsuyasu RT, Golde DW. Clinical role of granulocyte-macrophage colony-stimulating factor. Hematol Onc Clin N Am 1989; 3: 411..

82. Golde DW, Gasson JC. Hormones that regulate blood cell production. Scientific American 1988; 259: 62.

83. Hebert JC, O'Reilly M, Gamelli RL. Protective effect of recombinant granulocyte colony-stimulating factor against pneumococcal infections in splenectomized mice. Arch Surg 1990; 125: 1075.

84. Baldwin GC, Gasson JC, Kaufman SE, Quan SG et al. Nonhematopoietic tumor cells express functional GM-CSF receptors. Blood 1989; 73: 1033.

85. Donahue RE, Emerson SG, Wang EA, Wong GG et al. Demonstration of burst-promoting activity of recombinant human GM-CSF on circulating erythroid progenitors using an assay involving the delayed addition of erythropoietin. Blood 1985; 66: 1479.

86. Weisbart RH, Golde DW. GM-CSF/G-CSF physiology. Hematol Oncol Clin N Am 1989; 3: 369.

87. Weisbart RH, Golde DW, Gasson JC. Biosynthetic human GM-CSF modulates the number and affinity of neutrophil f-Met-Leu-Phe receptors. J Immunol 1986; 137: 3584.

88. Fleischmann J, Golde DW, Weisbart RH, Gasson JC. Granulocyte-macrophage colony-stimulating factor enhances phagocytosis of bacteria by human neutrophils. Blood 1986; 68: 708.

89. Lopez AF, Williamson J, Gamble JR, Begley CG et al. Recombinant human granulocyte-macrophage colony-stimulating factor stimulates in vitro mature human neutrophil and eosinophil function, surface receptor expression, and survival. J Clin Invest 1986; 78: 1220.

90. Weisbart RH, Golde DW, Clark SC et al. Human granulocyte-macrophage colony-stimulating factor is a neutrophil activator. Nature 1985; 314: 361.

91. Dipersio J, Billing P, Kaufman S, Egtesady P et al. Characterization of the human granulocyte-macrophage colony-stimulating factor. J Biol Chem 1988; 263: 1834.

92. Antin JH, Smith BR, Holmes W, Rosenthal DS. Phase I/II study of recombinant human granulocyte-macrophage colony-stimulating factor in aplastic anemia and myelodysplastic syndrome. Blood 1988; 72: 705.

93. Eschbach JW, Egrie JC, Downing MR et al. Correction of the anemia of end-stage renal disease with recombinant human erythropoietin. N Engl J Med 1987; 316: 73, 1987.

94. Johnson GR. Erythropoietin. Brit Med Bull 1989;

45: 506.

95. Gabrilove JL, Jakubowski A, Scher H, Sternberg C et al. Effect of granulocyte colony-stimulating factor on neutropenia and associated morbidity due to chemotherapy for transitional-cell carcinoma of the urothelium. N Engl J Med 1988; 318: 1414.

96. Furukawa T, Takahashi M, Moriyama Y et al. Successful treatment of chronic idiopathic neutropenia using recombinant granulocyte colony-stimulating factor. Ann Hematol 1991; 62: 22.

97. Vadhan-Raj S, Jeha SS, Buescher S et al. Stimulation of myelopoiesis in a patient with congenital neutropenia: biology and nature of response to recombinant human granulocyte-macrophage colony-stimulating factor. Blood 1990; 75: 858.

98. Brandt SJ, Peters WP, Atwater SK et al. Effect of recombinant human granulocyte-macrophage colony-stimulating factor on hematopoietic reconstitution after high-dose chemotherapy and autologous bone marrow transplantation. N Engl J Med 1988; 14: 869.

99. Groopman JE, Mitsuyasu RT, DeLeo MJ et al. Effect of recombinant human granulocyte-macrophage colony-stimulating factor on myelopoiesis in the aquired immunodeficiency syndrome. N Engl J Med 1987; 317: 593.

100. O'Reilly M, Gamelli RL. Recombinant granulocyte-macrophage colony-stimulating factor inproves hematopoietic recovery after 5-fluorouracil. J Surg Res 1988; 45: 104.

101. Devereux S, Linch DC, Campos Costa D et al. Transient leukopenia induced by granulocyte-macrophage colony-stimulating factor. Lancet 1987; 1: 1523.

102. Antman KS, Griffin JD, Elias A et al. Effect of recombinant human granulocyte-macrophage colony-stimulating factor on chemotherapy-induced myelosuppression. N Engl J Med 1988; 319: 593.

103. Jaiyesimi I, Giralt SS, Wood J. Subcutaneous granulocyte colony-stimulating factor and acute anaphylaxis. N Engl J Med 1991; 325: 587.

CHAPTER 25

ISSUES IN GERIATRIC TRAUMA

David J. Dries
Richard L. Gamelli

INTRODUCTION

Effective management of trauma patients includes the care of elderly persons. The progressive aging of American society carries with it the prospect that the injured elderly will be an expanding focus of trauma care in subsequent years. The geriatric population, in addition to increasing in number and longevity, are more active than in past generations. Normally, elderly persons find themselves in living situations that increase the likelihood of injury. Despite an increasing incidence of cancer and cardiovascular disease with aging, trauma remains a leading cause of death in the geriatric population. Susceptibility to injury in the elderly is in part a consequence of chronic disease or medication which may impair perception, reaction time, coordination and judgement.

Blunt injury is common in the elderly. Falls and motor vehicle trauma represent two leading causes of injury in the elderly and vehicular trauma is associated with age related increase in fatality rate. Death after falls predominates in the elderly, often secondary to complications related to previous medical status. In the elderly, ability of the body to absorb injury forces is reduced. Changes in the bony skeleton increase the likelihood of a given event, such as a fall, causing a fracture. Alteration in elasticity and plasticity of the chest wall may lead to a higher probability of rib fractures and injury to underlying thoracic and abdominal organs.

Recognition that physiologic reserve is age-dependent is essential to effective management of the elderly trauma victim. The geriatric patient is less tolerant of hemorrhage and requires early intervention to avoid even brief periods of hypoperfusion which may cause late complications. Elderly patients are often less capable of handling large volumes of resuscitation fluid and rapid volume shifts. Management of skeletal injury in the elderly is complicated by pre-existing medical problems, particularly cardiopulmonary insufficiency.

Thermal injuries highlight the difference in tolerance to injury among the elderly. While a patient in the second decade of life with a moderate size body surface area burn should invariably survive injury, a 70-year-old burn victim may not manifest the hyperdynamic physiologic response that is a consequence of injury and fail to tolerate this insult. Finally, a (real) problem is that the elderly suffer abuse and neglect. While this problem has been widely recognized in the pediatric age group, it is clear that abuse is becoming a common problem presenting in the geriatric population as well. Ongoing neglect may be manifest as nutritional deficiencies and often complicated by chronic alcoholism.

Pattern of Injury

Among elderly persons, falls, vehicular trauma, and burns are the most common forms of injury. Among patients aged 65 to 74 years, one-third of injury-related deaths are due to vehicular trauma and one-fourth are related to falls. In individuals greater than 75 years of age, more than 50% of trauma is due to falls and 20% is related to motor vehicle use.

Vehicular trauma causes 18% to 36% of injury-related deaths in the elderly. As noted in the recent review by Schwab and Kauder, in 1983 there were 13.3 million licensed drivers over the age of 65. This represents approximately 9.3% of all U.S. drivers. As the elderly population increases, this number is expected to rise. Older drivers frequently do not drive as well as their younger counterparts and have a correspondingly higher collision rate. This exceeds all groups except those under 25 years.

Unlike younger drivers, the elderly experience motor vehicle collisions in good weather, during daytime, and close to home. The majority of incidents are not related to high speed or alcohol but rather to errors in perception and judgement or to delayed reaction time. The effect of chronic medical conditions on vehicular trauma in the elderly is unclear, but drivers suffering from diabetes, seizure disorders, alcoholism and cardiovascular disease appear to have higher crash rates than those without these impairments.

Elderly pedestrians also account for a significant portion of the injury-related motor vehicle deaths. In 1985, patients over the age of 65 had the highest pedestrian fatality rate of any group studied and contributed over 20% to all pedestrian deaths due to trauma. Elderly patients involved in pedestrian incidents are often injured in crosswalks (while the young are typically involved in less predictable behaviors). People over the age of 60 experience a forward shift in the body center of gravity due to kyphosis and muscular skeletal changes. Changes in gait and stance contribute to a slower pace. These individuals are less likely to monitor traffic flow and traffic signals effectively. They also have alterations in gait and a slower pace contributing to difficulty with walking at the rate required to clear crosswalks before traffic signals change.

Falls comprise 50% to 70% of unintentional deaths among the elderly. One-third of elderly persons have at least one fall per year. Most of these falls do not result in significant injury, though one in 40 requires hospitalization. Fractures are common, often of the femur, forearm and hip. The elderly who fall do so during normal activities of living. They are susceptible to falling due to affects of aging and interaction with environmental hazards. Gait is wider-based in the old than in the young. Strength, coordination and ability to maintain balance decrease with age, thus impairing the ability to avoid a fall after tripping. Poor vision, impaired hearing and memory loss may also increase the risk of falling due to failure to recognize environmental hazards. Syncope is also implicated in falls. Decreased cerebral blood flow may be related to cardiac dysrhythmia, autonomic insufficiency, venous pooling, metabolic derangement or medications. Inciting incidents must be evaluated in these patients. Frequently, complications of coexisting medical problems and therapy may be related to neurologic, cardiovascular and metabolic instability.

The elderly also suffer a disproportionately high rate of burn injury. Older people sustain larger and deeper burns than the young, and their mortality rate is inordinately high. Scalds are most common, usually associated with prolonged contact with hot tap water. Falling and losing consciousness in the shower or bath can produce scald injuries. Contact burns associated with cooking and ignition of clothing are also frequently reported.

There are a variety of physiologic reasons for increased susceptibility of elderly persons to thermal injury and their poor outcome. The protective barrier of the skin is compromised due to decreased epidermal cell proliferation and dermal deterioration making full thickness injury in the elderly more likely than in a younger person given the same degree of insult. In addition, elderly persons have more difficulty separating themselves from a source of burning due to limitations in mobility and alteration in perception. Decreased sensation may also contribute to prolonged exposure to burning substances and increased injury. Preexisting medical conditions including cardiovascular disease contribute to high mortality in elderly persons. These inherent problems of the elderly contribute to complicated critical care and difficulty in surgical treatment of thermal injury. A young person with a 40% thermal injury can expect 80% survival while an individual aged 60 to 74 years has a 30% chance of survival with a comparable injury.

SYSTEM ISSUES IN GERIATRIC TRAUMA

Most of the issues raised in this text have not been addressed specifically in the traumatized elderly. Below, we will briefly review where this work exists or deficits appear as they relate to themes already raised.

TRAUMA SYSTEMS AND INJURY ASSESSMENT

The most common method for evaluating the traumatized patient employs the TRISS methodology. TRISS utilizes a combination of the Revised Trauma Score and Injury Severity Score to assess degree of injury and predict survival. The revised trauma score is a field index of physiologic derangement. A specific age factor has not been established for the trauma score, although it is thought to reliably reflect injury severity in patients over 12 years of age. This physiologic score is combined with an index of injury severity based on known anatomic injury to complete patient assessment. The Major Trauma Outcome Study (MTOS), is a retrospective study of more than 120,000 patients treated at trauma centers which serves as a basis for national norms of trauma care. Survival probability (Ps) outcome norms have been generated using the TRISS severity index. Data obtained from the MTOS demonstrated an increase in mortality for patients aged 60 years and greater. Longer hospital and ICU stay also accompanied increasing age. Perhaps the most important data from the MTOS is related to patients at the extremes of the survival probability scale. Many of the unexpected deaths had excellent admission physiology. In a group of over 800 unexpected deaths, 246 of these patients (27.8%) were more than 65 years old, although the elderly constituted only 10.1% of MTOS patients. In addition, over 50% of these unexpected deaths had significant head or neck

and thoracic injuries. These unexpected deaths may represent failure of present injury severity scoring methodology to accurately recognize severity and predict outcome from injures in these areas, particularly in older patients.

The MTOS elderly population has been a focus for trauma system planning. In a comparative study of elderly MTOS patients and younger counterparts whose data was submitted before 1987, older patients had a higher mortality rate (19% vs 9.8%), more frequent complications and a longer length of hospital and ICU stay. Increased mortality among older patients is thought consistent with lower average TRISS estimated survival probability for elderly patients even though injury severity in the elderly and younger individuals when measured by Revised Trauma Score and Injury Severity Score are similar. Increased vulnerability of the elderly to injury has been demonstrated and is only now being represented in MTOS norms accounting for reduced survival probability in patients 55 years of age and older.

An example of local implementation of injury analysis and control is the Queens Boulevard Pedestrian Safety Project which began in New York City in 1985. The New York City Police Department began a systematic examination and intervention program in the city's pedestrian injury program at that time. The unit reviewed police accident reports on fatal and severe pedestrian injuries from 1982-84. When these data were examined, 39 severe and fatal injuries were found to have occurred in one 2.5-mile stretch of Queens Boulevard. Seventy-five percent of all pedestrian injuries in this area were to persons over the age of 65 years. Eighty-five percent of the pedestrians killed along this stretch were over the age of 65, while only 30% of pedestrians killed in the city as a whole were in that age group.

The Traffic Safety Unit then undertook an indepth study to investigate why injuries were occurring. Queens Boulevard, at the point in question, was a wide roadway with pedestrians crossing distances of 150 feet. The traffic volume was high particularly during morning and evening rush hours. Among the study findings was routine violation of the 30 MPH speed limit and failure of elderly persons to walk across the boulevard in the 35 seconds allowed by the electrical walk signs. Due to the boulevard's width and vision loss among the elderly, pedestrians were unable to read the "walk" and "don't walk" signs. Vision loss and uncertainty of elderly pedestrians often caused these individuals to step off the curb and into the path of oncoming vehicles due to confusion regarding the direction in which to look for oncoming traffic.

The unit designed and implemented an intervention effort including resetting of "walk" and "don't walk" signs to allow additional time to cross the street and decreasing the distance between signs, so that vision impaired elderly could see them better. In addition, large arrows were painted on the pavement to indicate the direction from which traffic was coming and oversized speed limits signs were installed. Police increased enforcement of the speed limit in this area. These procedures were combined with an extensive public education campaign on pedestrian safety for senior citizens in the area.

Comparison of injury data in this area for the five years before intervention with the data for the 30 months afterward revealed a 44% decrease in the death rate and a 77% decrease in the rate of severe injuries. There was a 60% overall reduction in the rate of fatal and severe injuries (from 7.8 to 3.2 per 100,000). This project is an example of public health benefits resulting from carefully designed and implemented injury analysis and prevention programs.

INFECTION AND IMMUNITY

Epidemiologic studies point to age as a predictor of infectious complications resulting from trauma. Infection plays a major role in determining outcome after trauma with multisystem organ failure being the ultimate cause of 80% of late deaths due to injury. While the population sustaining trauma is generally young, trauma patients with infectious complications had a mean age of 53 years while the general population hospitalized patients with infection had a mean age of 33 years. A high risk group which has been identified is the elderly female. Injury is commonly the result of a fall. In one recent review, most of the elderly women developing infectious complications had sustained hip fracture and were placed at bed rest with traction. A high rate of urinary tract infections

was seen, probably due to the fact that urinary catheters were inserted during the stabilization period prior to surgery.

Patterns of immune response are incompletely characterized in the extremes of life. A recent review describes the differences in flow cytometry findings among immune competent cell subsets in the pediatric age group. Comparable data in the elderly, particularly the injured elderly, does not exist.

ORGAN SYSTEM FAILURE

Patients with organ system dysfunction are likely to be involved in the syndrome of multiple organ failure. This type of patient consumes a large portion of health care dollars, technical resources and physician effort. Despite this resource use, these individuals often do not survive. In univariate screening of variables comparing survivors and nonsurvivors of renal insufficiency for example, nonsurvivors had increasing transfusion therapy, a greater number of organ systems that failed and the unique presence of cardiac failure. Assessment of continuous variables by t-test methods in the same study suggested that age was significantly associated with poor outcome.

WOUND HEALING

Wound healing has been evaluated in studies comparing young and older animals. In mice receiving similar dorsal incisions, wound tensile strength was increased significantly at the six-week point in elderly as opposed to young animals. Old healed wounds appeared to regain baseline disruption strength earlier than similar wounds in younger animals. Histologic sections of animals from these studies suggests a greater fibrous component in the older wound whereas wounds in younger animals appear to be more vascular. A variety of other factors have not been compared in assessment of age-related wound healing. These include endocrine, nutrition and immune factors which may favor growth in young as opposed to old animals. Host tissue response to a variety of angiogenesis or other growth factors may also differ greatly with aging or tissues themselves may be lacking in factors essential for optimal healing.

Unfortunately, not all age-related changes in wound healing appear to be beneficial. Fibroblasts in the young appear to be more contractile than those in adulthood. This is seen in a variety of human and animal studies of full-thickness wound contraction which confirm that with aging the time before contraction is lengthened, the rate of wound contraction is lower, and the ultimate degree of contraction is less. In addition, while incisional wound breaking strength may plateau earlier in older animals (explaining the above animal work), the degree of maximal tension tolerated appears to be less. In general, the age-dependent response to injury is characterized by delayed cellular migration and proliferation along with reduced metabolic response and delayed biosynthetic activity. The rate of operative wound dehiscence is two to three times higher in patients more than 60 years of age. The impact of new wound healing developments including the recent recognition of growth factors is unknown in the elderly age group.

RESOURCE ALLOCATION IN GERIATRIC TRAUMA

Pories and coworkers[13] recently sought to predict more accurately the hospital charges related specifically to the trauma population. They examined the Trauma Score, Abbreviated Injury Scale, age, number of body areas injured and DRG assignments in relation to hospital charges using a regression analysis. The best prediction of hospital charge was obtained using DRG assignment, Injury Severity Score and age. Inclusion of the Trauma Score did not improve predictive ability. Failure to increment trauma reimbursement, utilizing age and ISS in addition to DRG compensation, resulted in a significant loss relative to hospital charge for the treatment of injured patients.

In an age of decreasing health care resources, however, every expenditure must be evaluated for efficacy. Some authors suggest that provision of trauma care in the injured elderly has been questioned in the past on the assumption that such care may be fruitless. The economic implications of aggressive treatment in geriatric trauma patients have been incompletely investigated.

A frequently cited report is that of Oreskovich and associates[7] from 1984. These authors reviewed 100 consecutive patients over 70 years of age with multiple injuries seen over a two-year period at a metropolitan trauma center. These patients were assessed for injury pattern and factors affecting survival. Analysis incorporated mechanism of injury, body region affected, injury severity, shock, change from level of prehospital function and mortality. Overall mortality was 15%. The Injury Severity Score was not predictive of survival in these patients. Central nervous system injury and hypovolemic shock were strongest predictors of in-hospital mortality. Eighty-five percent of the patients survived. However, 88% of the individuals reviewed did not return to their previous level of independence. From this review, these authors suggested a profile of a patient unlikely to survive. Ninety-three percent of nonsurvivors in this study required prehospital intubation. All were in shock at some interval before hospital admission and all required intubation longer than five days. Eighty percent of these individuals developed pulmonary infection with associated sepsis. When these authors extended followup to one year to determine change in level of function from preinjury status, they found that 96% of patients were independent at the time of injury while only 8% of individuals maintained this level of function one year following trauma. While only 10% of the population of the United States over the age of 70 was in nursing homes, 72% of the patients in the study of Oreskovich et al were in nursing homes at one year following injury.

A similar study was done by Gann and associates[8] at the Rhode Island Hospital Trauma Center and reported in 1987. This group followed 63 consecutive patients over the age of 65 years, all victims of blunt multiple trauma. Outcome status of each individual was assessed at hospital discharge and at long-term followup nine to 38 months after injury. Variables included age, injury severity, gender and need for emergency or delayed surgery. Ninety-seven percent of the patients in Gann's study were independent, living on their own at home prior to injury. One-third of injured individuals returned directly to independent living after discharge. Another 37% of patients required some

Heart disease	48%
Cancer	19%
Other	21%
Stroke	10%
Injury	2%

Table 1. Cause of death in people over 65.

- 11% of population
- 24% of trauma fatalities
  (24,000 deaths/year)
- Death rates from injury
  - age 15-24 = 64/100,000
  - age 75-84 = 166/100,000

Table 2. Injury in the elderly.

- Lesser tolerance and greater
  complication risk
- Physical changes and comorbid factors
- Cardiovascular disease
- Osteoporosis
- Pulmonary disease
- Nutrition—metabolism
- Senescence of the immune system
- Delays in access and treatment

Table 3. Reasons for higher fatality.

Falls	9,600(40%)
Motor Vehicle	6,000(25%)
Driver-passenger	4,000
Pedestrian	2,000
Fire, burns	1,700 (6%)
Firearms	1,200 (5%)
Suffocation ingested objects	1,200
Suffocation mechanical	600
Poisoning (solid, liquid)	400
Poisoning by gas	300
Other	3,000
Total	24,000

Table 4. Etiology of fatal injuries.

- 80% of people killed by falls are over 65
- 74% of hospital discharges for persons older
  than 65 were due to falls
- 45% of fatal falls occur in the home
- 15% in residential institutions

Table 5. Falls in the elderly.

assistance after discharge but could still be sent home. Thirty percent of individuals required nursing home admission. These individuals tended to be older and sustained more complications with longer hospital stays. Persons requiring nursing admission had sustained more severe head and neck trauma and more frequently required operative procedures after injury. Of interest, mechanism of injury, number of body regions injured and the presence of preexisting cardiopulmonary disease did not appear to be predictive of nursing home admission.

Of the patients initially sent to nursing homes, the majority returned home with a mean nursing home stay of 3.1 months. A number of additional individuals receiving support while at home also returned to independent status. Thus, 89% of surviving patients ultimately returned home. Of this 89%, 57% were considered independent, and the remaining 32% lived at home with some outside help. Only 11% of the patients followed by Gann et al required long term nursing home care at followup. There was no difference in injury severity between patients requiring permanent nursing home care and those able to return home. In the assessment of these authors, factors contributing to increased risk of mortality were age, injury severity and presence or absence of cardiac and infectious complications.

As complications play a critical role in increasing risk of mortality after trauma in the elderly, their prevention must be a primary goal of effective trauma care. In view of the generally favorable outcome for patients surviving trauma, liberal intensive care unit monitoring, aggressive pulmonary therapy and basic cardiac monitoring may prevent complications and decrease mortality rates.

It is sobering to realize that if, as has been proposed, costs for geriatric trauma are reimbursed under a DRG system, total reimbursement will approach 50% of the actual cost. In further discussion of this issue, Gann and associates delineate two distinct groups among the elderly. The younger elderly aged 65 to 79 years represent 8% of the total population and generate 8.5% of total hospital cost. The old elderly representing 3% of the total population generated 7% of total cost and 11% of total cost reimbursement deficit. Projected reimbursement in the old elderly subgroup allowed recovery of only 39% of hospital cost. In part this relates to increased hospitalization and hospital cost for elderly patients regardless of Injury Severity Score. The more severely injured elderly had hospital cost up to 80% higher than in those with lower Injury Severity Scores. Prospective reimbursement, however, rose only 38% in these individuals. Complications, as expected, had the single largest impact on increase cost. If more than one complication occurred in an elderly patient, average hospital cost rose over 300%. Despite this dramatic increase, reimbursement rose only 8%.

If the Medicare reimbursement system does not accurately reflect the true cost of providing care, the inevitable result will be to limit access to care for high cost groups. This would be a disaster for injured elderly patients whose tolerance for complications and delay in provision of care is limited. Perhaps age, injury severity and complications should promote factors increasing Medicare reimbursement for elderly trauma victims. Financial constraints have already closed a number of trauma centers. We must define health care priorities in general and trauma care in particular in order to prevent further erosion in the emergency care available to the injured elderly. The consumption of health care resources by bluntly injured elderly patients can be justified if outcome after trauma is good. Definitive data is unavailable to answer this question at this time. A number of studies suggest that aggressive treatment is rewarded by improved outcome in the elderly. Further clinical study will be required to justify this assertion.

To minimize mortality and morbidity, elderly trauma victims should be triaged to trauma centers at a lower threshold than similarly injured younger patients. Aggressive care recognizing the physiologic differences between the elderly and other portions of the trauma population should be applied with minimal delay. An expanded, rather than restricted, trauma system should be available to the elderly along with aggressive utilization of developments discussed earlier in this book. Further study is required to determine whether more rigorous infection prophylaxis, immunomodulation, pulmonary therapy and improvements in wound care will augment survival in elderly trauma patients

REFERENCES

1. Gamelli RL. Geriatric and pediatric trauma. In: Moore EE, Ducker TB, Edlich RF et al, eds. Early Care of the Injured Patient. Toronto: BC Decker, Inc., 1990:315.
2. Schwab CW, Kauder D, Geriatric trauma. In: Moore EE, Ducker TB, Edlich RF et al, eds. Early Care of the Injured Patient. Toronto: BC Decker, Inc., 1990:328.
3. Martin RE, Teberian G. Multiple trauma and the elderly patient. Emerg Med Clin North Am 1990; 8(2):411-420.
4. Champion HR, Copes WS, Buyer D et al. Major trauma in geriatric patients. Am J Public Health 79(9):1278-1282.
5. Smith DP, Anderson BL, Maull KI. Trauma in the elderly: Determinants of outcome. South Med J 1990; 83(2):171-177.
6. McCoy GF, Johnstone RA, Duthie RB. Injury to the elderly in road traffic accidents. J Trauma 1989; 29(4):494-497.
7. Oreskovich MR, Howard JD, Copass MK, Carrico CJ. Geriatric trauma: Injury patterns and outcome. J Trauma 1984; 24(7):565-572.
8. DeMaria EJ, Kenney PR, Merriam MA et al. Aggressive trauma care benefits the elderly. J Trauma 1987; 27(11):1200-1206.
9. Kenney PR, DeMaria EJ, Gann DS. Trauma care for the elderly? R I Med J 1991; 22(2):127-131.
10. Finelli FC, Jonsson J, Champion HR et al. A case control study for major trauma in geriatric patients. J Trauma 1989; 29(5):541-548.
11. The National Committee for Injury Prevention and Control. Injury Prevention: Meeting the challenge. New York: Oxford University, Press, 1989.
12. Denny T, Yoger R, Gelman R et al. Lymphocyte subsets in healthy children during the first five years of life. JAMA 1992; 267:1484-1488.
13. Pories SE, Gamelli RL, Vacek P et al. Predicting hospital charges for trauma care. Arch Surg 1988; 123:579:582.
14. Champion HR, Lopes WS, Sacco WJ, et al. The major trauma outcome study: establishing national norms for trauma care. J Trauma 1990; 30:1356-1365.
15. Pories SE, Gamelli RL, Mead PB et al. The epidemiologic features of nosocomial infections in patients with trauma. Arch Surg 1991; 126:97-99.
16. Cioffi WG, Ashikaga T, Gamelli RL. Probability of surviving postoperative acute renal failure: development of a prognostic index. Ann Surg 1984; 200:205-211.
17. Ershler WB, Gamelli RL, Moore AL et al. Experimental tumors and aging: local factors that may account for the observed age advantage in the B16 murine melanoma model. Exp Gerontol 1984; 19:367-376.

INDEX

A

Abbreviated Injury Scale (AIS), 15
Abel FL, 31
Acrolein, 49, 50
Acute phase proteins, 129
Acute Physiology and Chronic
    Health Evaluation (APACHE),
    18
Adhesion peptides, 159
Adhikari M, 165
Adult respiratory distress syndrome
    (ARDS), 36-43. See acute
    respiratory distress syndrome.
    inhalation injury, 51-52
    neutrophil, 87-88
    pathophysiology, 36-38
    therapy, 38-43
Acyloxyacyl hydrolases (AOAH), 83
Advanced Trauma Life Support
    (ATLS), 9
Alanine, 107
Albumin, 128
Aldehydes, 50
Alpha-1-acid glycoprotein (AAG),
    129
Alpha-1-antitrypsin, 129
Alpha 1 proteinase inhibitor, 87
Ambrose NS, 116
Ammonia, 49
Amylase, 23-24
Anatomic Profile (AP), 15
Anderson HV, 26
Angiotensin-converting enzyme
    (ACE), 48, 52, 172-173
Antibody-dependent cell-mediated
    cytotoxicity (ADCC), 180, 183,
    184
Antibiotics
    inhalation injury, 55-56
Antigen presenting cells, 75
Antin JH, 185
Antiphospholipid antibody (APA)
    syndrome, 173
Antithrombotics, 175-177
Arachidonic acid
    ARDS, 37
    hematopoiesis, 183, 184
    inhalation injury, 47, 49
A Severity Characterization of
    Trauma (ASCOT), 16
Ashbaugh DG, 52
Asphyxiants, 48
AT III, 169
ATP-MgCl, 27
Aub JC, 44
Avalos BR, 184

B

Bacterial translocation (BT), 37, 51,
    53, 74, 113
    experimental evidence, 114-116
    intestinal barrier, 113-114
Bactericidal permeability increasing
    (BPI) proteins, 82-82
Baker CC, 66, 180
Basal metabolic rate (BMR), 109
Basement membrane zone (BMZ),
    140, 141, 142
B-cell
    dysfunction, 69-70, 76-78
    T-cell interactions, 74-76
Beck RR, 31
Beutler B, 103
Bile salts, 114
Boosalis MG, 128
Border JR, 112, 117
Brandt SJ, 185
Braude A, 103
Bronchiectasis, 55
Bronchiolitis obliterans, 55
Brown GL, 144, 154
Bullous pemphigoid antigen (BPA),
    141
Bystander CPR, 2

C

C5a, 86, 87, 88, 89, 90
Ca^{2+} transient, 132
Calciosome, 132
Calcium
    agonist mediated activation of
    the intracellular Ca^{2+} signal,
    132-133
    intracellular binding proteins,
    133-134
    intracellular Ca^{2+}
        altered, 134
        homeostasis, 132
        mediator of cell injury, 134
    ionophore (A23187), 134
    sepsis, 135-138
        liver, 135-137
        skeletal muscle, 137
Calcium-calmodulin-dependent
    kinases, 134
Calmodulin, 134
Candida albicans, 116
Carbon monoxide (CO), 48
Carboxypeptidase N, 86

Catabolism
    acute phase response, 127-130
    skeletal muscle, 108
Catalase, 48
CD3$^+$ lymphocytes, 64, 67
CD4$^+$ lymphocytes, 64, 67, 75, 76
CD8$^+$ lymphocytes, 70, 75, 76, 78,
    79
CD11, 87
CD14, 82-83, 89
CD18, 87
Cerami (no initial given), 103
Ceruloplasmin, 87, 129
Chemotactic factor inactivator, 86
Chemotaxis, 86
Chiu CJ, 115
Chlorine, 49
Chondroitin-6-sulfate, 159
Christou NV, 66
Cimetidine, 39
Cioffi WG, 56, 57
Citral, 148
Clark SC, 182
Clark WR, 51
Coagulation, 168-170. See
    Hemostasis.
    colloids, 23, 24
    wound healing, 139
Coccia MT, 27
Collagen, 140, 147
    gel, 160
    glycosaminoglycans, 159-160
    type I, 141, 142
    type IV, 141, 142
    type V, 142
Collegenase, 142
Colloids, 21-24
Complement, 53, 129
    neutrophil, 86
Cowley MJ, 26
CR1, 87
CR3, 87
Craig RW, 142
C-reactive protein, 129
Crystalloids, 20-21, 24
Cuono CB, 160
Cuthbertson (no initial given), 106
Cyclosporin A, 148
Cyclooxygenase pathway, 38, 67
Cytochrome oxidase, 48
Cytokines
    acute phase response, 129-130
    hemostasis, 173
    sepsis, 66-67, 81-84
    thermal injury, 175

D

Defibrotide, 176
Dermatan sulfate, 159, 176
D-erythro-neopterin, 68
Deuel T, 151
Development of Trauma Systems (DOTS), 12
Devereux S, 186
Dextran, 22-23, 24
    hypertonic saline, 21-22
1,2-Diacyglycerol DAG), 132-133
Diagnosis Related Group (DRG), 17
Diltiazem, 136, 137
Dinarello (no initial given), 103
Diphenhydramine, 39
Disseminated intravascular coagulation, 167, 174-175
Dobrescu C, 122
Donahue RE, 183

E

E5, 98
Eicosanoids, 53-54, 83
ELAM-1, 87
Elastin, 142
Endobronchial polyposis, 55
Endothelial-derived relaxing factors, 172
Endothelium
    hemostasis, 172-173
Endotoxin, 69, 163, 165. See Lipopolysaccharide (LPS).
    bacterial translocation, 115, 116-117
    calcium regulation, 135-136
    glucose transport, 124-125
    tolerance, 166
Enteral feeding, 109, 117
Eosinophils, 183
EPI, 169
Epidermal growth factor (EGF), 143, 144, 151, 154
Enterobacter sp, 51
Erythropoietin (Epo), 181-183
Escherischia coli, 31, 51, 69, 70, 78, 92, 96, 115, 137, 165
Extracorporeal CO₂ removal (ECCO₂R), 42, 58
Extracorporeal membrane oxygenation (ECMO), 42, 58

F

Faist E, 64, 67
Fat metabolism, 107-108
Fibrin-fibrinogen, 141
Fibrinogen, 129, 170

Fibrinolysis, 170-171
Fibroblast
    collagen gel, 160
    cultures, 160
    hematopoeisis, 181
Fibroblast growth factor, 67, 139, 143, 153-154
Fibronectin, 47, 87, 88, 141, 142, 143
Filkins JP, 66
Fine J, 112
Finley RK, 160
Fluosol-DA-20% (Fluosol), 24-25
FMLP, 86, 87, 89
Furukawa T, 185

G

Gabrilove GL, 185
Gamelli R, 185
Gann DS, 196
Gattinoni L, 58
Gene expression
    shock, 104
Gene transfer, 71-72
Gibson (no initial given), 160
Gillio AP, 182
Glasgow Coma Scale (GCS), 15
Glucagon, 108
Glucose, 107
    metabolism, 121-125
    transport, 122-125
        sepsis, 124-125
Gluconeogenesis, 107
ß-Glucuronidase, 47
Glycerol, 107
Glycoproteins
    platelet membrane, 172
Glycosaminoglycans, 159-160
Granulocyte colony stimulating factor (G-CSF), 88, 154, 180-181, 182, 183-184
Granulocyte-macrophage colony-stimulating factor (GM-CSF), 180-181, 182, 183
Group-specific component (Gc) globulin, 86
Growth factors, 142-143
    wound healing, 143-145, 151-155
        hyperbaric oxygen, 155
Growth hormone (GH), 154
Guanine nucleotide binding protein (G-protein), 89, 132, 136
Gut-associated lymphoid tissue (GALT), 113-114

H

HA-1A, 97, 98, 165
Haptoglobin, 129
Harris-Benedict equations, 110
HC II, 169
Heat shock protein genes, 71
Hematopoiesis, 180
    colony-stimulating factors
        therapeutic potential, 185-186
    growth factors, 180-181
Hemoglobin, 48
Hemorrhage
    B-cell, 76-78
Hemostasis, 167-178
    coagulation, 168-170
    endocrine, 172-173
    fibrinolysis, 170-171
    platelet, 171-172
    thermal injury, 173-175
Heparin, 175, 176
Herndon DN, 51, 116, 144, 154
Hetastarch. See Hydroxyethyl starch (HES).
High frequency ventilation (HFV), 41-42, 58
H. influenzae, 164
Histamine, 47
HLA-DR, 64, 68, 69
Hull BE, 160, 161
Hunt-Schilling chamber model, 153
Hunt TK, 104, 144
Hydrogen chloride, 49
Hydrogen cynanide (HCN), 48, 49
Hydroxyethyl starch (HES), 23
Hyperbaric oxygen, 155
Hypermetabolism, 108
Hypertonic saline, 21
    dextran, 21-22

I

Ia antigen, 69
Ibuprofen, 38, 39
ICAM-1, 87
Ikebuchi K, 183
Immune response
    B-cell, 69-70, 74-76
    cell-mediated immunity, 64-65, 69-70, 74-80
    cytokine, 66-67
    prostaglandins, 67-68
    T-cell, 74-76, 78-79
    thermal injury, 65-66
Immune stimulation, 68-69
Immunization
    bacterial antigen, 77-78
Immunoglobulin A (IgA), 74-75, 77, 113-114
Immunoglobulin M (IgM), 114

Immunosuppression
    postinjury, 179-180
Immunotherapy. See Monoclonal
    antibody therapy.
Indirect calorimetry, 110
Indomethacin, 68, 147
Inhalation injury, 44-59
    acute respiratory distress
        syndrome, 51-52
    antibiotics, 55-56
    asphyxiants, 48-50
    barotrauma, 54
    ciliary dysfunction, 50
    classification, 44-45
    cutaneous thermal injury, 49-50
    endothelial cell, 52
    endotoxin, 52-53
    fluid management, 54
    infection, 50, 54
    long term sequelae, 55
    lower airway injury, 47-48
    neutrophil, 52
    oxygen toxicity, 54
    pathogens, 51
    pulmonary alveolar macrophage
        (PAM), 50, 51
    pulmonary toilet, 55
    steroids, 56
    surfactant, 50-51
    treatment, 55-58
    upper airway injury, 46-47
    ventilator management, 56-58
Injury Severity Score (ISS), 15, 193,
    195
Inositol 1,4,5,-triphosphate (IP$_3$),
    132-133, 136-137
Insulin 106, 107
    -mediated glucose uptake,
        121-122, 124
Insulin growth factor binding
    protein, 154
Insulin-like growth factor I (IGF$_1$),
    143, 144, 154
Insulin-like growth factor II (IGF$_2$),
    143
Integrins, 78, 87
Interferon gamma, 64, 67, 68, 69,
    76, 78, 142, 143, 148, 149
Interleukin-1 (IL-1), 28, 35, 37, 38,
    64, 67, 76, 78, 82, 87, 93, 104,
    108, 129, 130, 148, 154, 163,
    173, 179-180, 183
Interleukin-2 (IL-2), 28, 35, 64, 76,
    78, 149, 154, 173, 180
Interleukin-3 (IL-3), 78, 149, 180,
    181
Interleukin-4 (IL-4), 70, 76, 149,
    181, 182
Interleukin-5 (IL-5), 78, 181

Interleukin-6 (IL-6), 28, 35, 38, 67,
    70, 76, 78, 82, 93-94, 129,
    130, 163, 173, 181
Interleukin-8 (IL-8), 38, 78, 82, 87,
    88
Interleukin-1 receptor antagonist
    protein, 83
Intravenous oxygen/carbon dioxide
    exchange (IVOX), 42-43
Inverse ratio pressure-controlled
    ventilation (IRV), 41, 57

J

Jaiyesimi I, 186
Jurkovich GJ, 69

K

Kass EH, 103
Kauder D, 192
Keratinocyte, 140-141, 142
    cultures, 158
Keratinocyte growth factor, 153,
    154
Ketaserin, 39
Klebsiella pneumoniae, 69, 78
Knighton DR, 144
Kohler G, 102, 103
Krause W, 116
Krausz MM, 21
Kudsk KA, 117

L

Lachman C, 96
Lactated Ringer's solution, 21
Laminin, 87, 141, 143
Lang CH, 122
Leary AG, 181
Lee MT, 185
Lefer, 34
Leibovich SJ, 139, 140
Leuconostoc mesenteroides, 22
Leukocytes
    hemostasis, 173
Leukotriene B$_4$, 54, 88
Leukotrienes, 37, 38, 87, 172
Levine (initial not given), 157
Levine BA, 56
Lipooxygenase pathway, 37, 38
Lipopolysaccharide (LPS), 37, 70,
    90
Lipopolysaccharide binding (LPB)
    proteins, 82-83
    host response, 92-94
    structure, 92
Lipoprotein associated coagulation
    inhibitor (LACI). See EPI.
Liposomes
    hemoglobin, 27-28
    polysaccharide antigens, 78

Liquid ventilation, 43
Lopez EF, 181
Lymphocyte
    wound healing, 148-149
Lymphotoxin, 148
Lynch SE, 144

M

Macrophages. See Neutrophil.
    antigen presentation, 75, 76
    bacterial translocation, 116
    cytokine production, 76, 83
    immunosuppression, 179-180
    wound healing, 139, 143,
        147-148
Macrphage colony-stimulating
    factor (M-CSF), 181
Major Trauma Outcome Study
    (MTOS), 16, 193
Marshall JC, 116
Martinet N, 141
Mattox KL, 28
Meakins JL, 66, 70, 112
Mechanical ventilation
    ARDS, 40-41
Medawar P, 160
Mesenteric lymph node (MLN)
    complex, 114, 115
Metabolic response to injury, 106-
    107
    estimation of energy expendi-
        ture, 109-110
    nutritional requirements, 110-
        111
    substrate metabolism, 107-108
Methylprednisolone, 39
f-Met-Leu-Phe (f-MLP), 184
Michie HR, 67
Miller SF, 160
Milstein C, 102, 103
Mochizuki H, 117
Monoclonal antibody (mAbs)
    therapy
        ARDS, 38
        CD8$^+$, 78
        E5, 98
        endotoxin, 67, 70-71, 94-100
        HA-1A, 97, 98, 165
        monokine abrogation, 97-98
        synthesis, 103
Monocyte colony stimulating factor
    (M-CSF), 184-185
Mooney DP, 186
Moylan JA, 45, 56
Multiple organ failure (MOF), 53
    bacterial translocation, 112-113,
        116-117

Myocardial depressant factor (MDF), 34-35
Myocardial depression, 30-35
    adrenergic unresponsiveness, 34
    cardiac chamber dynamics, 30-34
Myoglobin, 48

N

Naloxone, 34
Nathanson, 31
Neutrophil
    ARDS, 37
    complement, 86
    endotoxin, 89-90, 92
    priming, 86-87
    pulmonary, 47-48, 50, 52
    signal transduction, 88-89
    surface receptors, 88-89
Nickoloff BJ, 141
Niemann GF, 50
Ninnemann JL, 65, 66
Nitrogen oxide, 49
Noninsulin-mediated glucose uptake (NIMGU), 121-122
Nohr CW, 70
Nutritional support, 108-109
    index of repletion, 127-130

O

Ogawa M, 181, 183
Ohlsson K, 103
O'Reilly M, 185
Oreskovich MR, 195
Oxidative burst, 87
Oxygen free radicals, 27, 37, 47-48, 52

P

PAF (1-0-alkyl-2-acetyl derivative of phosphorylcholine), 172
Parker MM, 31
Patient Management Categories (PMC), 17
PDWHF, 155
Pentastarch. See Hydroxyethyl starch (HES).
Pentoxifylline, 27, 38
Perfluorochemical emulsions (PFC), 24-26, 40, 43
Peroxidase, 48
Peschel C, 183
Phosgene, 49
Phosphoinositol phosphatase C, 89
Phospholipase C (PLPC), 132, 136
Phosphitidyl inositol bis-phosphate (PIP$_2$), 132-133

Plasma volume expanders. See Colloids and Crystalloids.
Plasmin, 170-171
Plasmin-antiplasmin, 175
Plasminogen, 170
Platelet
    hemostasis, 171-172
Platelet activating factor (PAF), 28, 37
Platelet derived endothelial cell growth factor, 154
Platelet derived growth factor, 67, 139, 143, 147, 151, 152-153, 155, 172
Platelet factor IV (PF$_4$), 139, 172
Polk HC Jr, 64, 66, 69, 180
Pollack (no initial given), 96
Polyclonal antibodies
    sepsis, 95, 96-97
Polymorphonuclear leukocyte (PMN), 146
Polysaccharide antigens, 75, 77-78
Polyurethane, 49
Polyvinyl alcohol (PVA) sponges, 147, 148
Polyvinyl chloride, 49
Pories SE, 195
Positive end-expiratory pressure (PEEP), 40, 56-57
Prealbumin (PA), 128, 129
Pressure controlled ventilation (PCV), 57
Prostacyclin, 52
Prostaglandin
    E$_1$ (PGE$_1$)
        ARDS, 38
    E$_2$ (PGE$_2$), 54, 64, 67-68
        platelets, 172
Protein C, 169, 172, 175
Protein S, 169, 175
Protein kinase C (PKC), 89, 132-133
Pseudomonas aeruginosa, 51, 77, 78, 96, 98, 186
Pulmonary alveolar macrophage (PAM), 50, 51, 53
Pyrolysis, 45-46

Q

Queens Boulevard Pedestrian Safety Project, 193-194

R

Rabbit ear dermal ulcer model, 153, 154
Rasmussen H, 135
Ras protein, 89
Ras-related protein, 84
Registries, 7-9
Reilly JM, 35

Reimbursement, 17-18
Rennick D, 183
Reperfusion injury, 27, 86
    ARDS, 37
    neutrophil, 88
Resource allocation, 16
Resting energy expenditure (REE), 109-110
Resuscitation solutions, 20-28
Retinoic acid, 148
Retinol binding protein (RBP), 128
Revised Trauma Score (RTS), 15, 193
Rhee P, 27
Rho protein, 89
Ross R, 139
Rush BF Jr, 116

S

Salmonella enteritidis, 124, 135, 136
Salmonella sp, 92
Sanderson CJ, 183
Saponin, 137
Sarcoplasmic/endoplasmic reticular (SR/ER) membrane, 132
Sartorelli KH, 186
Schulman KA, 73
Schultz GS, 144
Schwab CW, 192
Second messenger, 89
Selectins, 78
Sepsis, 103
    calcium metabolism, 131-138
    cytokines, 66-67, 81-84
    glucose metabolism, 121-125
    hemodynamics, 31
    hemostasis, 72
    immunotherapy, 67, 70-71, 94-100, 164-166
    pediatric, 163-164
Serum amyloid A, 129
Show, 31
Sieff CA, 181
Silver GM, 181, 186
Silver sulfadiazine cream, 144
Simultaneois independent lung ventilation (SILV), 41
Sittig K, 54
Skin substitutes
    allograft, 160-161
    biologic
        natural, 157-158
        processed, 158
    bilaminate, 157
    dermal replacements, 159
    epidermal, 158-159
    requirements, 156
    synthetic, 157
    unilaminate, 157

Slade CL, 66
S. minnesota, 96, 98
Somatomedin C, 143
Sporn M, 151
Staphylococcus sp, 51
Steroids
    inhalation injury, 56
Stomach
    stress bleeding, 117
Stone HH, 55, 56
Streptoccocal pneumonia, 186
Stroma-free hemoglobin, 26-27, 40
Sucralfate, 117
Sulfur dioxide, 49
Superoxide, 184. See Reperfusion
    injury.
Surfactant, 43, 50-51
Swinburn WR, 34

T

T-cell
    alterations after trauma, 78-79
    B-cell interaction, 74-76
    wound healing, 148-149
Technical Assistance Program, 12
Teng NNH, 103
Teule GJJ, 31
Tharrat RS, 57
Thrombin, 169, 170
Thromboplastin, 173
Thrmbosis
    thermal injury
        treatment, 176-178
Thrombospondin, 141, 143
Thromboxane A_2, 37, 38, 47, 52
Thymopentin, 67
Thymopoietin, 148
Thymosin fraction V (TF5), 148
Thymulin, 148
Thymus
    wound healing, 148
Till GO, 52
Toxophore, 95
Tracey KJ, 103
Tracheal stenosis, 55
Transferrin (TF), 128, 129
Transforming growth factor
    (TGF-ß), 84, 139, 143-144,
    147, 148, 149, 151, 152, 154,
    155

Transthyretin. See Prealbumin.
Trauma
    geriatric, 191-198
Trauma care systems
    access, 2-3
    data collection and manage-
        ment, 7-9
    development, 11-12
    failure, 12-13
    hospital care, 5-6
    legislation, 10-11
    medical control, 4-5
    personnel, 3-4
    prevention, 9
    quality assurance, 6-7
    research, 10, 16
    societal components, 9
    system funding, 10
    transportation, 3
    triage, 4
Trauma Care Systems Planning and
    Developemnt Act (PL-101-590),
    10
Trauma Related Groupings, 17
Trauma scoring
    anatomic indices, 15
    combination indices, 15-16
    elderly, 195
    ICU indices, 18
    physiologic indices, 1
Tremper KK, 25
TRISS, 16, 193
Tumor necrosis factor (TNF), 27,
    28, 142
    acute phase response, 129, 130
    ARDS, 37, 38, 53, 54, 88
    endotoxin, 92-93, 164
    hematopoiesis, 180, 183
    hemostasis, 173
    myocardial depression, 35
    neutrophil, 87, 88
    sepsis, 64, 72, 82, 92-93, 103,
    163
    wound healing, 140, 147
Tyrosine kinase, 143

V

Vaccinia growth factor, 144
Vadhan-Raj S, 185
van der Poll T, 72
van der Waaij D, 113
Vascular permeability factor (VPF),
    154
Vassar MJ, 22
Virchow R, 135
Voelkel NF, 53

W

w statistic, 17
Waxman K, 25
Wells CL, 116
West JG, 2
Wilmore DW, 117
Wolfe, 31
Wolochow H, 113
Woodley DT, 142
Wound healing, 139-145
    collagen and glycosaminogly-
        cans, 159-160
    cutaneous, 140-142
    elderly, 194-195
    fetal, 159
    growth factors, 143-145
    lymphocyte, 148-149
    macrophage, 147-148
Wound Healing Centers, 155

Y

Yang YC, 182
Yurt, 66

Z

Zapol WM, 58
Ziegler EJ, 97, 103, 165
z statistic, 17